# GENETICS AND PATHOPHYSIOLOGY OF ESSENTIAL HYPERTENSION

Edited by **Madhu Khullar**

**Genetics and Pathophysiology of Essential Hypertension**
Edited by Madhu Khullar

**Published by InTech**
Janeza Trdine 9, 51000 Rijeka, Croatia





**Publishing Process Manager** Dejan Grgur

**Technical Editor** Teodora Smiljanic

**Cover Designer** InTech Design Team

Additional hard copies can be obtained from orders@intechopen.com

Genetics and Pathophysiology of Essential Hypertension, Edited by Madhu Khullar
p. cm.
ISBN 978-953-51-0282-3

For EU product safety concerns:
IN TECH d.o.o., Prolaz Marije Krucifikse Kozulić 3, 51000 Rijeka, Croatia,
info@intechopen.com or visit our website at intechopen.com.

# Meet the editor

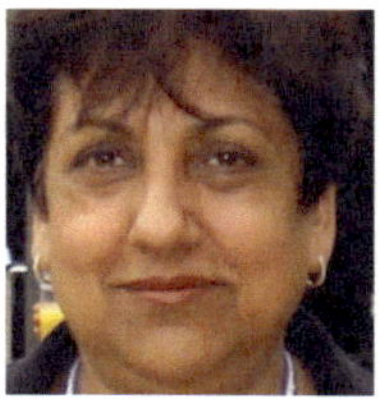

Dr Madhu Khullar is a Professor of Experimental Medicine and Biotechnology at Post Graduate Institute of Medical Education and Research, Chandigarh, India. She did her the Post Doctorate in Hypertension Research at the Henry Ford Hospital, Detroit, USA in 1985. Dr Khullar has keen research interest in genetics of hypertension and is currently studying pharmacogenetics of hypertension.

# Contents

# Preface

Hypertension or high blood pressure is one of the most common chronic diseases affecting more than 1 billion people worldwide, and by the year 2025, the global prevalence of hypertension is projected to increase to 29.2% of adult population (Kearney et al., 2005). High blood pressure where the medical cause of the disease is not known is defined as Essential hypertension and is the most common form of hypertension. Essential hypertension is a major risk factor for myocardial infarction, stroke, heart failure and renal failure. The cause of essential hypertension remains largely unknown and is an area of active research. It appears to have multifactorial and complex etiology where genetic and environmental factors play an important role. The current book addresses some of the research issues related to the pathophysiology, genetics and genomics of hypertension.

This book is divided into two main sections: Pathophysiology, and Genetics and Genomics. In pathophysiology, topics such as pathophysiology of resistant hypertension, target organ damage in hypertension, Baroreflex sensitivity and an interesting hypothesis on music as a therapy for lowering blood pressure are described. Genetics and genomics section provides an overview of different aspects of genetics research in hypertension, including genetic susceptibility markers, mitochondrial mutations and pharmacogenetics of hypertension. A chapter on microarray technology details the technique and identifies expression of altered genes. Role of TGF-β and other inflammatory genes has been portrayed in another chapter. This book provides comprehensive information on some of the important topics and issues related to pathophysiology of essential hypertension and it is hoped that it will be useful to researchers and clinicians with an interest in Essential hypertension.

**Dr Madhu Khullar**
Department of Experimental Medicine & Biotechnology
Post Graduate Institute of Medical Education and Research
Chandigarh,
India

# Part 1

## Pathophysiology of Hypertension

# 1

# Harmful or Helpful Hypertension – Pathophysiological Basis

M. Kasko[1], M. Budaj[2] and I. Hulin[2]
[1] *2nd Department of Internal Medicine, University Hospital and Faculty of Medicine, Comenius University, Bratislava,*
[2]*Department of Clinical Pathophysiology, Institute of Pathophysiology, Faculty of Medicine, Comenius University, Bratislava, Slovakia*

## 1. Introduction

The analytic approach does not always give an unambiguous response to the question as to why the disorder has developed. Rather, it rather clarifies the mechanisms responsible for the disorder. There is a great difference between the two following questions:

1. How the disorder has appeared?
2. Why the disorder has appeared?

In order to understand complex mechanisms, both questions need to be considered.

By analyzing the individual parts of mechanisms, we assume them to have equal importance. But in reality, this is not true. Even in most difficult systems consisting of individual parts, their role, value, and participation are in hierarchy. Some elements may be superior to the others.

Usually not all the very difficult mechanisms lying very deep within cells are apparent. However, this can not excuse the assumption that none of phenomena can be determined only by intracellular processes. If we admit that we are the result of the huge evolution of life, our primeval substance is then represented by cells. The cells can be the hidden motor forcing the organism to fulfill the cellular needs. According to this view, blood pressure is not the only part of a functioning circulation.

Life has been formed in water which serves as the medium, procuring everything from the reception of energy to the elimination of unneeded substances. The changes in pressure might represent a simple mechanism allowing the functioning of cells. Even more simple are however the alterations in osmotic concentration of internal water environment. Is this not a phylogenetically conserved regulation? The increase in blood pressure in human organisms brings about an increase in the elimination of water together with natriuresis. Nevertheless, the question of regulation can be posed the other way round. So far, we used to say that blood pressure is influenced by defined factors. We usually suppose that blood pressure is regulated by known and lesser-known mechanisms. Might the order not be reversed? Could not the blood pressure serve as a cellular tool that optimizes the osmotic factors? Such mechanisms can not be isolated, and are probably more complex. Subsequently the complexity raises the possibility that undesired anomalies will develop. This is the reason why many disorders can occur and they can not be easily included in a single scheme.

In the far past, at the beginning of evolution of difficult biological systems, water, osmotic factors, and pressure factors occurring in layers separating two interfaces represented the mechanisms that determined entirely everything. Perhaps we should see the phylogenetic residue in the fact that the activity of organism can be associated with a change in these values on the level of all cells. The optimization of osmotic and pressure factors can be achieved in various ways. These mechanisms can very effectively manage new situations in each cell, preferably in selected cells. The activation of organism that is associated with the activity of the sympathoadrenal system (SAS) triggers complex pathways. The long-lasting activation of these mechanisms may lead to their fixation, enabling the pressure to serve as a tool for increasing the natriuresis at general load.

Biological systems, which are considered to be our primeval predecessors, had to develop their own mechanisms to improve their ability to retain sodium. At the same time, they had to develop mechanisms that could basically help them to eliminate the excessive sodium. Moreover, a perfect system necessarily needs to develop mechanisms to gain sodium. In this aspect, we can operate with three facts. The first is the ability to save sodium, the second is to eliminate its excess, and the third is to gain sodium.

People living in warm geographical latitudes of the Earth needed to save sodium to retain water, and to procure its return. Later, when it got colder and people moved to territories with milder climate, a new situation had consequently emerged that did not require one to guard the stored sodium. The mechanisms used for its gaining became excessive. The fact that Afro- American people are more sensitive to salt-intake than Caucasians can be a 'message from our premedieval past'. This assumption is supported by the polymorphisms of the gene for angiotensinogen (ATG gene), beta$_2$ adrenergic receptors, and epithelial sodium channels in some African populations. Perspiration and infectious diarrhea were the reasons of permanent loss of sodium [1]. Therefore the long-lasting evolution preferred genotypes, which were better equipped to save sodium. This notion can be acceptable; however, it does not necessarily need to be correct.

There exists a negative correlation between the risk of hypertension and birth weight. Low weight at birth in babies of mothers living under dire social and economic conditions is a strong predisposition for the development of hypertension in adulthood of their offspring. The reason can also reside in the fact that during their intrauterine life, these individuals have not reached the full glomerular count, resulting in a smaller filtration area. Lower filtration rate is then compensated by increased pressure in order to achieve optimal natriuresis. If these facts were proved, it would be possible to eliminate the possible risks incurred by intrauterine development of kidneys by changing the system of nutrition in children with low birth weight.

The genetic determination applies when appropriate conditions or mechanisms playing the role of triggers are present. This gives the basis for the conception that hypertension can never originate from one single cause. Moreover, all biologic systems show great plasticity. The possible maladaptation of some mechanisms however, can function as the factor responsible for the consequences leading to hypertension.

Hypertension is an extraordinarily difficult pathophysiologic problem. It has very often devastating consequences; however many times it is only asymptomatic and remains such for a long time before an acute crisis occurs. Hypertension mainly leads to negative conditions as follows: disorder of coronary bed, renal failure, and changes in peripheral vessels in limbs. Hypertension is going to be the largest risk of premature deaths [2].

Nevertheless, the basic question of the origin of hypertension is to be raised, or rather the justness of our used conceptions should be called into question. We can question whether hypertension is actually caused solely by changes in mechanisms, molecules, or some structures. Could we not assume that hypertension is an inevitable adaptation to provide adequate oxygenation in tissues? In that case, reducing the blood pressure would protect one from catastrophic consequences; however at the same time it would particularly inconvenience oxygenation on the level of microcirculation. Does the decrease in pressure procure optimal oxygenation of brain in hypertensive patients? Can it not be assumed that successful treatment of hypertension on one hand eliminates the risks of catastrophe though at the same time, it accelerates chronic degenerative processes [3]? An increase in pressure to a certain limit might improve the oxygenation of tissues. A marked increase in pressure brings about a decrease in perfusion due to induced vasoconstriction. Therefore, there can be a positive correlation with neurodegenerative diseases [4].

In general, it is accepted that hypertension is a complex disorder determined by several factors. It is assumed that it occurs as a result of interactions between genetic factors predisposing to development of hypertension and external environment (diet habits, obesity, hyperlipidemia, smoking, stress).

## 2. Functional anatomy of the circulation

The circulation (Table 1) can perform its basic function in an optimal way only when the amount of blood flowing through the capillaries of each tissue, or organ per a time unit is fair enough to keep the homeostasis of that organ, so that it can perform its function adequately. The blood flow per minute via the capillaries of the given tissue or organ is the most important parameter of the blood flow (haemodynamics).

The vessels from the functional point of view can be devided into:

1. Compliance vessels, that form the large and intermediate arteries. Their function is to provide a continuous flow of blood. Ensure a fast transport of blood to the peripheries.
2. Resistant vessels are the major determinants of the general peripheral vascular resistance and by this even the regional blood flow. The whole peripheral vascular resistance is an important factor upon which the intermediate arterial blood pressure depends. It includes: The elastic resistance in the arterial system, the peripheral resistance of the resistant vessels, and the resistance which is imposed by the pre-capillary sphincter. We recognize two types of the resistant vessels:

a. pre-capillary resistant vessels - small arteries and arterioles - which form about one half of the value of the peripheral vascular resistance.
b. post-capillary resistant vessels - venules and small veins - that form a small part of the resistance. They participate in the changes of the potential volume of the capacity field.

3. pre-capillary sphincter is that part of the vessel that regulates blood flow into the capillaries and selectively distributes blood into those capillaries. By opening and closing these segments we can determine the number of transition capillaries in a given organ or tissue. The pre-capillary sphincter undergoes systemic and local effects. That determines the metabolism of the tissue or organ.
4. capacitance vessels (volume) are mainly the large systemic veins. They represent the reservoir for heart filling.
5. exchange vessels are the true blood capillaries. They mediate the contact between the blood field and the interstitial place.
6. shunt vessels of the arterio-venous shunts. These vessels provide a fast flow of blood from the arterial to the venous side without passing through the capillaries (bypassing the capillaries). They exist in certain tissues such as skin and lungs.

The primary function of the cardiovascular system is to provide adequate flow of blood through different tissues. The power that provides this is the mean arterial pressure. There is a physical relation between the mean arterial pressure, the minute volume of the heart, and the total peripheral resistance.

The mean arterial pressure = minute volume multiplied by the total peripheral resistance.

| | |
|---|---|
| aorta | 2.5 $cm^2$ |
| small arteries | 20.0 $cm^2$ |
| arterioles | 40.0 $cm^2$ |
| capillaries | 2500.0 $cm^2$ |
| venules | 250.0 $cm^2$ |
| small veins | 80.0 $cm^2$ |
| vena cava | 8.0 $cm^2$ |

Table 1. Area of the calibres of different vessels of the circulation.

## 3. Regulation of blood pressure to its optimal level

Under the headline the arterial (systemic) blood pressure we understand the lateral hydrostatic pressure that acts on the arterial wall during the ventricular systole. The perfusion of organs and tissues is dependent upon the mean arterial pressure. The value of which depend on:

1. The volume of blood pumped by the left ventricle in a time unit. The cardiac output.
2. The resistance to the blood flow laid down by the vessels in the peripheries of the vascular field.

The minute cardiac output is regulated by four factors:

a. The end diastolic volume of the left ventricle (preload)
b. The myocardial contractility
c. The resistance against which the left ventricle pumps the blood (afterload)
d. The frequency of the heart.

All these factors affecting the minute cardiac output are affected by the autonomic nervous system: that activates adrenergic receptors in the SA (sinoatrial) node, the myocardium, the smooth muscle in the arterial wall, venules, and veins.

Regulation of vascular tonus. The value of the tonus depends on the structural and functional characteristics of the individual vessels. This value is under the effect of many systemic and local factors.

Systemic factors regulating the vascular tonus are mainly nervous mechanisms, sympathicoadrenal system, renin-angiotensin-aldosterone system, and the vasopressin system.

Local factors can be devided into three groups:

1. the vascular myogenic reaction to tension
2. chemical factors having metabolic origin
3. humoral factors

i. The caliber of blood vessels is determined by two physical antagonizing factors. These are the transmural distending pressure and the tangentially acting tension on the vascular wall. In the state of equilibrium the relation between these two and the diameter of the vessel is defined by Laplace law. According to this law the smaller is the vascular diameter the lower is the pressure needed to close the vessel. This is why as soon as the pre-capillary sphincter starts to contract and its translucency is decreased (the wall thickness increases) the tendency of this sphincter to close the vessel is increasing. This magic circle tends to close the vessels completely.
ii. An increase in the tissue metabolism is accompanied by an increase in the regional blood flow, which is known as functional hyperemia. The regional vascular tonus is decreasing and the blood flow is increasing. Contraversly in non functioning organs or tissues the blood flow drops down. Functional hyperemia is related to the effects of local chemical factors, either by the accumulation of metabolic products or by the depletion of nutrients. Intensive hyperemia occurs during muscular exertion: there is a marked dilatation of the pre-capillary and post-capillary resistant vessels. According to the vasodilatatory theory the vascular tonus is regulated by factors that originate during the exertion in the contracted muscle fibers, released to the interstitium and can affect the vascular tone directly: $CO_2$, lactate, other carbohydrate metabolites, decrease in pH, acetylcholin, (ATP – adenosine triphosphate) that evoke active vasodilatation such as histamine and bradykinin, and eventually leading to an increase of capillary permeability. According to the oxygen theory - vascular vasodilatation in active tissues is caused by inadequate $O_2$ supply. Attention is given mainly to three factors: Hypoxia, regional increase of the extracellular concentration of potassium, and regional hyperosmolarity. Changes in the extracellular concentration of potassium and osmolarity probably influence the vascular tone via the $Ca^{2+}$ influx into the muscle fiber.
iii. Humoral factors: a group of vasoactive substances - kinins that have the character of local hormones. Their main function is the regulation of microcirculation. These are mainly: acetylcholin, histamine, 5-hydroxytryptamine - serotonin, prostaglandin, endothelium derived relaxing factor - EDRF, endothelin.

Direct regulation of blood pressure is provided by three reflexes:

- baroreceptor reflex
- chemoreceptor reflex
- ischemic reaction CNS (central nervous system) – (Cushing reflex)
  - Baroreceptors are situated in the carotid sinus, aortic arch, pulmonary arteries and less frequently in other large arteries in the upper chest. Any increase in arterial blood pressure stimulate the baroreceptors, these will depress the activity of the vasomotor center that is followed by lowering the sympathetic tonus: resulting in peripheral vasodilatation lowering cardiac activity and normalization of blood pressure. An opposite effect could be achieved when there is an initial drop in blood pressure.
  - Chemoreceptors react to changes in $pO_2$ of blood flowing towards the aortic and carotid bodies and they exert their action on blood pressure that ranges between 40-100 mmHg. When there is decrease in the blood flow there is a consequent drop in oxygen supply and a resulting conduction of activity to the vasomotor center will aim to return the pressure back to its original level.
  - Reaction of CNS to ischemia is a defensive mechanism against the extreme drop of blood pressure. This is about a mechanism that ensures an adequate blood flow to the brain. When the blood pressure drops down or the brain is badly perfused due to other reason, the vasomotor centrum suffers and starts to be exclusively active. It starts to send sympathetic vasoconstricting impulses to the vessels and cardiac accelerating impulses to the heart. This mechanism is activated only when the arterial blood pressure drops below 60 mmHg.

The vasomotor center is mainly controlled by the hypothalamus, which posterolateral part increases the activity of the vasomotor center, the anterior part inhibits it.

The central and peripheral sympathetic nervous systems regulate the cardiovascular function via adrenoreceptors. The mediator is noradrenaline, which is produced by the nerve endings. Sympathetic vasoconstricting agents (eg. psycho-emotional stress) stimulate the chromaffin system of the adrenals as well, that leads to the production of adrenaline and low amounts of noradrenaline. Adrenaline leads to an increment in the cardiac output, evokes tachycardia, and increases the systolic blood pressure. The total peripheral resistance is basically not changed. Noradrenaline increases the systolic and diastolic blood pressure by increasing the peripheral vascular resistance. Catecholamins lead to a decrement of the vascular blood flow through the kidneys, and hence a decrement of sodium and water excretion by the kidneys. There is also activation of the renin-angiotensin system.

The renin-angiotensin system is composed of a multistep cascade of on each other dependent substances. The key substance and a limiting factor is the enzyme renin. This enzyme is produced in the juxtaglomerular apparatus of the kidneys. The renin-angiotensin system exists in other tissues too. This extrarenal system is subjected to an intensive study mainly in the vessels.

Angiotensin II binds to the cellular membrane receptors and stimulates $Ca^{2+}$ influx, but do not activate adenylcyclase. Angiotensin as well stimulates the biosynthesis and proliferation of smooth muscle. It causes constriction of the systemic arterioles (by its direct effect on the pre-capillary resistant vessels). During physiological conditions there is a dynamic equilibrium between the pressor and the depressor mechanism, this equilibrium keeps the blood pressure in the optimal range. (Arterial hypertension can be the consequence of the disorder of the mentioned equilibrium being either due to the relative or the absolute excess of the pressing factors or the inadequacy of the depressing factors).

Differing from the nervous regulatory mechanisms that can react within few seconds, other regulatory mechanisms need longer time for exerting their effect.

1. Transcapillary shift of fluids (the flow of fluid out of the capillaries or into the capillaries): With blood pressure change there will be a change in the capillary pressure. When the arterial blood pressure drops down there will be a consequent drop of fluid filtration through the capillary membrane into the interstitial space and hence increasing the amount of circulating blood. Contraversly, in cases of increased blood pressure there will be fluid escape into the interstitial space. This mechanism reacts slowly.
2. Mechanism of vascular adaptation: For example after a massive blood transfusion there will be an initial raise in blood pressure, yet after certain time - from 10 minutes to one hour - and due to vascular relaxation the blood pressure returns to normal range even though the blood volume increases by nearly 30% over the normal level. Contraversly after a massive bleeding this mechanism can lead to vasoconstriction enclosing the remaining blood volume and by this keeping normal haemodynamics. This mechanism has its restriction by which it can correct only changes ranging between +30% and -15% of the blood volume.

Long lasting regulation of blood pressure is obtained mainly by the kidneys as an organ. Aldosterone limits water and salt loss.

The renal mechanisms of sodium and water excretion have the greatest importance for long lasting regulation. With raising blood pressure there is a consequent raise of perfusion pressure in the kidneys and sodium and water excretion into urine. The raise in blood pressure that results from the raise of cardiac output (for e.g.: in cases of expansion of the body fluids) at normal renal function will evoke pressure diuresis and natriuresis and hence decrease in volume and blood pressure. In renal function disturbance e.g. in low blood flow through the kidneys, which results from the general drop of blood pressure, or from a loss of functional kidney parenchyma there will be sodium and water retention in the organism that will consequently lead to raise in the venous return, cardiac output, and blood pressure.

There will be an establishment of a new state of equilibrium (high blood pressure, high peripheral resistance, normal cardiac output, and normal volume of body fluids) that characterizes most of the hypertension cases. This condition modifies the function of baroreceptors, sympaticoadrenergic mechanisms, renin-angiotensin system, mineralocorticoids and other factors.

Blood pressure is a relative variable and a continuous physiologic value. The level of blood pressure deserves attention because it has been found that it almost directly increases the cardiovascular risk. As the increase is continuous, arbitrary values of arterial hypertension (hereinafter hypertension), at which we can consider the cardiovascular risk to be increased, have been assessed. These values are currently 90 mmHg for the diastolic and 140 mmHg for the systolic blood pressure. According to this criterion, approximately 25% of the world population suffers from hypertension. It seems that the risk of complications depends more on the increase in systolic pressure than diastolic pressure, and it is higher in some specific groups, for example, in Afro-Americans. As opposed to the latter, a decrease in blood pressure in hypertensive patients markedly decreases the incidence of ischemic disease of the heart, heart failure, brain attack, and the incidence of lethal attacks.

It is necessary to understand the regulation of blood pressure and especially the molecular pathways of its regulation, to be able to treat it. Despite our persistent struggle, we still do not know the details of many of its mechanisms.

We are successful in assessing the etiology of hypertension only in 5%—15% of patients. Secondary hypertension most often develops on the basis of primary hyperaldosteronism, Cushing's syndrome, feochromocytoma, atherosclerotic narrowing of renal artery (renovascular hypertension) or other disorders.

In 80%-95% of patients, the cause of hypertension is unknown. So far, the efforts to find the factor that is responsible for the origin of this 'essential hypertension' have failed. Individual physiological components as cariac output, volume of extracellular fluid, or plasmatic renin activity differs among patients, implying that essential hypertension is not a disease, but rather a syndrome that is common in several diseases based on variable etiology. The interconnection of difficult mechanisms regulating the blood pressure however leads to the fact that even if there is one factor primarily responsible for the origin of hypertension, others are responsible for its maintenance. It shows that environmental factors as stress, lack of exercise, smoking, alcohol, fat intake, and especially sodium intake in food have to find a sufficiently 'fertile' genetic substrate.

## 4. Analytical view of blood pressure regulation and factors leading to hypertension

The analytical view of any problem resides in the breakdown of the entire system right down to its individual parts. The latter can be further broken down until we achieve a simplification that can be easily understood. This approach is fully justified in the process of scientific research. However, it is necessary to note that after losing the associations of individual parts with the entire unit, this procedure can lead to a dead end.

Etiology and pathogenesis of essential hypertension is only partially understood. Due to a large number of factors and pathogenic mechanisms that participate in the development and progression of hypertension its pathogenesis is rather complicated. The heterogenesity of the factors which lead to the eventual effect - increasing the systemic arterial blood pressure - is the cause of the fact that has not been unified yet. It seems that it is not even possible, because according to the newest information essential hypertension is a common name for regulatory disturbances of blood pressure, which might have various causes of development and therefore different pathogenic mechanism. Most of the theories which try to explain the pathogenesis do agree on that there is a disorder in blood pressure regulation (this disturbance may probably affect any parts of the regulating chain), that is due to some internal (endogenous) or external (exogenous) factors.

The endogenic factors are multifactorial, including genetic ones. The exogenous factors are the realizators of the genetic propensity, and they include primarily a high salt intake, high energy provision and some psychogenic factors.

### 4.1 Genetic and familiar affects

It is known, that hypertension usually affects more than one member of the family. The blood pressure, similarly as other quantitative constitutional signs, is to a certain limit similar in all members of the same family.

The decisive factor yet is considered to be the inheritance of those factors that have some importance in the etiology and the pathogenesis of essential hypertension. It was proven that some biochemical and other markers, and even some reactions to different stimuli - that are present in people with essential hypertension - can be noticed also in still healthy normotensive members of hypertensive families:

- There might be some genetically conditioned changes of the metabolism and the release of catecholamines.
- Fast release of noradrenaline from the thrombocytes, can be one of the genetic markers (the place of noradrenaline storage are even the thrombocytes).
- Low contents of kallicrein (a depressor factor) were found in some children of hypertensive families.
- Apart from the discovered high systolic and diastolic blood pressure as well as the body weight in children of the hypertensive families, they also have a significantly low level of plasma aldosterone.
- There is also a genetically based high sensitivity to $Na^+$ expected in people with essential hypertension.
- There might be a genetic factor that is expressed even due to stress (e.g. normotensive people react differently to various psychogenic stimuli by increasing the blood pressure and a long lasting increment of the blood pressure).
- Meanwhile there is an intensive study about some enzyme transport systems, mainly for $Na^+$, $K^+$, $Ca^{2+}$ (in the kidneys and the vascular wall, in erythrocytes, leukocytes, and lymphocytes). The genetic determinant of these transport abnormalities in patients suffering from essential hypertension was shown.

The question of genetic markers is very important for the practical field - mainly for the future. As markers blood and serum groups are being studied before all. Meanwhile it is the HLA system and other systems that influence the immunity. For hypertension they are important only for its familiar predilection and also for prognosis of atherosclerosis development and its complications. The hereditary factors basically participate in the variability of the blood pressure and in the genesis of essential hypertension. The type of inheritance is most probably polygenic, additive and it further more interacts with exogenic factors.

### 4.2 Factors of external environment

SALT: The relation between salt and hypertension development has been known since the beginning of this century. Its role in the pathogenesis is based partly on many epidemiological studies (from different regions of the world), from which it was clear that the prevalence of hypertension is directly related to the amount of salt intake. And partly due to some clinical studies, that refer to that that lowering the blood pressure is parallel with decreasing the extracellular fluid that may be accomplished by diet containing markedly low quantities of salt or by continuous diuretic therapy.

Increasing the salt intake will result in increased volume of extracellular fluid. This fact results in a larger venous return to the heart, that will consequently cause an increase of the cardiac output and due to autoregulation peripheral vessel resistance will be secondarily increased. According to Guyton the peripheral tissues protect themselves in this way from high perfusion, if they are not functioning. Another possibility is a primary increase of the peripheral resistance. During an abnormally high sodium intake there will be an increase of sodium concentration in the muscle cells of the vascular wall that will consequently result in the retention of more $Ca^{2+}$ ions leading to higher vascular wall sensitivity to vasoconstricting agents.

According to the latest studies concerning the pathogenesis of essential hypertension the genetic defect of kidneys to excrete salt plays a very important role. Yet, the exact mechanism that results in increasing of the blood pressure is still not exactly understood or proven. One of the possible explanations that are accepted nowadays are the changes of the cation transport across the cellular membrane. To maintain a constant low $Na^+$ concentration of $Na^+$ intracellularly, the $Na^+$ has to be expelled out across the cellular membrane using these active transport mechanisms:

- $Na^+$-$K^+$ pump: actively expels $Na^+$ extracellularly against the concentration gradient. The needed energy for this active process is supplied from the hydrolysis of ATP with the aid of the $Na^+$, $K^+$ dependent ATPase. The activity of the $Na^+$-$K^+$ ATPase is a measure of the sodium pump activity. From the quantitative point of view sodium pump is responsible for about 80 % of the active transport of sodium from the cell, the action of which is inhibited by ouabain or digoxin.
- $Na^+$-$K^+$ cotransport mediates a simultaneous unidirectional transport of $Na^+$, and $K^+$ and may be also chlorides intra- or extracellularly.

In physiological conditions these and other transport systems form an optimal electrolyte composition of the intracellular fluid. A disorder of these transport mechanisms can decrease the active transport of sodium from the cell. This means that during an unchanged passive intracellular transport the content of intracellular $Na^+$ will rise. This rise of the intracellular $Na^+$ concentration causes rise of the concentration of free intracellular $Ca^{2+}$ as well (due to the fact that there is close relation between the intracellular $Ca^{2+}$ concentration and a transmembrane $Na^+$ gradient due to the presence of $Ca^{2+}$-$Na^+$ exchange mechanism. Even a slight rise of the intracellular sodium concentration leads to an increment of $Ca^{2+}$ transport intracellularly.)

These transport systems do exist even in the formed blood elements such as erythrocytes, leukocytes, and lymphocytes. This provides us with the chance to study the activity of those transport systems for $Na^+$ also in human and not only in experimental animals. The activity of $Na^+$-$K^+$ ATPase was proven to be low in erythrocytes, leukocytes, and even lymphocytes of patients with essential hypertension.

Low $Na^+$-$K^+$ ATPase activity is more prominent in patients with high or normo renin essential hypertension (according to the plasma renin activity we classify hypertension as: low-, normo-, and high renin hypertension). Upon increasing the volume of extracellular fluid and hence increasing the extracellular $Na^+$ content the organism will compensate this by increasing the level of natriuretic substances, mainly, the atrial natriuretic peptide (ANP), which is formed in the cardiac atria and its function is realized in the kidneys where ANP increases the excretion of $Na^+$ by increasing the glomerular filtration and inhibiting its tubular reabsorption. It also lowers the aldosterone production. An other of the natriuretic substances is a natriuretic hormone that inhibits $Na^+$-$K^+$ ATPase, which will consequently lead to a limited transport into cells or to expulsion of $Na^+$ outside the cells, and hence to an increase of the intracellular $Na^+$ content followed by an increase of intracellular $Ca^{2+}$ content as well (as explained previously). It is not clear yet whether the natriuretic hormone and digitalis-like endogenous substances (digitalis-like compounds) are the same and the only $Na^+$-$K^+$ ATPase inhibitors.

As a consequence of all above mentioned is that there might be a congenital primary defect of the transmembranous $Na^+$ transport caused by a high level of humoral substance - that is supposed to be the natriuretic hormone.

What is more important here is that during the mentioned exchange mechanisms intracellular $Ca^{2+}$ concentration increases, which is then a trigger mechanism for muscular contraction of vessels. By this mechanism the increased $Na^+$ concentration in the myocytes of the vascular wall could lead to an increased susceptibility for vasoconstriction stimuli, and by this to become an important pathogenic mechanism for the development of hypertension.

Potassium ($K^+$) There is a lot of evidence that a high $K^+$ intake is protective against hypertension and maybe even against other hurtful effects of high sodium intake. High potassium intake results in drop of the blood pressure. (Individuals that consume mainly vegetarian food have low blood pressure). The combination of low $Na^+$ intake and higher $K^+$ intake is more effective than low $Na^+$ intake alone.

There are many possibilities of the hypotensive effect of potassium:

1. It causes diuresis and hence lowers the plasma volume.
2. In patients treated with $K^+$ there is a drop in the body weight and there is a decrease of $Na^+$ content in the organism.
3. It inhibits the plasma renin activity.
4. It can cause vasodilatation due to a direct effect on the arteriolar smooth muscle.

Magnesium ($Mg^{2+}$) It was found that adding $Mg^{2+}$ (in the form of aspartate hydrochloride) increases the depressor effect of the diuretics. Any disturbance of $Mg^{2+}$ metabolism may result in generalized muscular contraction and hence affecting the blood pressure. $Mg^{2+}$ is a $Na^+$-$K^+$ ATPase activator and it is a $Ca^{2+}$ antagonist. When the level of $Mg^{2+}$ is low it causes an increase of the intracellular $Ca^{2+}$ concentration and hence promotes vasoconstriction.

Obesity practically all the epidemiological studies point to that there is a direct relationship between the level of the blood pressure and the body weight. This relationship concerns the primitive as well as the developed polulations, and also concerns both children and adults.

To explain the relationship between obesity and blood pressure we noticed that obese people who expend more energy need as well a higher expenditure of salt per day. In obese people there might be hyperinsulinemia and as well as insulin resistance. Insulin enhances the retention of sodium in the kidneys. Too much eating is also accompanied by an increase of the sympathetic tonus and an increased noradrenaline turnover.

Psychoemotional stress In the interaction with other mechanisms the neurovegetative system also takes part in the regulation of blood pressure. Also its function arises from the basic circulatory functions - in any case to ensure the supply of oxygenated blood under the required blood pressure to all organs and tissues according to their actual needs.

The CNS reacts to exogenous stress factors (stressors of the outside environment) actually via a dual efferent stereotype which affects also the blood pressure:

1. Activating the sympathetic system that leads to the release of catecholamines from the adrenal medulla and this is characterized by some known reactions.
   - fight (associated with vasodilatation in all limbs)
   - flight (vasodilatation only in lower limbs)
2. Activating of the adenohypophysis and via the adrenocorticotropic hormone the stimulation of the adrenal cortex.

In the initial phase of stress there will be an activation of antidiuretic hormone (ADH) that is formed in the hypothalamus. After its release from the neurohypophysis (where it is only stored) into the circulation, it acts on the distal and the collecting tubules of the kidneys. Its action lies in enhancing the reabsorption of water. Apart from this it shares the modulation of blood pressure. In the beginning of the stress situation and as a result of the peripheral vasoconstriction there will be a lowered renal perfusion that leads to the activation of the renin-angiotensin-aldosterone system.

Aldosterone increases the volume of body fluids by the reabsorption of $Na^+$ and hence water in the distal tubules. Angiotensin II is a pressor factor. It stimulates vasoconstriction via direct mechanism. It enhances the synthesis and the release of noradrenaline from the nerve endings and it also blocks its uptake by the nerve terminals. Apart from this it stimulates adrenaline and aldosterone release from the adrenals as well as the vasopressin from the neurohypophysis, what will consequently lead into an increased vascular susceptibility to vasoconstricting agents.

Along with the stimulation of the sympathetic nervous system and the adrenal medulla, there will also be release of hormones of the anterior lobe of the pituitary (adenohypophysis), from which the most important one in stressful situations is the adrenocorticotropic hormone (ACTH).

The accepted fact meanwhile is that high blood pressure is associated with certain personality characters as well as with certain type of occupation. From this point of view there are some interesting studies that classify people according to their behavior and reactivity into two types: type A and type B. Type A people - who are predisposed to hypertension are characterized by high agility, ambition, psychological instability that might turn into aggressive and impulsive behaviour, the person is despotic and egocentric. People of type B are characterized as phlegmatic, psychologically stable, with no personal ambitions.

From the mechanistic point of view, blood pressure is proportionate to the cardiac output and peripheral resistance. Therefore, all factors involved in the development or maintenance of hypertension must be associated with changes in one or both of these two physiological values.

In a majority of patients with incipient essential hypertension, there is an increase in cardiac output, whereas the peripheral resistance and the extracellular fluid volume stay normal. Later, as blood pressure increases, the cardiac output decreases again to physiological or mildly increased values just as well as the volume of extracellular fluid (with the exception of the disorder in renin-angiotensin-aldosterone system), whereas the peripheral resistance increases. In advanced stages of the disease as a result of the damage incurred to target organs, the glomerular filtration decreases (the extracellular volume increases), and the perfusion of the brain and coronary vessels also decreases. In this phase, the maintenance of high blood pressure is inevitable in order to procure sufficient perfusion of brain and kidneys (to maintain the glomerular filtration at a decreased filtration surface). Hypertrophic heart muscle without the respective growth in coronary perfusion, however, is not able to provide sufficient perfusion pressure against the increased vascular resistance. The activation of renin-aldosterone system and the retention of fluids theoretically improve this state, yet eventually they bring about further fixation and progression of hypertension. As a result of progressive damage to nephrons, a decrease in glomerular filtration takes place in advanced stages of the disease and further contributes to the retention of sodium and extracellular fluid.

Consequent comprehension of the pathomechanism of hypertension needs to take into account all the possible disorders in regulation of individual physiological components, determining the development and maintenance of increased blood pressure, cardiac output, and peripheral resistance.

## 5. Factors determining the peripheral resistance and its role in blood pressure regulation

*Haemodynamic changes in essential hypertension*

During the initial stage of the essential hypertension the cardiac output is increased and tachycardia is present. The causes and the mechanism of an increased cardiac output in hypertensive patients with the initial stage of essential hypertension are due to an increased sympathetico-adrenal activity. It acts directly on the heart and the vascular structure, where there is an increased tension of the vascular wall in the resistant and the capacitive (venous) field. Narrowing the venous field will increase the preload and could be the primary cause of increased cardiac output.

But more marked haemodynamic changes can be seen in people with essential hypertension during physical activity. During the early stages of hypertension there will already be a drop in cardiac output due to the drop of systolic output. However, the resistance of arteries increases. In the late stages the signs of hypokinetic situation due to the subnormal systole become even more prominent.

In patients with long lasting hypertension high blood pressure is the result of high peripheral resistance in case of low functioning myocardium, or a marked cardiac insufficiency. The first change occurring in the vessels can be functional vasoconstriction or some structural changes in the vascular wall.

During vasoconstriction that is caused by high sympathetic tonus, concentration of $Na^{+}$, $Ca^{2+}$ and water content in the vascular wall also increase. Later on there will be some structural changes in the wall of the vessels: Thickening of the wall due to the hypertrophy of the media and hyperplasia of the collagen fibers. That is the cause of the changes in the relation between the thickness of the vascular wall and its lumen. Narrowing of the lumen alone can increase peripheral resistance. In patients with developed hypertension the high peripheral resistance is caused by vasoconstriction and by structural changes in vascular walls.

The arteriolar vasoconstriction and the vascular resistance do not occur in all organs equally in essential hypertension. The most affected are the vessels of the skin and kidneys, whereas the skeletal muscles are perfused normally.

Peripheral resistance is determined especially by the lumen of resistant arterioles, and to a lesser extent, by the lumen of medium and large arteries. These can be changed either by active contraction of smooth muscles, or passively by remodeling. Both mechanisms are influenced by hemodynamic load and neurohumoral regulation (balance between vasoconstrictors and vasodilators), as well as by concentrations of sodium and potassium ions.

Further, it is necessary to note that on one hand the vascular bed perfusion is directly proportional to pressure difference; on the other hand however, it is inversely proportional to peripheral vascular resistance. In other words, the increased blood pressure under the condition of increased peripheral resistance does not necessarily have to improve the perfusion. On the contrary, increased peripheral resistance means that in order to maintain the same perfusion, it is necessary to increase the systemic pressure; thus greater cardiac work is needed. If the increase in blood pressure is inappropriate in relation to the increase in vascular resistance, then the microcirculation can even deteriorate by forming a further requirement to increase the blood pressure. In this way a vicious circle develops, leading to further fixation and progression of hypertension.

## 6. The role of microcirculation

A great problem resides in microcirculation. The perfusion of blood via capillary bed is regulated by physical laws. We can quantify neither the details of myogenic tonus of arterioles, nor the transmural pressure within capillaries [5-7].

It is very probable that the capillary bed functions as a modular system. The blood does not flow instantly through all capillaries. The fluctuation of perfusion and nonperfusion forms a complex system that has not yet been investigated. The diameter of capillaries ranges from 4 to 12 μm; erythrocytes achieve the diameter of 7.2 μm. This fact implies that the perfusion of blood through capillaries has no analogy in the flow of water through an elastic system. Probably it would be very illusory to imagine that in the capillarized organism, the processes of filtration and reabsorption take place very near each other, and at the same time. The argument can be seen in the structure of kidneys. The arterial end of capillary with filtration is represented by capillaries within glomeruli and the venous end of capillaries is represented by peritubular capillaries.

When imagining the modular system of microcirculation the filtration takes place, with subsequent reabsorption in the same capillaries. The exchange of filtration and reabsorption is probably a complex system, the changes of which compel the inflow of blood to take place under higher pressure.

The increased heart rate represents another problem. The pulse waves crash into one another, possibly resulting in decreased perfusion. Each increase in heart rate causes an increase in the filling of the system; however not an increase in microcirculation via capillaries. In adrenergic situations, the increase in blood pressure with no increase in heart rate would be more advantageous for the organism. The entire process is however a matter of the complex system of regulation and participation of the sympathetic nerves, enabling the circulation to adapt to various stimuli.

## 7. Pathophysiologic outcome for the possible therapeutic benefit

The vessels supplying the tissues with blood and thus with oxygen can be regarded as an elastic system that is submerged within the elastic environment (e.g. myocardium). Two elastic systems are involved. A change in pressure within the tissue surrounding the vascular bed influences the blood perfusion [8, 9]. The impact of pressure on vessels and perfusion is in close relation to their diameter. An increase in outer pressure decreases the perfusion within arterioles and shifts the blood into the capillary bed [8]. It is very probable that Hook's law can also be applied in this situation. Despite the great progress achieved in medicine, and two centuries of investigation, the exchange of substances on the capillary level remains a problem for both physiologists and philosophers [10].

In their biomechanic studies, Wang et al. [11] applied the Hook's law to intravascular blood circulation. A decrease in compliance and elasticity (increased rigidity, or increased pressure) within the surrounding tissue can decrease the blood perfusion even in an entirely intact vascular bed. Current clinical studies as well as experimental investigations are focused on the vascular system, especially its distributing part. These measurements provide many valuable parameters. The changes in structures and tissues surrounding the capillary bed however still elude our understanding. We lack precise parameters and have only a mosaic notion of them. We can only assume that within these tissues plasticity and elasticity decrease with age.

Animal experiments prove our conception of the possible impact that changes occurring within the perivascular tissue pressure have on blood perfusion [12]. The latter authors however admit that in large vessels also the tunnel-in-gel concept is justified. In compliance with this conception, a change in elastic properties of tissues, namely a decrease in their elasticity decreases the blood perfusion within these tissues. This notion is in accord with experimental measurements of Golub et al. [13]. By using a special technique of phosphorescence quenching microscopy they found that the decrease in partial oxygen pressure in the course of arterioles is negligible. They found that there is a measurable difference between partial oxygen pressure present in small arterioles and that in venules. By means of the latter technique, they discovered local differences in tissue $pO_2$ and the dependence of $O_2$ consumption on local pressure changes. Wilson et al. [14] used this technique to measure the partial oxygen pressure and stated a hypothesis that the capillary wall had no impact on the diffusion of oxygen from plasma into pericellular space.

It is generally known that electrophysiological measurements of intracellular and pericellular values of oxygen pressure range from 0 mmHg to 5 mmHg, and within the mixed venous blood it ranges between 30 mmHg and 40 mmHg. The normal function of both isolated cells and cells within tissues requires pressure exceeding 2 mmHg [15]. The most significant moment appears to be the difference between vascular and intracellular values of oxygen pressure. We assume that a decrease in diastolic pressure can bring about a decrease in intracellular and pericelluar values of oxygen pressure. The mechanisms of processing this information within the body are still not known. A decrease in pericellular and intracellular oxygen can be a consequence of decreased diastolic and hydrostatic pressure (Fig. 1). This phenomenon is facilitated by the fact that pericellular and intracellular values of oxygen pressure are already under very low physiological conditions. This conception can possibly be an acceptable explanation of adverse effects that appear as a consequence of therapeutic decrease of blood pressure down to the level of 70 mmHg or lower [16, 17, 18].

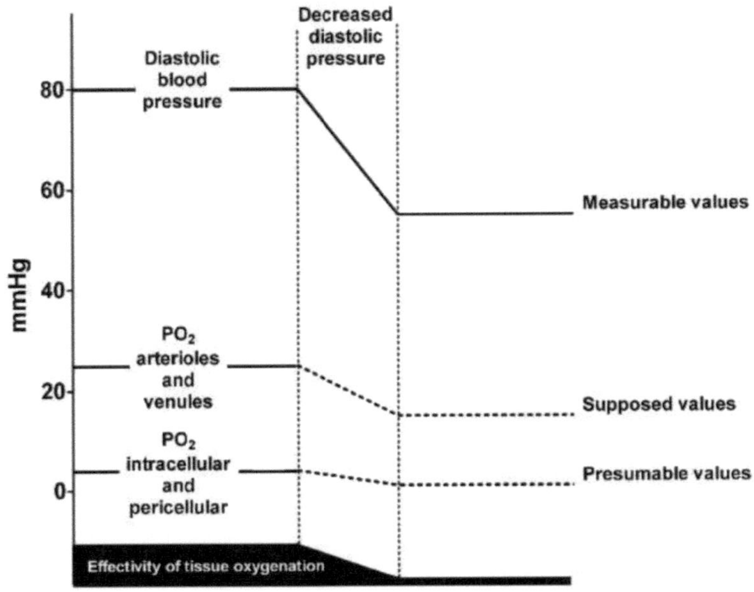


Fig. 1. Probable changes of oxygen pressure caused by decreased diastolic pressure.

## 8. Conclusions

Essential hypertension is a consequence of complex multifactorial disorders. In some cases it can be the mutation of one gene in a large population. Most probably essential hypertension is a result of a combination of mutations and polymorphisms of some genes influencing the blood pressure in interaction with various environmental factors.

Most probably, even in the future it will still not be possible to assess all polymorphisms and altered molecular mechanisms responsible for the origin of hypertension. However, a more detailed knowledge about the molecular pathways involved in blood pressure regulation would most probably help us to understand the development of hypertension in more details. We assume that the origin of hypertension can be inevitable to ensure sufficient oxygen delivery under higher pressure because it is necessary due to the hypertension-induced alteration in the structure of microcirculation. On the contrary, a therapeutic decrease in blood pressure can deteriorate tissues oxygenation at least, for a particular time until a new balance is formed and until new remodeling takes place (Fig. 2).

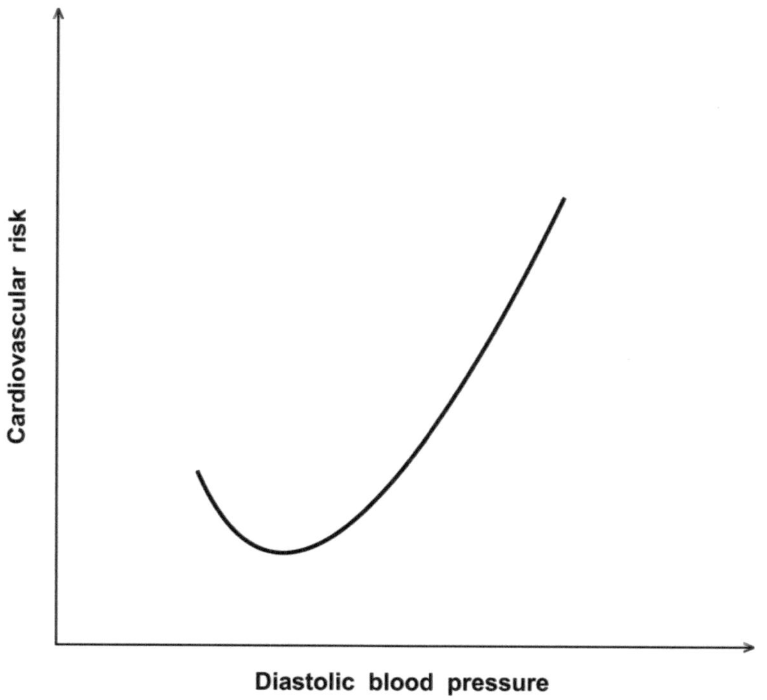


Fig. 2. J-curve as a possible consequence of insufficient tissues oxygenation.

## 9. Learning points

- The cells can be the hidden motor forcing the organism to fulfill the cellular needs. In this view blood pressure is not only a part of a functioning circulation.
- The optimization of osmotic and pressure factors can be achieved in various ways. These mechanisms can very effectively manage new situations in each cell, preferably in selected cells. The long-lasting activation of these mechanisms may lead to their fixation enabling the pressure to serve as a tool for increasing natriuresis at general load.
- Essential hypertension is a consequence of complex multifactorial disorders. Most probably, essential hypertension is a result of a combination of mutations and polymorphisms of some genes influencing the blood pressure in interaction with various environmental factors.
- We assume that the origin of hypertension can be essential to ensure sufficient oxygen delivery under higher pressure because it is necessary due to hypertension-induced alteration in the structure of microcirculation.
- Therapeutic decrease in blood pressure can deteriorate tissue oxygenation, at least for a particular time until a new balance is formed and until new remodeling takes place. Does the decrease in pressure procure optimal oxygenation of brain in hypertensive patients?
- It is an established fact that about hypertension has accumulated a lot of information. Hypertension can be treated successfully. Drug therapy reaches approximately physiological blood pressure. Hypertonic patients with approximately normal blood pressure in spite of this fact die due to hypertension. Successfully treated patients

compared with untreated live a little longer. But they die on the same consequences as untreated patients with hypertension.

## 10. References


[1] Weder AB. Evolution and hypertension. Hypertension 2007;49:260-5.

[2] Kaplan NM. Clinical trials for hypertension: expectations fulfilled and unfulfilled. Hypertension 2007;49:257-9.

[3] Vimo A, Winblad B, Angero-Torres H, von Strauss E. The magnitude of dementia occurrence in the world. Alzheimer Dis Assoc Disord 2003;17:63-7.

[4] Staessen JA, Richart T, Birkenhäger VH. Less atherosclerosis and lower blood pressure for a meaningful life perspective with more brain. Hypertension 2007;49:384-400.

[5] Feihl F, Liaudet L, Waeber B, Levy BI. Hypertension. A disease of the microcirculation. Hypertension 2006;48:1012-7.

[6] Jeong JH, Sugii Y, Minamiyama M, Okamoto K. Measurement of RBC deformation and velocity in capillaries in vivo. Microvasc Res 2006;71:212-7.

[7] Williams DA. Change in shear stress (Deltatau)/hydraulic conductivity (Lp) relationship after pronase treatment of individual capillaries in situ. Microvasc Res 2007;73:48-57.

[8] Hulin I, Slavkovsky P. Segmental blood flow through intamyocardial coronary arteries during ventricular systole. Med Hypotheses 1994;43:312-4.

[9] Hulin I, Kadlec O, Grigel M, Niks M, Brozman B, Kratochvilova E. Pathogenesis of hypertension in Masugi's nephritis. Bratisl Lek Listy 1974;61:149-68.

[10] Hwa C, Aird WC. The history of the capillary wall: doctors, discoveries, and debates. Am J Physiol Heart Circ Physiol 2007;293:H2667-79.

[11] Wang C, Zhang W, Kasab GS. The validation of generalized Hook's law for coronary arteries. Am J Physiol Heart Circ Physiol 2008;294:H66-73.

[12] Liu Y, Dang C, Garcia M, Gregersen H, Kassab GS. Surrounding tissue affect the passive mechanics ofthe vessel wall: theory and experiment. Am J Physiol Heart Circ Physiol 2007;293:H3290-330.

[13] Golub AS, Barker MC, Pitman RN. Microvascular oxygen tension in the rat mesentery. Am J Physiol Heart Circ Physiol 2008;294:H21-8.

[14] Wilson DF, Lee WMF, Makonen S, Finikova O, Apreleva S, Vinogradov S. Oxygen pressure in the interstitial space and their relationship to those in the blood plasma in resting skeletal muscle. J Appl Physiol 2006;101:1648-56.

[15] Wilson DF. Quantifying the role of oxygen pressure in tissue function. Am J Physiol Heart Circ Physiol 2008;294:H111-3.

[16] Hulin I, Duris I, Sapakova E, Paulis L, Mravec B. Essential hypertension - Syndrome or Compensatory mechanism. Cas Lek Cesk 2008;147:14-24.

[17] Hulin I, Duris I, Paulis L, Sapakova E, Mravec B. Dangerous versus useful hypertension (A holistic view of hypertension). Eur J Intern Med 2009;20:226-230.

[18] Hulin I, Kinova S, Paulis L, Slavkovsky P, Duris I, Mravec B. Diastolic blood pressure as a major determinant of tissue perfusion: potential clinical consequences. Bratisl Lek Listy 2010;111(1):54-6.

2

# Target Organ Damage in Essential Hypertension

Bogomir Žižek
*Department of Angiology, University Medical Centre, Ljubljana, Slovenia*

## 1. Introduction

Epidemiological data suggests that hypertension remains a major modifiable risk factor for cardiovascular disease in Western countries. The prevalence of the disease among adults in Slovenia aged 25–64 years is between 40–50% (CINDI, 2006). The early detection and severity of typical target organ damage and secondary diseases are key determinants of cardiovascular prognosis in patients suffering from arterial hypertension (Mancia et al., 2009). The classic manifestations of hypertensive target organ damage include: damage in the conduit arteries (atherosclerosis), kidney (nephrosclerosis) and heart (left ventricular hypertrophy, diastolic dysfunction, reduction of coronary reserve). The recommendations of medical societies specializing in hypertension do not base risk stratification solely on blood pressure (BP), but rather take into account concomitant cardiovascular diseases as well (Mancia et al., 2009). Early detection and adequate management of hypertensive target organ damage can slow or prevent damage, or even allow disease regression where organ damage is still at reversible stage. Therefore, the diagnosis of hypertensive target organ damage is of decisive importance. The purpose of this review is to summarize current and emerging approaches to the pathophysiology, early detection and treatment of hypertensive disease.

## 2. Etiopathogenesis of essential hypertension

In spite of intensive investigation, etiology of essential hypertension (EH), which accounts for 90-95% of all cases of arterial hypertension remains poorly understood. Heredity is a predisposing factor (Sagnella & Swift, 2006), but environmental factors (e.g., dietary $Na^+$, obesity, sedentary lifestyle, stress, alcohol intake) seem to increase the risk of developing hypertension (Kyrou et al., 2006; Lackland & Egan, 2007).

Pathogenesis is also not known. Because BP equals cardiac output (CO) × total peripheral vascular resistance (TPR), pathogenic mechanisms must involve increased CO, increased TPR, or both. Many theories have been proposed to explain this equation; the microcirculation theory is the most attractive among them. In accordance with this theory the primary defect involves small resistance vessels, leading to increased TPR and sustained elevated BP. Several basic studies support this theory as functional and morphological abnormalities in the microcirculation may appear very early in evolving EH. Functional changes (endothelial dysfunction) could be the first event; later on, morphological changes of the vasculature ensue. The latter include increased media/lumen ratio due to hypertrophy and/or hyperplasia of myocytes in the vessel wall and decreased density (rarefaction) of blood vessels on biopsy (Mark, 1984; Schiffrin, 1992; Sivertsson et al., 1979; Takeshita & Allyn, 1980). Plethysmographic studies suggest that TPR is increased even in normotensive young men with a familial predisposition to hypertension (Takeshita et al., 1982).

Endothelial cells (EC) have a pivotal role in the maintenance of the basal tone and modulation of TPR. In the endothelium releases several biologically active substances, which maintain the homeostasis between circulating blood and arterial wall via autocrine and paracrine mechanisms. Vasoconstricting factors (endothelin-1, thromboxane $A_2$, angiotensin II) on one side and vasorelaxing factors (prostacyclin, nitric oxide /NO/) on the other are secreted by EC (Lüscher, 1994; Vane et al., 1990) (Figure 1.). In their pioneer work Furchgott and Zawadzki 1980 reported that EC stimulated by a neurotransmitter (acetylcholine) can evoke vasodilation (Furchgott & Zawadzki, 1980). The mediator of these responses is a diffusible substance with a half-life of few seconds, the so-called *endothelium derived relaxing factor* – EDRF, which is chemically identical to NO and is continuously secreted upon shear stress forces (produced by blood flow) from EC (Hutchinson & Palmer, 1987; Ignarro et al., 1987). Basal generation of NO keeps arterial circulation in an actively dilated state (Schiffrin, 1992). The intracellular mechanism by which NO causes dilation in vascular smooth muscle cells involves formation of cyclic 3′,5′-guanosine monophosphate (cGMP) via the enzyme soluble guanylyl cyclase, intracellular $Ca^{++}$-ion depletion and consequently relaxation of myocytes (endothelium-dependent dilation) (Palmer et al., 1987; Rubany et al., 1986; Wennmalm, 1994). Indeed, many experimental studies have shown that NO could contribute to TPR and to modulation of BP (Persson et al., 1990; Rees et al., 1989; Vallance et al., 1989). In addition, NO appears to be an endogenous inhibitor of norepinephrine in animal studies and thus a modulator of the sympathetic nerve system, a mechanism which could also be involved in the pathogenesis of EH (Cohen & Weisbrod, 1988; Greenberg et al., 1990).

## 3. Target organ damage

### 3.1 Vascular abnormalities (endothelial dysfunction) in EH

Recently, works related to the association between EH and sustained endothelial damage has gained popularity among hypertension scientists. It remains unclear however whether endothelial changes precede the development of hypertension or whether such changes are mainly due to long standing elevated BP.

The term endothelial dysfunction describes several pathological conditions, including altered anticoagulant and anti-inflammatory properties in the endothelium, impaired modulation of vascular growth, and deregulation of vascular remodeling, decreased production of NO and unbalanced production of other different vasoactive substances (endothelin-1, thromboxane $A_2$, and angiotensin II) (Moncada et al., 1991). In the literature

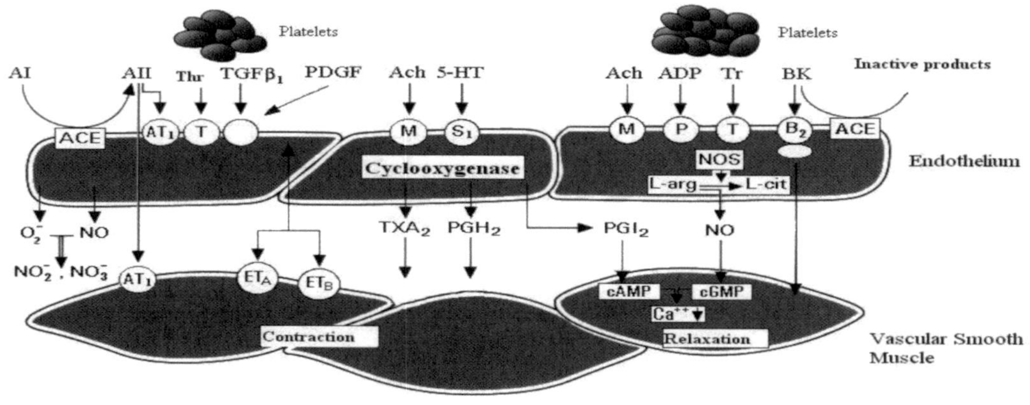


Fig. 1. Endothelium derived vasoactive substances. The endothelium is a source of relaxing (*right*) and contracting factors (*left*). *$AT_1$*, angiotensin receptor; *A II*, angiotensin II; *ACE*, angiotensin-converting enzyme; *Ach*, acetylcholine; *ADP*, adenosine diphosphate; *BK*, bradykinin; *cAMP/cGMP*, cyclic adenosine/guanosine monophosphate; *5-HT*, 5-hydroxytryptamine (serotonin); *ET-1*, endothelin-1; *L-arg*, L-arginine; *NO*, nitric oxide; *$NO_2^-$/$NO_3^-$*, nitrite/nitrate; *$O_2^-$*, superoxide radical; *$PGI_2$*, prostacyclin; *$TGF\beta_1$*, transforming growth factor $\beta_1$; *Thr*, thrombin; *$TXA_2$*, thromboxane $A_2$; *Circles* represent receptors; Modified from Lüscher, 1994.

however, the term specifically refers to an impairment of endothelium-dependent vasodilation caused by decreased NO bioavailability in the vessel wall (Poredoš, 2002). Endothelial dysfunction has been demonstrated in subjects with different risk factors for atherosclerosis including arterial hypertension, and in coronary atherosclerotic disease (Egashira et al., 1995; Zeiher et al., 1993). We shall now focus on evidences which indicate that endothelial dysfunction is a characteristic finding in patients with EH (Taddei & Salvetti, 2002).

Under basal conditions, whole-body NO bioavailability is diminished in hypertension (Moncada et al., 1991). With few exceptions (Cockcroft et al., 1994), hypertensive patients have shown to have impaired endothelium-dependent vasodilative response of the peripheral resistance arteries (usually measured by forearm blood flow using venous occlusion plethysmography) to NO stimulants (acetylcholine) (Panza et al., 1993; Panza et al., 1990; Taddei et al., 1993), but not to endothelium-independent vasodilators such as nitroprusside (Panza et al., 1993). Using B-mode ultrasound the impairment of dilation capability of systemic conduit arteries during reactive hyperemia was demonstrated, as was reduced vasodilative response to acetylcholine in coronary vessels of patients with EH (Treasure et al., 1993; Zeiher et al., 1993; Žižek et al., 2001a; Žižek & Poredoš 2001b). Authors postulate that EH like other risk factors for atherosclerosis (hypercholesterolemia, diabetes and smoking) damage and change the function of EC (Drexler et al., 1991; Zeiher et al., 1991). The evidence for a role of defective NO-mediated vasodilation in the etiopathogenesis of arterial hypertension has been further strengthened by its recognition in still normotensive children of hypertensive parents (Žižek et al., 2001a, Žižek & Poredoš, 2001b). As impaired endothelium-dependent vasodilation precedes and predicts the future development of hypertension, one could reasonably speculate that endothelial dysfunction is causally related to EH (Rossi et al., 2004). Moreover, it seems that endothelial dysfunction is partly inherited but deteriorates further in evolving hypertension – thus suggesting that endothelial dysfunction in established hypertension could be the cause and the consequence of hypertensive disease (Calver et al., 1992; Žižek et al., 2001a).

There are relatively few data, albeit controversial, on mechanisms leading to decreased production of NO in EH. The majority of investigators attach weight to inherited or acquired decreased activity of a key enzyme, NO synthase (Bogle et al., 1995; Mehta et al., 1994). Recent reports have shown that reduced NO bioactivity may be linked to increased circulating level of the endogenous NO synthase inhibitor, asymmetric dimethyl L-arginine (Achan et al., 2003). In sustained EH decreased vasodilation was explained by a deficiency of L-arginine, the precursor of NO (Panza et al., 1993), inactivation of NO due to free radicals formation (Mechta et al., 1994), impeding diffusion to smooth muscle cells (Van de Voorde & Leusen, 1986), blunted response of the smooth muscle to pharmacological and physiological stimuli (Robinson et al., 1982), and increased production of vasoconstricting factors (endothelin-1, angiotensin II) (Lüscher, 1994).

In addition to NO, prostacyclin ($PGI_2$) is released by EC in response to shear stress, hypoxia and to several substances (acetylcholine, substance P, serotonin) which are also released by NO (Figure 1.). $PGI_2$ is synthesized by cyclo-oxygenase from arachidonic acid (Vane et al., 1990). Prostacyclin increases cyclic 3′,5′-adenosine monophosphate (cAMP) in smooth muscle cells and platelets. Its platelet inhibitory effects are probably more important than its contribution to endothelium-dependent relaxation (Vane et al., 1990). The synergistic effect of both $PGI_2$ and NO enhances the antiplatelet and anticoagulant activity of the EC (Pearson & Wheeler-Yones 1997; Yang et al., 1994).

The family of endothelins consists of three closely related peptides: endothelin-1 (ET-1), endothelin-2, and endothelin-3 (Figure 1.). EC produce exclusively endothelin-1, which is the strongest vasoconstricting factor (Rossi et al., 1999). The release of the peptide is modulated by shear stress, epinephrine, angiotensin II, thrombin, inflammatory cytokines (tumor necrosis factor-α, interleukin-1, -2) and hypoxia (Moncada et al., 1991). There are well known interactions between ET-1 and other vasoactive substances. After inhibition of the endothelial L-arginine pathway, thrombin and angiotensin II induced ET-1 production is augmented (Moncada et al., 1991). ET-1 can release NO and $PGI_2$ from EC, which as a negative feedback mechanism reduces peptide production in endothelium and its vasoconstrictor action in smooth muscle (Moncada et al., 1991; Rossi et al., 1999). Infusion of an ET-1 receptor antagonist in healthy humans leads to vasodilation, indicating a role of ET-1 in the maintenance of basal vascular tone (Haynes et al., 1996). In some severe hypertensive patients ET-1 gene expression and vascular hypertrophy in small resistance arteries were reported (Schiffrin et al., 1997).

Oxidative stress plays an important role in the development of endothelium injury found in EH. It is defined as imbalance between production of reactive oxygen species (ROS) and antioxidants that neutralize them (Landmesser & Drexler, 2007; Spieker et al., 2000). Formation of ROS, resulting in scavenging of NO and reduced NO bioavailability, has been suggested as a hallmark of endothelial dysfunction and a pathogenetic mechanism in several cardiovascular diseases, including hypertension (Figure 1.) (Schulz et al., 2011). Indeed, increased production of ROS has been observed in human hypertension (Higashi et al., 2002;

Redon et al., 2003) as well as evidenced in animal models, such as in angiotensin II (Landmesser et al., 2002) or in genetically defined hypertension (Nishiyama et al., 2004).

Increased production of vascular ROS, especially superoxide anion ($O_2^-$) contributes significantly to functional and morphological alterations in hypertension (Touyz et al., 2004). Exaggerated superoxide production and low NO bioavailability lead to endothelial dysfunction and hypertrophy of vascular cells promoting atherosclerosis (Figure 1.). It has been reported that the enzyme NAD(P)H oxydase plays a major role as the most important source of superoxide anion in vascular cells (Zalba et al., 2001). Experimental observations indicated an enhanced superoxide generation as a result of the activation of vascular NAD(P)H oxydase in hypertension (Griendling et al., 2000). During pulsatile stretch of the arterial wall expression of the enzyme is increased, thus enabling a positive feedback mechanism between oxidative stress and hypertension (Hishikawa et al., 1997). Although NAD(P)H oxydase responds to stimuli such as vasoactive factors, growth factors, and cytokines, some recent data suggest a genetic background modulating its expression (Landmesser & Drexler, 2007). Oxidative excess is also linked to a pro-inflammatory state of the vessel wall. Adhesion and chemotactic molecules upregulated by ROS seem to play a key pathophysiological role in the process of atherogenesis (Touyz, 2004). In particular, increased $O_2^-$ production is associated with NO bioinactivation, which influences afferent arteriolar tone, tubuloglomerular feedback responses, and sodium reabsorption - all of which is paramount in long-term BP regulation (Wilcox, 2002). Moreover, ROS are known to quench NO with formation of peroxynitrite, which is a cytotoxic oxidant. Peroxynitrite leads to degradation of NO synthase cofactor of tetrahydrobiopterin leading to uncoupling of endothelium NO synthase in hypertension and secretion of ROS rather than NO (Landmesser et al., 2003).

The best known regulator of BP and determinant of target organ damage in hypertension is the renin-angiotensin-aldosterone system (RAAS). The basic scheme of function has been known for a long time; however, recent evidence shows that apart from circulating RAAS, tissue RAAS also exists and may well be of greater importance (Hsueh & Wyne, 2011). Tissue RAAS is most important in the vessel wall, the heart and the kidney. Constituents of RAAS could enter the endothelium or could originate from it (Hsueh & Wyne, 2011). The role of angiotensin II in neurohumoral modulation is very well investigated. Angiotensin II modifies the vascular tone either directly by activation angiotensin 1 ($AT_1$) receptors in vessel wall myocytes or indirectly by stimulation of norepinephrine secretion from the nerve endings (Kim & Iwao, 2000; Williams, 2001). Although acute hemodynamic effects of angiotensin II are useful, its chronic elevation could have deleterious non-hemodynamic consequences. Angiotensin II can cause endothelial dysfunction, vascular stiffness and accelerated atherogenesis independently from BP (Williams, 2001). It is proposed that in the condition of low plasma renin level for its non-hemodynamic effects an increased expression of $AT_1$ receptors could play a role (Figure 1.). Namely, in hypertension expression is increased due to pulsatile stretch of arterial wall leading to increased local effects of $AT_1$ receptors. This inaugurates increased angiotensin II effects and other constituents of RAAS, especially aldosterone (Kim & Iwao, 2000; McMahon, 2001). Harmful effects of the latter extend from endothelial dysfunction, fibrosis and inflammation of arterial wall to systemic electrolytes and hemodynamic imbalance (Brasier et al., 2002; Duprez, 2006). In particular, convincing evidence exist that overactivation of RAAS, or at least part of it, may induce ET-1 production and increase angiotensin-converting enzyme

(ACE) activity, which splits bradykinin, an important endothelium-derived relaxing factor (Watanabe et al., 2005). Angiotensin II has been shown to increase secretion of vascular NAD(P)H oxydase and formation of ROS (Hitomi et al., 2007). Indeed, increased production of ROS has been observed in human hypertension (Higashi et al., 2002; Redon et al., 2003).

Endothelial dysfunction is the earliest measurable disturbance in arterial wall function, which could be measured *in vivo*. Early detection of endothelial dysfunction in EH can be achieved by the abovementioned methods - namely, measurement of hemodynamic changes by ultrasound, measurement of hemodynamic changes by occlusive plethysmography, and measurement of circulating markers of defective EC function (ET-1, adhesion molecules, tumor necrosis factor–TNF-α, von Willebrand's factor, plasminogen activator inhibitor-1, asymmetric dimethyl L-arginine) (Achan et al., 2003; Devaraj et al., 2003; Treasure et al., 1993; Yang et al., 2010; Žižek et al., 2001a). Detailed description of these methods exceeds the purpose of this paper.

Endothelial dysfunction could be improved or even restored with preventive measures. Different studies showed that elimination or management of risk factors (for example treating hypercholesterolemia with statins) results in improvement of endothelial dysfunction (Wassmann et al., 2001). Considerably less interventional data, albeit controversial, are available concerning treatment of EH and endothelial dysfunction of the large conduit arteries. Studies on animal models and in humans have shown that normalization of BP can restore impaired endothelium-dependent vascular responses (Iwatsubo et al., 1997; Lüscher & Vanhoutte, 1987). Conversely, another group of investigators failed to show normalization of endothelial dysfunction in conduit arteries treated with the same drug (ACE inhibitor) (Eržen et al., 2006). Thus, several questions still remain unanswered - it is not clear whether endothelial dysfunction can be completely normalized, whether normalization of endothelial function is related to adequacy of antihypertensive treatment, and whether antihypertensive drugs importantly differ in their ability to improve endothelial dysfunction. In this regard, ACE inhibitors seem to be the most appropriate class of antihypertonic agents (Virdis & Ghiadoni, 2011). Endothelial dysfunction could also be improved by substances with protective function on endothelium such as L-arginine, low-cholesterol diet, exercise and antioxidants (vitamin C) (Kabat & Dhein, 2006). Significance of the measures taken in the improvement of endothelial function is of greater importance when we consider the results from studies showing that cardiovascular morbidity and mortality very much depends on the severity of endothelium dysfunction (Kitta et al., 2005).

### 3.2 Morphological changes of the large arteries – atherosclerosis

EH is an important risk factor for atherosclerosis. As the cellular and molecular pathogenetic mechanisms of atherosclerosis and the effects of hypertension are being more clearly defined, it becomes apparent that the two processes have certain common mechanisms. The endothelium is a likely source of interaction between both diseases. NO acts as a vasodilator and inhibits platelet adherence and aggregation, smooth muscle proliferation, and endothelial cell-leukocyte interaction. Furthermore, a decrease in NO activity may contribute importantly to the initiation and progression of atherosclerotic lesions. It is proposed that several interrelated cellular and molecular processes such as inflammation are a likely consequence of mechanical and chemical damage of the endothelium by different risk factors, including hypertension (Badimon & Fuster, 1993; Bondjers et al., 1991; Fuster et al., 1992; Landmesser & Drexler, 2007). However, recent observations favour the hypothesis that endothelial dysfunction in EH could be a primary defect and as such directly inherited (Bondjers et al., 1991; Vane et al., 1990; Žižek et al., 2001a; Žižek & Poredoš 2001b). Irrespective of the sequence of events, endothelial dysfunction promotes atherogenesis through different mechanisms: expression of adhesions molecules, increased adherence of monocytes and platelets, enhanced permeability of the endothelium layer to monocytes/macrophages and lipoproteins, which then accumulate in the vessel wall. As the atherosclerotic process progresses to plaque formation growth factors secreted by macrophages stimulate smooth muscle cells migration, proliferation and interstitial collagen synthesis. In the late stages of disease, the event that initiates the development of the majority of myocardial infarctions is the rupture of the fibrous cap of the plaque inducing thrombus formation. (Fuster et al., 1998; Ross, 1993).

It must be emphasized that risk factors for atherosclerosis tend to cluster, and therefore EH is rarely the only risk factor found in an individual patient. Hypertension is often accompanied by the metabolic syndrome, which encompasses a cluster of risk factors: obesity, dyslipidemia, glucose intolerance, a pro-thrombotic (high levels of fibrinogen and plasminogen activator inhibitor-1) and a pro-inflammatory state (high levels of tumor necrosis factor-$\alpha$, interleukin-1, -2, C-reactive protein) (Devaraj et al., 2003; DeFronzo & Ferrannini, 1991; Tamakoshi et al., 2003). It is proposed that these heterogeneous groups of clinical conditions favor atherogenesis. People with the metabolic syndrome are at increased risk of coronary heart disease and other diseases related to plaque buildups in the arterial wall (e.g., stroke and peripheral vascular disease) (Olijhoek et al., 2004).

Assessment of the earliest morphological abnormalities in the arterial wall by B-mode ultrasound has been reported two decades ago. Diffuse thickening of the inner layer of arterial wall could be measured and followed by this non-invasive method (Pignoli et al., 2006). However, the method does not differentiate intima from media. Therefore both entities are measured together as the intima-media thickness (IMT) (Salonen et al., 1993). IMT of large peripheral arteries, especially carotid arteries, can be assessed by B-mode ultrasound in a relatively simple way. Due to tight associations between atherosclerotic changes in the carotid arteries and in other parts of the circulation, especially coronary arteries, carotid arteries could be regarded as a gateway enabling us to estimate the progression of arterial disease (Poredoš, 2004). Carotid arterial IMT is used in studies as a surrogate endpoint to measure progression of atherosclerosis. Several studies have shown a significant relationship between IMT and cardiovascular risk factors, such as age, male gender, cholesterol levels, BP, diabetes mellitus and smoking habits (Poredoš et al., 1999; Salonen et al., 1993; Žižek & Poredoš, 2002). Thicker IMT could be detected in healthy normotensive offspring of parents with EH, thus implying that morphological changes could be directly inherited (Žižek & Poredoš, 2002).

The relation between IMT and EH was confirmed in interventional studies. One of the largest studies, ELSA (European Lacidipine Study on Atherosclerosis) assessed IMT in EH patients. It showed that slowing of progression of the thickening could be achieved only by some drugs irrespective of the comparable lowering of the BP (Tang et al., 2000). This finding is important because in recent years we got strong evidence that IMT is an independent risk factor for cardiovascular events and is a better predictor of events than all other known single conventional risk factors. In a Finnish study, ultrasonographic assessment of 1,257 men was compared with diagnostic information obtained from a prospective registry for acute myocardial infarction; it concluded that for each 0.1 mm of the common carotid IMT, the risk for a myocardial infarction increased by 11% (Salonen et al., 1993).

Recently, ample interest has been devoted to the relationship between arterial stiffness and cardiovascular disease. Pulse pressure and pulse wave velocity, surrogate measurements of arterial stiffness, indicate that arterial stiffness increases both with age and in certain disease states that are themselves associated with increased cardiovascular risk, including hypertension, diabetes mellitus and hypercholesterolemia (Glasser et al., 1997). Arterial stiffness may be measured using a variety of different techniques, mainly ultrasound based. Applanation tonometry pulse wave velocity is the most commonly used parameter in detecting central arterial stiffness (Nichols, 2005). Arterial stiffening has been particularly implicated in the development of isolated systolic hypertension and heart diseases leading to increased cardiovascular morbidity and mortality (Laurent et al., 2001).

### 3.3 Hypertensive nephropathy

EH is the main cause of the chronic kidney disease; however, morphologic evidence on the subject remains poorly understood (Fournier et al., 1994). A perennial problem in understanding the interaction between kidney and hypertension is the poor correlation between hypertension, and vascular and glomerular lesion. This is in part due to these lesions being present to a greater or lesser degree in the normotensive, aging kidney, with racial differences in severity further confounding the problem. Recent experimental and clinical data suggest that functional impairment and vasoconstriction in afferent arterioles (renal autoregulation) precede morphologic lesions. Progression of the endothelial dysfunction and consequent alterations in autoregulation of renal blood flow at higher pressures enable to dilate afferent arterioles transferring elevated BP to the glomeruli. The latter mechanism finally leads to glomerulosclerosis. Histological changes in the arterioles (stiffness) are present as intimal thickening, afferent arteriolar hyalinosis and smooth muscle atrophy. Loss of renal autoregulation with glomerular hypertrophy, hyperfiltration, and focal segmental glomerulosclerosis is now recognized to contribute significantly to nephrosclerosis, particularly in the black population. However, ischemic glomerulosclerosis may ultimately be the most important lesion, with consequent hypoxia in the parenchyma leading to tubular atrophy and interstitial fibrosis. Pathomorphological changes contribute variably to renal failure according to the level of hypertension (Freedman et al., 1995; Hill, 2008)

Recent studies provided convincing evidence that overactivation of RAAS, or part of it, may play a key role in functional and morphological abnormalities found in hypertensive nephrosclerosis (Volpe et al., 2002). In line with this statement, interventional studies showed that ACE inhibitors, $AT_1$ receptor blockers (ARBs) and direct renin inhibitors such aliskiren may slow down or stop progression of chronic kidney disease (Momback & Toto, 2009; Riccioni, 2011).

Hypertensive nephropathy often results in chronic renal failure, which mostly occurs unnoticed and without clinical symptoms. It has been shown that even a minimal reduction of renal function could be regarded as an independent risk factor for cardiovascular mortality and morbidity (Ruilope & Bakris, 2011; Segura et al., 2004). Hypertensive nephropathy can be detected by means of early signs such as the occurrence of mild albuminuria and reduced glomerular filtration rate, both of which are easily measured parameters. Albuminuria can be traced to functional and morphological transformational processes in the glomeruli that are associated with increased permeability (Hill, 2008). A recent study demonstrated that increasing albuminuria is associated with an exponential increase in the risk of developing chronic renal failure and cardiovascular complications (Levey et al., 2009).

Rigorous, mostly multidrug antihypertensive therapy can prevent the progression of chronic renal failure and albuminuria/proteinuria and thereby improve both, renal and cardiovascular prognosis (Ruilope & Bakris, 2011). Hence, treatment with ARB (losartan) as shown in the LIFE study reduction of albuminuria in hypertensive patients with left ventricular (LV) hypertrophy is associated with fewer cardiovascular complications (Ibsen et al., 2005).

### 3.4 Hypertensive heart disease

The heart in EH is affected very often and sometimes very early. LV hypertrophy, diastolic dysfunction and reduced coronary vasodilation reserve are direct manifestations of cardiovascular target organ damage in patients with arterial hypertension and signify hypertensive heart disease. Coronary artery disease, afflicted by atherosclerotic processes is another indirect consequence of hypertension. All these pathophysiological conditions are interrelated and may end in myocardial infarction, heart failure and arrhythmia (Schmieder, 2010).

#### 3.4.1 Abnormalities in left ventricular diastolic function

The term diastolic dysfunction is used to describe abnormalities of ventricular filling, including decreased diastolic distensibility and impaired relaxation. LV is not able to accept adequate blood volume without compensatory increase of the filling pressure (Zile & Brutsaert, 2002). Diastolic dysfunction is thought to represent an important pathophysiological intermediate between hypertension and heart failure, especially in heart failure with normal ejection fraction (Sanderson, 2007). Up to 50% of patients with history of hypertension have evidence of diastolic dysfunction, which represents an attractive target for heart failure prevention (Fischer et al., 2003). However, to date no specific treatments have been definitively shown to improve diastolic function and clinical outcome (Solomon et al., 2007).

Diastolic dysfunction is considered the earliest functional change in evolving hypertension and could be measured before morphological abnormalities (hypertrophy) ensue. We reported that LV filling abnormalities were detected in normotensive offspring of hypertensive families suggesting that diastolic dysfunction is affected by factors other than BP (Žižek et al., 2008). Diastolic filling abnormalities in hypertensive heart disease result from a delayed LV relaxation and in the later stages from a reduced LV compliance due to increased myocardial fibrosis (Zile & Brutsaert, 2002). Systemic/local RAAS or parts of it and ET-1 have been reported as factors influencing fibrosis (Böhm et al., 2011; Hart et al.,

2001). The mechanisms involved in delayed relaxation are not completely understood, but altered myocardial metabolism of energy-rich phosphates has been proposed (Lamb et al., 1999). In hypertensive patients decreased concentration of ATP and increased concentration of other phosphates leading to disturbances in $Ca^{++}$ homeostasis have been reported (Lamb et al., 1999). Decreased levels of $Ca^{++}$ in sarcoplasmic reticulum not only impair LV systolic function but also delay relaxation, which may ultimately end in abnormalities in LV filling properties and heart failure (Piacentino et al., 2003).

Recent experimental studies have firmly established that NO released from coronary endothelial cells and from myocytes exerts several specific effects on myocardial function, analogous to endothelial regulation of vascular wall function (Paulus & Shah, 1999). In particular, these include selective enhancements of myocardial relaxation (Cotton et al., 2001) and reduction in myocardial oxygen consumption (Xie et al., 1996). Several other paracrine and autocrine effects of NO on myocardial function have been described, e.g. modulating inotropic state (Cotton et al., 2001), modulating sarcolemmal $Ca^{++}$ homeostasis (Piacentino et al., 2003) and inhibiting growth-promoting effects of norepinephrine in myocites and fibroblasts (Calderone et al., 1998; Ruetten et al., 2005).

Echocardiography is now the most commonly used noninvasive tool for assessment of cardiac function. Detailed information can be obtained by standard pulsed Doppler echocardiography and from recent developed tissue Doppler-, strain rate- and speckle tracking imaging (Wang & Nagueh, 2009).

### 3.4.2 Left ventricular hypertrophy

An increase in peripheral vascular resistance is the hallmark of established hypertension. Following sustained hypertension the heart develops concentric hypertrophy that is characterized by thickening of LV walls. Hypertrophic process is initially adaptive and enables the heart to neutralize wall stress associated with increased impedance to ventricular emptying (afterload) (Grossman, 1980). Moreover, this thickening process is accompanied by a series of maladaptive changes that occur in the extracellular matrix as well as in cardiac myocytes. The presence of LV hypertrophy is clinically important because it is associated with an increased incidence of myocardial infarction, heart failure, ventricular arrhythmias and sudden cardiac death (Muiesan et al., 1996).

Pathogenetic mechanisms leading to LV hypertrophy and dysfunction in EH are not completely understood. It seems that they are results of various interrelated hemodynamic and non-hemodynamic factors. Sometimes hypertrophy can be detected in the prehypertensive period of evolving hypertension implying that a genetic background could also play a role (Žižek & Poredoš, 2008). One fundamental component of cardiomyocyte response to pressure overload of the LV is a slowing of maximum shortening velocity ($V_{max}$). Diminution of $V_{max}$ is beneficial at the cardiomyocyte level, allowing the cardiac fiber to contract at a normal energy cost. However, at the LV level the diminution of $V_{max}$ is the first step that will finally lead to heart failure (Swynghedauw et al., 2010). Another component of the response of the myocyte to pressure overload includes increased cell size, caused by multiplication of contractile units and, according to the law of Laplace this will normalize wall stress and preserve LV chamber function (Frohlich et al., 2011). An additional component of the cardiomyocyte response involves a shift in substrate oxidation from fatty acids (FAs) toward carbohydrates (Akki & Seymour, 2008). Although in terms of oxygen cost, the oxidation of glucose is more efficient than that of FAs, in absolute terms the oxidation of one molecule FAs yields far more ATP than glucose. Accordingly, the hypertrophied heart is an energy-compromised organ with a diminished ATP production. On the other hand, a sustained decline in FAs oxidation may cause inappropriate accumulation of lipids in the hypertrophied cardiomyocyte resulting in contractile dysfunction (Neubauer, 2007).

The re-expression of the cardiomyocyte fetal gene program is essential for the abovementioned pathophysiological responses to sustained hypertension (Barry et al., 2008). Activation of the fetal gene program allows coordinated synthesis of proteins necessary to bring about increased cardiomyocyte size and adjustment to the altered energy demands of these larger cells. Recent studies have revealed that in conditions of pressure overload both neurohumoral factors and physical stretch stimulate protein G and phospholipase C leading to activation of several signaling molecules including $Ca^{++}$-dependent proteins (i.e., $Ca^{++}$/calmodulin and calcineurin), protein kinases (i.e., protein kinase C and mitogen-activated protein kinases ERK, JNK and p38), and intracrine growth factors (i.e., angiotensin II) that result in altered gene expression associated with pathological cardiomyocyte hypertrophy (Baker et al., 2004; Dorn & Force, 2005).

Systemic/local RAAS is an important pathogenetic mechanism in development of hypertensive heart disease (Agabiti-Rosei & Muiesan, 2001, Schunkert et al., 1997). Experimental studies on hypertensive rat hearts and cell culture media confirm cardiotropic effects of angiotensin-II (Brilla et al., 1994). The angiotensin II has direct influences on various pathophysiological abnormalities in intracellular $Ca^{++}$ handling, metabolism of contractile proteins and myocardial remodeling (Agabiti-Rosei & Muiesan, 2001). Studies performed during the last two decades have provided evidence that complex changes in myocardial composition are responsible for the morphological remodeling of the myocardium in hypertensive heart disease beyond cardiomyocyte hypertrophy (Frohlich et al., 2011). Exaggerated deposition of collagen fibers types I and III promoting interstitial and perivascular fibrosis, which is a well recognized lesion in hypertrophied myocardium (Weber, 2000). The interstitial fibrosis increases myocardial stiffness, thus facilitating LV diastolic dysfunction and diastolic heart failure (Neubauer, 2007). Mounting evidence shows that fibrosis may be a reparative response of fibroblasts induced by pro-inflammatory and pro-fibrotic factors, such as aldosterone (Böhm et al., 2011; Young, 2008). In alignment with the latter statement, epidemiologic studies show that aldosterone is a predictor of future EH and cardiovascular complications (Blacher et al., 1997; Vasan et al., 2004).

Beyond hemodynamic and humoral factors, the genetic background may also influence myocardial composition in hypertensive heart disease. Up to 60% of the variance of LV mass may be due to genetic factors independent of BP. An increasing number of genes have been described, including members of the RAAS system, the type A human natriuretic peptide receptor gene, protein G gene affecting the $Na^{+}/H^{+}$ exchanger, as well as genes related to contractility and function such as the myosin-binding protein C and genes involved in the β-adrenergic system (Deschepper et al., 2002). Among them, the most strongly associated with LV hypertrophy is the polymorphism of genes that encode components of the RAAS system (Kuznetsova et al., 2004). These non-hemodynamic factors may be involved in the development of inappropriate LV mass, which is defined as the growth of the LV exceeding the individual needs to compensate hemodynamic load imposed by increased BP (Agabiti-Rosei & Muiesan, 2001). Moreover, increased LV mass may be associated with cardiac dysfunction and adverse cardiovascular prognosis (Muiesan et al., 1996).

Echocardiography is the gold standard test for LV hypertrophy. It can precisely estimate a patient's left ventricular mass and assess for other morphological cardiac abnormalities. Electrocardiography is more commonly used in everyday practice; it is more cost-effective and has high specificity, but lower sensitivity (Schmieder, 2010).

In recent years, many papers dealing with antihypertensive therapy have been published. Treatment of hypertension accompanied with LV hypertrophy has shown that each and every class of available antihypertensive drugs could diminish LV mass but with different efficacy. ACE inhibitors and ARBs seem to be superior to other classes of antihypertonic agents (Dahlöf et al., 1992; Oren et al., 1996). Later on the investigators demonstrated that reduction of the LV mass is associated with reduced cardiovascular risk (Verdecchia et al., 2003) and that observed clinical benefit with ACE inhibitors and ARBs tended to be greater than that expected from a decrease in BP. These potential effects "beyond BP control" are perhaps responsible for the protective properties of these drugs interfering with RAAS system-mediated myocardial remodeling (Devereux et al., 2004). However, data from the large ONTARGET/TRASCEND study has shown that treatment with an ARB (telmisartan) alone or in combination with an ACE inhibitor (ramipril) was associated with a lower prevalence of LV hypertrophy, but this was ultimately not translated into a prognostic benefit (Verdecchia et al., 2009). Whatever the causes of these unsatisfactory results, the unacceptably high residual risk still persisted in treated hypertensive patients in whom LV mass decreased with the treatment (Zanchetti, 2009).

Increasing evidence suggests that aldosterone receptor blockade (spirinolactone, eplerenone) may prevent myocardial fibrosis in patients with hypertensive heart disease independent of its effects on BP (Böhm et al., 2011; Jansen et al., 2009). In patients with EH, addition of low-dose spirinolactone to an ACE inhibitor (enalapril/trandolapril) or ARB (candesartan) resulted in a greater decrease in LV mass and fibrosis than any of these drugs alone (Sato et al., 2002; Taniguchi et al., 2006). The failure of ACE inhibition to achieve regression of LV hypertrophy might in part be caused by the phenomenon of aldosterone escape, which means the inability of ACE inhibitor therapy to reliably suppress aldosterone release (Sato & Saruta, 2001).

### 3.4.3 Reduced coronary reserve

Reduced coronary vasodilation reserve is a typical complication in patients with established hypertension and may be presented in the absence of angiographically demonstrable atherosclerotic disease (Antony et al., 1993). Reduced coronary microcirculatory reserve could be even detected in hypertensive patients without LV hypertrophy (Brush et al., 1988). Authors have reported that functional and morphological abnormalities in microcirculation may appear very early in evolving EH. Functional (endothelial dysfunction) changes could be the first event, with morphological changes of vessels ensuing later on (Schiffrin, 1992). Functional abnormalities of the vessels are evidenced by blunted response to pharmacological and physiological stimuli (Drexler & Zeiher, 1991). An interrelationship between endothelial dysfunction and microvascular angina (syndrome X) has been proposed. This clinical setting is characterized by angina-like pain and abnormal exercise electrocardiography changes in the presence of a normal coronary angiogram (Scheler et al., 1994). The role of endothelial dysfunction in this setting is controversial. It has been shown that patients with microvascular angina have endothelial dysfunction in the resistance vessels, possibly as result of diminished formation of NO. However, other studies on coronary arteries in patients with syndrome X were unable to find signs of endothelial dysfunction (Bøtker & Ingerslev, 2000).

Morphological changes in small arteries in hypertrophied LV and unbalance between increased LV mass and blood supply are the another pathophysiological mechanisms underlying a reduced coronary reserve in small arteries (Agabiti-Rosei & Muiesan, 2001). It has been suggested that morphological abnormalities (such as increased media/lumen ratio due to hypertrophy and/or hyperplasia of myocites in the vessel wall, and the rarefaction of blood vessels in the myocardium) represent adaptations to an increased hemodynamic load imposed by increased BP (Kozakova et al., 1997).

Some controversy in the literature exists whether endothelial dysfunction in small resistance vessels could be influenced by drugs. In experimental animal models, improvement or even normalization by ACE inhibitor (captopril) and ARB (losartan) were reported (Rodrigo et al., 1997). In human studies, improvement was only noticed after a single application of captopril (Hirooka et al., 1992). Conversely, months of therapy with ACE inhibitors and ARBs resulted in only a slight or no effect on endothelial function in resistance arteries (Ghiadoni et al., 2000; Kiowski et al., 1996).

## 4. Conclusions

The results of recent studies emphasize the key role of endothelial function in the pathogenesis of essential hypertension. In accordance with the microcirculation theory, functional and morphological changes in small resistance vessels are thought to be the cause and consequence of hypertensive disease. This condition is predisposed by abnormal endothelial cell function, which is characterized by decreased production of nitric oxide and unbalanced production of other vasoactive substances (angiotensin II, endothelin-1, prostacyclin, and aldosterone) and reactive oxygen species. The target organ damage in conduit arteries (atherosclerosis), kidney (nephrosclerosis) and heart (diastolic dysfunction, left ventricular hypertrophy, reduction of coronary reserve) are the consequence of elevated blood pressure. There is currently no effective treatment known for hypertension. It is important to treat hypertension in the early stages, when preventive measures and antihypertensive therapy (preferably angiotensin-converting enzyme inhibitors and angiotensin receptor blockers) are most effective. Nowadays, non-invasive ultrasound based methods can detect abnormalities in different organs, which predict the unfavorable course of hypertensive disease resulting in a worse cardiovascular prognosis.

## 5. References

Achan V, Broadhead M, Malaki M, et al. Asymmetric dimethylarginine causes hypertension and cardiac dysfunction in humans. *Arterioscler Thromb Vasc Biol* 2003; 23: 1455–59.

Agabiti-Rosei E, Muiesan ML. Hypertensive left ventricular hypertrophy: pathophysiological and clinical issues. *Blood Press* 2001; 10: 288–98.

Akki A, Seymour AM. Compensated cardiac hypertrophy is characterized by decline in palmitate oxidation. *Mol Cell Biochem* 2008; 311: 215–24.

Antony I, Nitenberg A, Foult JM, et al. Coronary vasodilator reserve in untreated and treated hypertensive patients with and without left ventricular hypertrophy. *J Am Coll Cardiol* 1993; 22: 514–20.

Badimon JJ, Fuster V, Chesebro JH, Badimon L. Coronary atherosclerosis, a multifactorial disease. *Circulation* 1993; 87 Suppl 2: S3–16.

Baker KM, Chernin MI, Schreiber T, et al. Evidence of a novel intracrine mechanism in angiotensin II-induced cardiac hypertrophy. *Regul Pept* 2004; 120: 5–13.

Barry SP, Davidson SM. Molecular regulation of cardiac hypertrophy. *Int Biochem Cell Biol* 2008; 40: 2023–39.

Blacher J, Amah G, Girerd X, et al. Association between increased plasma levels of aldosterone and decreased systemic arterial compliance in subjects with essential arterial hypertension. *Am J Hypertens* 1997; 10: 1326–34.

Bogle RG, MacAllister RY, Whitley GS, et al. Induction of $N^G$-monomethyl-L-arginine uptake: a mechanism for differential inhibition of NO synthases? *Am J Physiol* 1995; 269: C750–56.

Bondjers G, Glukhova M, Hansson GK, et al. Hypertension and atherosclerosis. Cause and effect, or two effects with one unknown cause? *Circulation* 1991; 84 Suppl 6: S2–16.

Böhm M, Reil JC, Bramlage P, Pitt B, Zannad F. Clinical efficacy of aldosterone-blocking agents. *Eur Heart J* 2011; 13 Suppl B: B36–9.

Bøtker HE, Ingerslev J. Plasma concentrations of von Willebrand factor in patients with angina pectoris secondary to coronary atherosclerosis or cardiac syndrome X. *Thromb Res* 2000; 97: 519-23

Brasier RA, Recinos A, Eledrisi MS. Vascular inflammation and the rennin-angiotensin system. *Arterioscler Thromb Vasc Biol* 2002; 22: 1257–66.

Brilla CG, Zhou G, Matsubara L, et al. Collagen metabolism in cultured adult rat cardiac fibroblasts: response to angiotensin II and aldosterone. *J Mol Cell Cardiol* 1994; 26: 809–820.

Brush JE, Cannon RO, Schenke WH, et al. Angina due to coronary microvascular disease in hypertensive patients without left ventricular hypertrophy. *N Engl J Med* 1988; 319: 1302–7.

Calderone A, Thaik CM, Takahashi N, Chang DLF, Colucci WS. Nitric oxide, atrial natriuretic peptide, and cyclic GMP inhibit the growth-promoting effects of norepinephrine in cardiac myocites and fibroblasts. *J Clin Invest* 1998; 101: 812–8.

Calver A, Collier J, Moncada S, Vallance P. Effect of local intra-arterial NG-monomethyl-L-arginine in patients with hypertension: the nitric oxide dilator mechanism appears abnormal. *J Hypertens* 1992; 10 : 1025-31.

CINDI (WHO Countrywide Integrated Noncommunicable Disease Intervention) Program Survey 2002/2003. *Slov Kardiol* 2006; 3: 106–14.

Cockcroft JR, Chowienczyk PJ, Benjamin N, et al. Preserved endothelium-dependent vasodilatation in patients with essential hypertension. *N Engl J Med* 1994; 330: 1036–40.

Cohen RA, Weisbrod RM. Endothelium inhibits norepinephrine release from adrenergic nerves of rabbit carotid artery. *Am J Physiol* 1988; 254: H871–8.

Cotton JM, Kearney MT, MacCarthy PA, et al. Effects of nitric oxide synthase inhibition on basal function and the force-frequency relationship in the normal and failing human heart in vivo. *Circulation* 2001; 104: 2318–23.

Dahlöf B, Pennert K, Hansson L. Reversal of left ventricular hypertrophy in hypertensive patients. A metaanalysis of 109 treatment studies. *Am J Hypertens* 1992; 5: 95–110.

DeFronzo RA, Ferrannini E. Insulin resistance. A multifaceted syndrome responsible for NIDDM, obesity, hypertension, dyslipidemia, and atherosclerotic cardiovascular disease. *Diabetes Care* 1991; 14: 173–94.

Deschepper CF, Boutin-Ganache I, Zahabi A, Jiang Z. In search of cardiovascular candidate genes. Interaction between phenotypes and genotypes. *Hypertension* 2002; 39: 332–6.

Devaraj S, Xu DY, Jialal I. C-reactive protein increases plasminogen activator inhibitor-I expression and activity in human aortic endothelial cells. Implications for the metabolic syndrome and atherothrombosis. *Circulation* 2003; 107: 398–404.

Devereux RB, Wachtell K, Gerdts E, et al. Prognostic significance of left ventricular mass change during treatment of hypertension. *JAMA* 2004; 292: 2350–6.

Dorn GW, Force T. Protein kinase cascades in the regulation of cardiac hypertrophy. *J Clin Invest* 2005; 115: 527–37.

Drexler H, Zeiher AM. Endothelial function in human coronary arteries in vivo. Focus on hypercholesterolemia. *Hypertension* 1991; 18 Suppl 4: S90–9.

Duprez DA. Role of the renin-angiotensin-aldosterone system in vascular remodeling and inflammation: a clinical review. *J Hypertens* 2006; 24: 983–91.

Egashira K, Suzuki S, Hirooka Y, et al. Impaired endothelium-dependent vasodilation of large epicardial and resistance coronary arteries in patients with essential hypertension. Different responses to acetylcholine and substance P. *Hypertension* 1995; 25: 201–6.

Eržen B, Gradišek P, Poredoš P, Šabovič M. Treatment of essential arterial hypertension with enalapril does not result in normalization of endothelial dysfunction of the conduit arteries. *Angiology* 2006; 57: 187–92.

Fischer M, Baessler A, Hense HW, et al. Prevalence of left ventricular diastolic dysfunction in the community. Results from Doppler echocardiographic-based survey of a population sample. *Eur Heart J* 2003; 24: 320–28.

Fournier A, El Esper N, Makdassi R, et al. Hypertension and progression of renal insufficiency. *Nephrol Dial Transplant* 1994; 9 Suppl 3: S28–34.

Freedman BI, Iskandar SS, Appel RG. The link between hypertension and nephrosclerosis. *Am J Kidney Dis* 1995; 25: 207–21.

Frohlich ED, González A, Díez J. Hypertensive left ventricular hypertrophy risk: beyond adaptive cardiomyocytic hypertrophy. *J Hypertens 2011;* 29 : 17–26.

Furchgott RF, Zawadzki JV. The obligatory role of endothelial cells in the relaxation of arterial smooth muscle by acetylcholine. *Nature* 1980; 288: 373–6.

Fuster V, Badimon L, Badimon JJ, et al. The pathogenesis of coronary artery disease and the acute coronary syndromes. *N Engl J Med* 1992; 326: 242–50.

Fuster V, Badimon JJ, Chesebro JH. Atherothrombosis: mechanisms and clinical therapeutic approaches. *Vasc Med* 1998; 3: 231–9.

Ghiadoni L, Virdis A, Maqaqua A, et al. Effect of the angiotensin II type 1 receptor blocker candesartan on endothelial function in patients with essential hypertension. *Hypertension* 2000; 35: 501–6.

Glasser SP, Arnett DK, McVeigh, et al. Vascular compliance and cardiovascular disease: a risk factor or a marker? *Am J Hypertens 1997*; 10: 1175–89.

Greenberg SS, Diecke FPJ, Peevy K, et al. Release of norepinephrine from adrenergic nerve endings of blood vessels is modulated by endothelium-derived relaxing factor. *Am J Hypertens* 1990; 3: 211–8.

Griendling KK, Sorescu D, Ushio-Fukai M. NAD(P)H oxydase: role in cardiovascular biology and disease. *Circ Res* 2000; 86: 494–501.

Grossman W. Cardiac hypertrophy: useful adaptation of pathologic process? *Am J Med* 1980; 69: 576–84.

Hart CY, Meyer DM, Tazelaar HD, et al. Load versus humoral activation in the genesis of early hypertensive heart disease. *Circulation* 2001; 104: 215–20.

Haynes WG, Ferro CJ, O'Kane KPJ, Somerville D, Lomax CC, Webb DJ. Systemic endothelin receptor blockade decreases peripheral vascular resistance and blood pressure in humans. *Circulation* 1996; 93: 1860–70.

Higashi Y, Sasaki S, Nakagawa K, Matsuura H, Oshima T, Chayama K. Endothelial function and oxidative stress in renovascular hypertension. *N Engl J Med* 2002; 346: 1954–62.

Hill GS. Hypertensive nephrosclerosis. *Curr Opin Nephrol Hypertens* 2008; 17: 266–70.

Hirooka Y, Imaizumi T, Masaki H, et al. Captopril improves impaired endothelium-dependent vasodilation in hypertensive patients. *Hypertension* 1992; 20: 175–80.

Hishikawa K, Oemar BS, Yang Z, et al. Pulsatile stretch stimulates superoxide production and activates nuclear factor-kappa B in human coronary smooth muscle. *Circ Res* 1997; 81: 797–803.

Hitomi H, Kiyomoto H, Nishiyama A. Angiotensin II and oxidative stress. *Curr Opin Cardiol* 2007; 22: 311–5.

Hsueh WA, Wyne K. Renin-Angiotensin-aldosterone system in diabetes and hypertension. *J Clin Hypertens* 2011; 13: 224–37.

Hutchinson PJA, Palmer RM, Moncada S. Comparative pharmacology of EDRF and nitric oxide on vascular strips. *Eur J Pharmacol* 1987; 141: 445–51

Ibsen H, Olsen MH, Wachtell K et al. Reduction in albuminuria translates to reduction in cardiovascular events in hypertensive patients: Losartan intervention for endpoint reduction in hypertension study. *Hypertension* 2005; 45: 198–202.

Ignarro LJ, Buga GM, Wood KS, et al. Endothelium-derived relaxing factor produced and released from artery and vein is nitric oxide. *Proc Natl Acad Sci USA* 1987; 84: 9265–9.

Jansen P, Danser AHJ, Imholz BP, van den Meiracker AH. Aldosterone receptor antagonism in hypertension. *J Hypertens* 2009; 27: 680–91.

Kabat A, Dhein S. L-arginine supplementation prevents the development of endothelial dysfunction in hyperglycemia. *Pharmacology* 2006; 76: 185–91

Kim S, Iwao H. Molecular and cellular mechanisms of angiotensin II-mediated cardiovascular and renal diseases. *Pharmacol Rev* 2000: 52: 11–34.

Kiowski W, Linder L, Neusch R, Martina B. Effects of cilazapril on vascular structure and function in essential hypertension. *Hypertension* 1996; 27: 371–6.

Kitta Y, Nakamura T, Kodama Y, , et al. Endothelial vasomotor dysfunction in the brachial artery is associated with late in-stent coronary restenosis. *J Am Coll Cardiol* 2005; 46: 648–55.

Kozakova M, Palombo C, Pratali L, et al. Mechanisms of coronary flow reserve impairment in human hypertension. An integrated approach by transthoracic and transesophageal echocardiography. *Hypertension* 1997; 29: 551–9.

Kuznetsova T, Staessen J, Thijs L, et al. Left ventricular mass in relation to genetic variation in angiotensin II receptors, renin system genes, and sodium excretion. *Circulation* 2004; 110: 2644–50.

Kyrou I, Chrousos GP, Tsigos C. Stress, visceral obesity, and metabolic complications. *Ann N Y Acad Sci* 2006; 1083: 77–110.

Lackland DT, Egan BM. Dietary salt restriction and blood pressure in clinical trials. *Curr Hypertens Rep* 2007; 9: 314–9.

Lamb HJ, Beyerbacht HP, van der Laarse A, et al. Diastolic dysfunction in hypertensive heart disease is associated with altered myocardial metabolism. *Circulation* 1999; 99: 2261–7.

Landmesser U, Drexler H. Endothelial function and hypertension. *Curr Opin Cardiol* 2007; 22: 316–20.

Landmesser U, Dikalov S, Price SR, et al. Oxidation of tetrahydrobiopterin leads to uncoupling of endothelial cell nitric oxide synthase in hypertension. *J Clin Invest* 2003; 111: 1201–9.

Landmesser U, Cai H, Dikalov S, McCann L, Hwang J, Jo H, Holland SM, Harrison DG. Role of p47(phox) in vascular oxidative stress and hypertension caused by angiotensin II. *Hypertension* 2002; 40: 511–15.

Laurent S, Boutouyrie P, Asmar R, et al. Aortic stiffness is an independent predictor of all-cause and cardiovascular mortality in hypertensive patients. *Hypertension* 2001; 37: 1236–41.

Levey AS, Cattran D, Friedman A et al. Proteinuria as a surrogate outcome in CKD: report of a scientific workshop sponsored by national Kidney Foundation and the US Food and Drug Administration. *Am J Kidney Dis* 2009; 54: 205–26.

Lüscher TF. The endothelium in hypertension: bystander, target or mediator? *J Hypertens* 1994; 12 Suppl 10: S105–16.

Mark AL. Structural changes in resistance and capacitance vessels in borderline hypertension. *Hypertension* 1984; 6 Suppl 3: S69–73.

Mancia G, Laurent S, Agabiti-Rosei E, et al. Reappraisal of European guidelines on hypertension management: a European Society of Hypertension Task Force document. *J Hypertens* 2009; 27: 2121–58.

McMahon EG. Recent studies with eplerenone, a novel selective aldosterone receptor antagonist. *Curr Opin Pharmacol* 2001; 1: 190–6.

Mehta JL, Lopez LM, Chen L, et al. Alterations in nitric oxide synthase activity, superoxide anion generation, and platelet aggregation in systemic hypertension, and effects of celiprolol. *Am J Cardiol* 1994; 74: 901–5.

Momback AS, Toto R. Dual blockade of the renin-angiotensin-aldosterone system: beyond the ACE inhibitor and angiotensin-II receptor blocker combination. *Am J Hypertens* 2009; 22: 1032-40.

Moncada S, Palmer RM, Higgs EA. Nitric oxide: Physiology, Pathophysiology, and Pharmacology. *Pharmacol Rev* 1991; 43: 109–42.

Muiesan ML, Salvetti M, Rizzoni D, et al. Persistence of left ventricular hypertrophy is a stronger indicator of cardiovascular events than baseline LV mass or systolic performance. A ten years follow-up. *J Hypertens* 1996; 14 Suppl 5: S43–51.

Neubauer S. The failing heart - an engine out of fuel. *N Engl J Med* 2007; 356: 1140–51.

Nichols WW. Clinical measurement of arterial stiffness obtained from noninvasive pressure waveforms. *Am J Hypertens* 2005; 18: 3S–10.

Nishiyama A, Yao L, Nagai Y, et al. Possible contributions of reactive oxygen species and mitogen-activated protein kinase to renal injury in aldosterone/salt-induced hypertensive rats. *Hypertension* 2004; 43: 841–8.

Olijhoek J, JK, van der Graaf Y, Banga JD, et al. The metabolic syndrome is associated with advanced vascular damage in patients with coronary heart disease, stroke, peripheral arterial disease or abdominal aortic aneurism. *Eur J Cardiol* 2004; 25: 342–8.

Oren S, Grossman E, Frohlich ED. Reduction in left ventricular mass in patients with systemic hypertension treated with enalapril, lisinopril, or fosinopril. *Am J Cardiol* 1996; 77: 93–6.

Palmer RM, Ferrige AG, Moncada S. Nitric oxide release accounts for the biological activity of endothelium-derived relaxing factor. *Nature* 1987; 327: 524–6.

Panza JA, Quyyumi AA, Brush JE, Epstein SE. Abnormal endothelium-dependent vascular relaxation in patients with essential hypertension *N Engl J Med* 1990; 323: 22–7.

Panza JA, Casino PR, Badar DM, et al. Effect of increased availability of endothelium-derived nitric oxide precursor on endothelium-dependent vascular relaxation in normal subjects and in patients with essential hypertension. *Circulation* 1993; 87: 1475–81.

Paulus WJ, Shah AM. NO and cardiac diastolic function. *Cardiovasc Res* 1999; 43: 595–606.

Pearson JD, Wheeler-Jones CPD. Platelet-endothelial cell interactions: regulation of prostacyclin and von Willebrand factor secretion. In: *Born GVR, Schwartz CJ eds.* Vascular endothelium: physiology, pathology, and therapeutic opportunities. Stuttgart, New York: Schattauer, 1997: p. 157–67.

Persson MG, Gustafsson LE, Wiklund NP, et al. Endogenous nitric oxide as a modulator of rabbit skeletal muscle microcirculation *in vivo. Br J Pharmacol* 1990; 100: 463–6.

Piacentino V, Weber CR, Chen X, et al. Cellular basis of abnormal calcium transients of failing human ventricular myocytes. *Circ Res* 2003; 92: 651–8.

Pignoli P, Tremoli E, Poli A, et al. Intimal plus medial thickness of the arterial wall: a direct measurement with ultrasound imaging. *Circulation* 1986; 74: 1399–406.

Poredoš P, Orehek M, Tratnik E. Smoking is associated with dose-related increase of intima-media thickness and endothelial dysfunction. *Angiology* 1999; 50: 201–8.

Poredoš P. Endothelial dysfunction and cardiovascular disease. *Pathophysiol Haemost Thromb* 2002; 32: 274–7.

Poredoš P. Intima-media thickness: indicator of cardiovascular risk and measure of the extent of atherosclerosis. *Vasc Med* 2004; 9: 46–54.

Redon J, Oliva MR, Tormos C, Giner V, Chaves J, Iradi A, Saez GT. Antioxidant activities and oxidative stress byproducts in human hypertension. *Hypertension* 2003; 41: 1096–101.

Rees DD, Palmer RM, Moncada S. Role of endothelium-derived nitric oxide in the regulation of blood pressure. *Proc Natl Acad Sci USA* 1989; 86: 3375–8.

Riccioni G. Aliskiren in the treatment of hypertension and organ damage. *Cardiovasc Ther* 2011; 29: 77–87.

Robinson BF, Dobbs RJ, Bayley S. Response of forearm resistance vessels to verapamil and sodium nitroprusside in normotensive and hypertensive men: evidence for functional abnormality of vascular smooth muscle in primary hypertension. *Clin Sci* 1982; 63: 33–42.

Rodrigo E, Maeso R, Munoz-Garcia R, et al. Endothelial dysfunction in spontaneously hypertensive rats: consequences of chronic treatment with losartan or captopril. J Hypertens. 1997; 15: 613–8.

Ross R. The pathogenesis of atherosclerosis: a perspective for the 1990s. *Nature* 1993; 362: 801–9.

Rossi GP, Colonna S, Pavan E, et al. Endothelin-1 and its mRNA in the wall layers of human arteries ex vivo. *Circulation* 1999; 99: 1147–55.

Rossi R, Churlia E, Nuzzo A, Cioni E, Origliani G, Modena MG. Flow-mediated vasodilation and the risk developing hypertension in healthy postmenopausal women. *J Am Coll Cardiol* 2004; 44: 1636–40.

Rubanyi GM, Romero CJ, Vanhoutte PM. Flow-induced release of endothelium-derived relaxing factor. *Am J Physiol* 1986; 19: 1145–49.

Ruetten H, Dimmeler S, Gehring D, Ihling C, Zeiher AM. Concentric left ventricular remodeling in endothelial nitric oxide synthase knockout mice by chronic pressure overload. *Cardiovasc Res* 2005; 66: 444–53.

Ruilope LM, Bakris GL. Renal function and target organ damage in hypertension. *Eur Heart J 2011*; 32: 1599–604.

Sagnella GA, Swift PA. The renal epithelial sodium channel: genetic heterogeneity and implications for the treatment of high blood pressure. *Curr Pharm Des* 2006; 12; 2221–34.

Salonen JT, Salonen R. Ultrasound B-mode imaging in observational studies of atherosclerotic progression. *Circulation* 1993; 87 Suppl 2: S56–65.

Sanderson JE. Heart failure with a normal ejection fraction. *Heart* 2007; 93: 155–8.

Sato A, Hayashi M, Saruta T. Relative Long-term effects of spironolactone in conjunction with an angiotensin-converting enzyme inhibitor on left ventricular mass and diastolic function in patients with essential hypertension. *Hypertens Res* 2002; 20: 837–42.

Sato A, Saruta T. Aldosterone escape during angiotensin-converting enzyme inhibitor therapy in essential hypertensive patients with left ventricular hypertrophy. *J Int Med Res* 2001; 29: 13–21.

Scheler S, Motz W, Strauer BE. Mechanism of angina pectoris in patients with systemic hypertension and normal epicardial coronary arteries by arteriogram. *Am J Cardiol* 1994; 73: 478–82.

Schiffrin EL. Reactivity of small blood vessels in hyprtension: relation with structural changes. *Hypertension* 1992; 19 Suppl 2: S1–9.

Schiffrin EL, Deng LY, Sventek P, Day R. Enhanced expression of endothelin-1 gene in endothelium in resistance arteries in severe human essential hypertension. *J Hypertens* 1997; 15: 57–63.

Schmieder RE. End organ damage in hypertension. *Dtsch Arztebl Int* 2010; 107: 866–73.

Schulz E, Gori T, Münzel T. Oxidative stress and endothelial dysfunction in hypertension. *Hypertens Res* 2011; 34: 665–73.

Schunkert H, Hense HW, Muscholl M, et al. Asociations between circulating components of the renin-angotensin-aldosterone system and left ventricular mass. *Heart* 1997;77: 24–31.

Segura J, Campo C, Gil P, et al. Development of chronic kidney disease and cardiovascular prognosis in essential hypertensive patients. *J Am Soc Nephrol* 2004; 15: 1616–22.

Sivertsson R, Andersson O, Hansson L. Blood pressure reduction and vascular adaptation. *Acta Med Scand* 1979; 205: 477–82.

Solomon SD, Janardhanan RJ, Verma A, et al. Effect of angiotensin receptor blockade and antihypertensive drugs on diastolic function in patients with hypertension and diastolic dysfunction: a randomized trial. *Lancet* 2007; 369: 2079–87.

Spieker LE, Noll G, Ruschitzka FT, et al. Working under pressure: the vascular endothelium in arterial hypertension. *J Hum Hypertens* 2000; 14: 617–30.

Swynghedauw B, Delcayre C, Samuel JL, Mebaza A, Cohen-Solal A. Molecular mechanism in evolutionary cardiology failure. *Ann N Y Acad Sci* 2010; 1188: 58–67.

Taddei S, Salvetti A. Endothelial dysfunction in essential hypertension: clinical implications. *J Hypertens* 2002; 20: 1671–4.

Taddei S, Virdis A, Mattei P, et al. Vasodilation to acetylcholine in primary and secondary forms of human hypertension. *Hypertension* 1993; 21: 929–33.

Takeshita A, Allyn ML. Decreased vasodilator capacity of forearm resistance vessels in borderline hypertension. *Hypertension* 1980; 2: 610–6.

Takeshita A, Imaizumi T, Ashihara T, et al. Limited maximal vasodilator capacity of forearm resistance vessels in normotensive young men with a familial predisposition to hypertension. *Circ Res* 1982; 50: 671–7.

Tamakoshi K, Yatsuya H, Kondo T, et al. The metabolic syndrome is associated with elevated circulating C-reactive protein in healthy reference range, a systemic low-grade inflammatory state. *Int J Obes* 2003; 27: 443–9.

Tang R, Henning M, Thomasson B, et al. Baseline reproducibility of B-mode ultrasonic measurement of carotid artery intima-media thickness: the Europe Lacidipine Study on Atherosclerosis (ELSA). *J Hypertens* 2000; 18: 197–201.

Taniguchi I, Kawai M, Date T, et al. Effects of spirinolactone during an angiotensin II receptor blocker treatment on left ventricular mass reduction in hypertensive patients with concentric left ventricular hypertrophy. *Circ J* 2006; 70: 995–1000.

Touyz RM. Reactive oxygen species, vascular oxidative stress, and redox signaling in hypertension: what is the clinical significance? *Hypertension* 2004; 44: 248–52.

Treasure CB, Klein LJ, Vita JA, et al. Hypertension and left ventricular hypertrophy are associated with impaired endothelium-mediated relaxation in human coronary resistence vessels. *Circulation* 1993; 87: 86–93.

Vallance P, Collier J, Moncada S. Effects of endothelium-derived nitric oxide on peripheral arteriolar tone in man. *Lancet* 1989; 2: 997–1000.

Van de Voorde JV, Leusen I. Endothelium-dependent and independent relaxation of aortic rings from hypertensive rats. *Am J Physiol* 1986; 250: H711–7.

Vane JR, Änggård EE, Botting RM. Regulatory functions of the vascular endothelium. *N Engl J* 1990; 323: 27–36.

Vasan RS, Evans JC, Larson MG, et al. Serum aldosterone and the incidence of hypertension in nonhypertensive persons. *N Engl J Med* 2004; 351: 33–41.

Verdecchia P, Angeli F, Borgioni C, Gattobigio R, de Simone G, Devereux RB, Porcellati C. Changes in cardiovascular risk by reduction of left ventricular mass in hypertension: a meta-analysis. *Am J Hypertens* 2003; 16: 895–9.

Verdecchia P, Sleight P, Mancia G, et al. ONTARGET/TRASCEND Investigators. Effects of telmisartan, ramipril, and their combination on left ventricular hypertrophy in individuals at high vascular risk in the Ongoing Telmisartan Alone and in Combination With Ramipril Global End Point Trial and the Telmisartan Randomized Assessment Study in ACE Intolerant Subjects With Cardiovascular Disease. *Circulation* 2009; 120: 1380–9.

Virdis A, Ghiadoni L, Taddei S. Effects of antihypertensive treatment on endothelial function. *Curr Hypertens Rep* 2011; 13: 276–81.

Volpe M, Savoia C, De Paolis P, et al. The renin-angiotensin system as a risk factor and therapeutic target for cardiovascular and renal disease. *J Am Soc Nephrol* 2002; 13 Suppl 3: S173–8.

Wang J, Nagueh SF. Current perspectives on cardiac function in patients with diastolic heart failure. *Circulation* 2009; 119: 1146–57.

Wassmann S, Laufs U, Baumer AT, et al. HMG-CoA reductase inhibitors improve endothelial dysfunction in normocholesterolemic hypertension via reduced production of reactive oxygen species. *Hypertension.* 2001; 37: 1450–7.

Watanabe T, Barker TA, Berk BC. Angiotensin II and the endothelium: diverse signals and effects. *Hypertension* 2005; 45: 163–9.

Weber KT. Fibrosis and hypertensive heart disease. *Curr Opin Cardiol* 2000; 15: 264–72.

Wennmalm Å. Endothelial nitric oxide and cardiovascular disease. *J Intern Med* 1994; 235: 317–27.

Wilcox CS. Reactive oxygen species: roles in blood pressure and kidney function. *Curr Hypertens Rep* 2002; 4: 160–6.

Williams B. Angiotensin II and the pathophysiology of cardiovascular remodeling. *Am J Cardiol* 2001; 87 Suppl 1: S10–17.

Xie YW, Shen W, Zhao G, Xu X, Wolin MS, Hintze TH. Role of endothelium-derived nitric oxide in the modulation of canine myocardial mitochondrial respiration in vitro. Implications for the development of heart failure. *Circ Res* 1996; 79: 381–7.

Yang Z, Arnet U, Bauer E, et al. Thrombin-induced endothelium-dependent inhibition and direct activation of platelet-vessel wall interaction. Role of prostacyclin, nitric oxide, and thromboxane $A_2$. *Circulation* 1994; 89: 2266–72.

Yang P, Liu F, Yang L, Wei Q, Zeng H. Mechanism and clinical significance of the prothrombotic state in patients with essential hypertension. *Clin Cardiol* 2010; 33: 81–6.

Young MJ. Mechanisms of mineralcorticoid receptor-mediated cardiac fibrosis and vascular inflammation. *Curr Opin Nephrol Hypertens* 2008; 17: 174–80.

Zalba G, Gorka SJ, Moreno MU, et al. Oxidative stress in arterial hypertension. Role of NAD(P)H oxydase. *Hypertension* 2001; 38: 1395–99.

Zanchetti A. Bottom blood pressure or bottom cardiovascular risk? How far can cardiovascular risk be reduced? *J Hypertens* 2009; 27: 1509–20.

Zeiher AM, Drexler H, Saurbier B, et al. Endothelium-mediated coronary blood flow modulation in humans. Effects of age, atherosclerosis, hypercholesterolemia, and hypertension. *J Clin Invest* 1993; 92: 652–62.

Zeiher AM, Drexler H, Wollschlaeger H, et al. Modulation of coronary vasomotor tone in humans. Progressive endothelial dysfunction with different early stages of coronary atherosclerosis. *Circulation* 1991; 83: 391–401.

Zile MR, Brutsaert DL. New concepts in diastolic dysfunction and diastolic heart failure: Part I and II: diagnosis, prognosis, and measurements of diastolic function. *Circulation*. 2002; 105: 1387–93, 1503–8.

Žižek B, Poredoš P, Videčnik V (2001a). Endothelial dysfunction in hypertensive patients and in normotensive offspring of subjects with essential hypertension. *Heart*; 85: 215–6.

Žižek B, Poredoš P (2001b). Insulin resistance adds to endothelial dysfunction in hypertensive patients and in normotensive offspring of subjects with essential hypertension. *J Intern Med*; 249: 189–97.

Žižek B, Poredoš P. Dependence of morphological changes of carotid arteries on essential hypertension and accompanying risk factors. *Int Angiol* 2002; 21: 70–7.

Žižek B, Poredoš P. Increased left ventricular mass and diastolic dysfunction are associated with endothelial dysfunction in normotensive offspring of subjects with essential hypertension. *Blood Press* 2007; 16: 36–44.

Žižek B, Poredoš P, Trojar A, Željko T. Left ventricular diastolic dysfunction is associated with insulin resistance, but not with aldosterone level in normotensive offspring of hypertensive families. *Cardiology* 2008; 118: 8–15.

# 3

# Resistant Hypertension, Elevated Aldosterone/Renin Ratio and Reduced RGS2: A Pathogenetic Link Deserving Further Investigations?

Andrea Semplicini, Federica Stella and Giulio Ceolotto
*Internal Medicine 1, SS. Giovanni e Paolo Hospital, Venice, and Department of Clinical and Experimental Medicine "G. Patrassi", University of Padua*
*Italy*

## 1. Introduction

Hypertension control is unsatisfactory in most countries and it carries an unacceptably high cardiovascular risk and death toll (Mancia et al., 2007) The reasons for the poor blood pressure control are different and interrelated (motivation of patients and physicians, costs, compliance, access to health care, secondary and resistant hypertension). Among them, resistant hypertension is receiving considerable attention, as it may be caused by unrecognized secondary hypertension, mainly primary aldosteronism (PA).

We have recently shown in patients with resistant hypertension elevated aldosterone / renin ratio (ARR) and reduced RGS2 expression. We, therefore, hypothesize that in many patients resistant hypertension is secondary to disproportionate aldosterone secretion caused by blunted inhibition of angiotensin II (Ang II) cellular effects due to low RGS2 expression.

## 2. Resistant or uncontrolled hypertension

Resistant hypertension is defined as blood pressure remaining above the goal levels in spite of the concurrent use of three antihypertensive agents of different classes at the same time, with diuretic as one of the three agents and all agents prescribed at optimal dose (Calhoun et al., 2008). This implies that also patients whose blood pressure needs four or more drugs to be controlled should be considered resistant to treatment. Resistant hypertension identifies patients who are at a high risk of having secondary and reversible causes of hypertension or patients who may benefit from further diagnostic and therapeutic work up. Uncontrolled hypertension is not synonymous of resistant hypertension as uncontrolled hypertension includes patients who do not reach blood pressure control due to poor adherence or an inadequate treatment regimen, as well as patients with true treatment resistance.

### 2.1 Prevalence

The prevalence of resistant hypertension is unknown, even if according to the literature it is not an uncommon condition: the majority of studies indicate that less than 40% of elderly patients reach a goal blood pressure with drugs. Among high risk populations and, in particular with application of the lowest blood pressures goal recommendation of the Seventh Report of the Joint National Committee on Prevention, Detection, Evaluation, and Treatment of High Blood Pressure (JNC 7) for patients with diabetes mellitus or chronic kidney disease, the percentage of uncontrolled hypertensive patients is even higher.

### 2.2 Prognosis

Prognosis of patients with resistant hypertension compared with patients with drug controlled hypertension is likely to be worse due to the long history of poorly controlled or uncontrolled hypertension and the presence of commonly associated cardiovascular risk factors, such as obstructive sleep apnea, diabetes, left ventricular hypertrophy and chronic kidney disease. Yet, no clinical trial has been conducted to specifically evaluate its associated increased risk.

The cardiovascular risk reduction associated to the treatment of resistant hypertension is unknown. The benefits of effective treatment, however, are supposed to be substantial, as suggested by several outcome studies, and, therefore, achievement of goal pressure levels should always be urged.

### 2.3 Patient characteristics

Populations who are at the highest risk of developing resistant hypertension have been investigated. The strongest predictors of treatment resistance are chronic kidney diseases, obesity and diabetes mellitus. Differences between races and genders have been reported, since blacks and women are at higher risk of resistant hypertension.

Blood pressure is considered uncontrolled most often because of persistent elevation of systolic values as patients treated with antihypertensive drugs reach correct diastolic more easily than systolic values. This diversity in systolic versus diastolic blood pressure control worsens with increasing age of patients, as arterial stiffness (strongly related with age) is the main cause of isolated systolic hypertension. This explains why the strongest predictor of the lack of blood pressure control is old age. High baseline systolic pressure was associated with increased risk of never reaching goal blood pressure (Lloyd-Jones et al., 2002). Other strong predictors of poor systolic blood pressure control are the presence of left ventricular hypertrophy and obesity (that is, body mass index [BMI] greater than 30 kg/m2). The prevalence of resistant hypertension is predicted to increase in older and heavier cohorts in association with the growing prevalence of diabetes and chronic kidney disease.

In terms of poor diastolic pressure control, the strongest negative predictor is obesity, with goal blood pressure reached one third less often in obese than in lean patients.

### 2.4 Genetics / pharmacogenetics

The genetics of hypertension is complex and there is no known single gene playing a major role, but rather many different genes contributing all together with different environmental factors in rising blood pressure. Due to its particular type, it is reasonable that in resistant hypertension genetic factors may play an even greater role than in the general hypertensive population. However, in resistant hypertensive population, genetic studies are limited and based on a very small number of patients, even if identification of genetic influences on resistance to current therapies might lead to development of new therapeutic targets. Gene variants of ENaC (epithelium sodium channel) (Hannila-Handelberg et al., 2005) and of CYP3A5 enzyme (11β-hydroxysteroid dehydrogenase type 2) (Givens et al., 2003; Ho et al., 2005) have been demonstrated, focusing attention on sodium homeostasis, and on cortisol and corticosterone metabolism but the clinical relevance of these mutations is unclear.

### 2.5 Pseudoresistance

Pseudoresistance is the condition of poor blood pressure control with no real treatment resistance and no coexisting factors causing persistently high blood pressure values. There are many causes of pseudoresistance that can be related either to medical or to lifestyle factors. These conditions should be kept in mind and carefully searched in resistant hypertensive patients to avoid incorrect classification of hypertension.

Among the medical related causes of pseudoresistant hypertension, the most frequent are poor blood pressure measurement techniques, poor adherence to therapy, white-coat effect and drug-related causes.

Poor blood pressure technique consists in inaccurate measurement of blood pressure, resulting falsely high. Blood pressure should be measured only after the patient has been sitting quietly for a few minutes and with the use of adequate size cuff, not too small as it often happens. (Pickering et al., 2005) Poor adherence to therapy is probably the main cause of the lack of blood pressure control (Yiannakopoulou et al., 2005): near 40% of newly diagnosed hypertensive patient discontinue therapy during the first year of drug treatment (Caro et al., 1999; Mazzaglia et al., 2005) and 60 % of patients at five and ten year follow up show poor adherence to the suggested treatment (Van Wijk et al., 2005) . It should be noticed that the percentage of poor adherence to therapy falls from 40 to 15 % when the patients are seen in hypertension specialist clinic rather then at primary care.

White-coat effect consists in clinic blood pressure values persistently elevated while out-of-office values are normal or significantly lower (Brown et al., 2005) . The prevalence of this condition is similar in patients with resistant hypertension and in the general hypertensive population, with values in the range of 20% to 30%. It can be identified with ambulatory blood pressure recording showing normal out of office blood pressure values (Redon et al., 1998; Muxfeldt et al, 2003; Pierdomenico et al., 2005).

Drug-related causes are due either to incorrect antihypertensive drug assumption or to drug interactions. Identification of poor adherence is clinically relevant to stop useless continuous modification of the treatment regimens and further investigations. Drug interactions should always be looked for, in particular in those patients assuming complex combination therapies. Several classes of drugs can increase blood pressure and contribute to treatment resistance:

- stimulants (dextroamphetamine, amphetamine, methamphetamine, methylphenidate, dexmethylphenidate) ;
- sympathomimetic agents (like nasal decongestants, diet pills and cocaine);
- NSAIDs - Nonsteroidal antiinflammatory agents, including selective COX-2 inhibitors;
- alcohol;

- glucocorticoids (such as prednisone);
- corticosteroids (mainly the ones with the greatest mineralcorticoid effect such as cortisone and hydrocortisone);
- oral contraceptives;
- cyclosporine and calcineurine inhibitors;
- erythropoietin;
- Natural products such as licorice (common in oral tobacco products) or herbal compounds (ephedra or ma huang).

The effect of these agents is highly variable with most patients manifesting little or no effect and other individuals showing severe blood pressure elevations (Radack et al., 1987; Conlin et al., 2000). Due to large use and wide distribution, non narcotic analgesics are probably the most common interacting medicaments with antihypertensive drugs (Dedier et al, 2005; Forman et al., 2005). NSAIDs induced blood pressure increase is modest but predictable, apart from patients with significant fluid retention and/or acute kidney disease in which there is subsequent sodium and fluid retention and rebound pressure relevant increase due to inhibition of renal prostaglandin production.

Among lifestyle factors the most relevant are obesity, excessive dietary salt and alcohol intake. Obesity is associated with the need for an increased number of antihypertensive medications, a more severe hypertension and increased probability of difficult achieving or never achieving appropriate blood pressure control (Bramlage et al., 2004). Mechanisms of obesity-induced hypertension are multiple, complex and not fully understood: activation of the renin-angiotensin-aldosterone system, impaired sodium excretion and increased sympathetic nervous system activity (Hall et al., 2003). As a consequence, obesity is a common feature of patients with resistant hypertension (Nishizaka et al., 2005).

Excessive dietary salt intake sustains resistant hypertension both by increasing blood pressure directly and by decreasing the effect of most classes of antihypertensive agents (Weinberger 1988; He & MacGregor, 2004; Luft & Weinberger, 1988;). These effects are mainly found in salt-sensitive patients, like the elderly, those suffering from chronic kidney disease (Boudville et al, 2005) and both African and American races.

Alcohol intake at high doses is associated with increased risk of hypertension and resistant hypertension. Epidemiological studies have shown a direct relationship between alcohol intake and blood pressure, which is particularly evident when 28 g of ethanol per day are exceeded (Henningsen et al., 1980; Aguilera et al., 1999; Wildman et al., 2005). All the subpopulations that have been analyzed (males, females, Caucasian and African race) show a blood pressure increase related to alcohol consumption, but the African race shows a blood pressure greater raise compared to Caucasians at the same intake. Chronic daily intake of alcohol it is not required for the hypertensive effect, since it has been proven that also consumption confined to only a few days a week is associated with increased blood pressure. Prospective studies have demonstrated that cessation of heavy alcohol ingestion reduced 24-hour ambulatory systolic blood pressure.

## 2.6 Secondary causes

Secondary causes of hypertension are common among patients with resistant hypertension, mainly in older patients due to high incidence of sleep apnea syndrome, renal parenchymal disease, diabetes mellitus, renal artery stenosis and primary aldosteronism. Uncommon causes of secondary resistant hypertension include pheochromocytoma, Cushing's syndrome, hyperparathyroidism, aortic coarctation.

### 2.6.1 Obstructive sleep apnea

Obstructive sleep apnea is strongly associated with hypertension. In normotensive subjects it predicts development of hypertension, and it is very common in patients with resistant hypertension (Nieto et al., 2000; Peppard et al., 2000). There is a significant gender distribution, with males more affected than females. The more severe and untreated is sleep apnea syndrome, the less likely is blood pressure controlled despite the use of polymedications (Grote et al., 2000; Lavie & Hoffstein, 2001) Sleep apnea seems to create and maintain hypertension by increasing sympathetic nervous system (SNS) activity generated by intermittent hypoxemia; the SNS hyperactivation increases cardiac output, peripheral vascular resistances and fluid retention (Grassi et al., 2005).

### 2.6.2 Renal parenchymal disease

Renal parenchymal disease is both cause and complication of uncontrolled hypertension. Serum creatinine higher than of 1.5 mg/dL is a strong predictor of failure to achieve blood pressure goal, due to increased sodium and water retention and intravascular volume expansion (Klahr et al., 1994; Buckalew et al., 1996).

### 2.6.3 Diabetes

Diabetes and hypertension are commonly associated, in particular in patients with resistant hypertension. Diabetes associated insulin resistance is supposed to contribute to the development of hypertension directly through sympathetic nervous activity, vascular smooth muscle cell proliferation, and increased sodium retention with intravascular volume expansion (Bakris, 2001) .

### 2.6.4 Renovascular disease

Renal artery stenosis is a common finding in resistant hypertension, with several studies suggesting a percentage of renovascular disease in resistant hypertension between 12 and 15%. More than 90% of renal artery stenoses have an atherosclerotic origin, with increased incidence in smokers, older patients, and widespread atherosclerotic disease (Aqel et al., 2003; Cuckson et al., 2004). Less than 10% of renal lesions are fibromuscular in etiology, developing particularly in young women. Specific diagnostic studies should be performed when renovascular disease is suspected, such as ultrasound, magnetic resonance angiography (MRA), renal scintigraphy, and computed tomography angiography (Leiner et al., 2005).

### 2.6.5 Pheochromocytoma

Pheochromocytoma accounts for a small number of secondary causes of resistant hypertension. Its prevalence is 0.1% to 0.6% among hypertensive patients, and even if the prevalence as a cause of resistant hypertension is unknown, it has to be underlined that 95% of pheochromocytomas show hypertension at clinical onset and 50% have resistant hypertension (Omura et al., 2004; Sinclair et al., 1987). It should be suspected in every hypertensive patient with headaches, palpitations, and sweating, typically occurring in an episodic way; not all pheochromocytomas show up with these typical symptoms, and this is the reason why there is often a delay between the initial symptoms and the final diagnosis, with an average delay of three years. Moreover, pheochromocytoma is characterized by increased blood pressure variability due to inconstant catecholamine release, which represents an additional independent risk factor beyond increased blood pressure itself for cardiovascular morbidity and mortality (Kikuya et al., 2000; Björklund et al., 2004; Zelinka et al., 2005).

### 2.6.6 Cushing's syndrome

The mechanism that causes hypertension in Cushing's syndrome is overstimulation of the nonselective mineralocorticoid receptor by cortisol (Moneva & Gomez-Sanchez, 2002; Ferrari, 2003) , even if other factors contribute to hypertension in this disease, such as sleep apnea and insulin resistance (McFarlane et al, 2001) .

Cortisol is the hormone which is mainly increased in Cushing syndrome and hypertension is present in 70-85% of patients suffering from this syndrome. Hypertension is often resistant because of the cortisol dependent pressor activity: the most common therapeutic agents (renin-angiotensin system blockers, calcium channel antagonists, adrenergic blockers, and diuretics) are frequently ineffective. The most effective antihypertensive agents are mineralocorticoid receptor antagonists (such as spironolactone or eplerenone), but frequently only surgical removal of an adrenocorticotropic hormone (ACTH) or another cortisol-producing tumor allows effective blood pressure control. Target organ damage and overall cardiovascular risk in Cushing's syndrome is more severe than in primary hypertension, because the disease is associated with other cardiovascular risk factors such as metabolic syndrome, diabetes mellitus, obesity, sleep apnea syndrome, and dyslipidemia (Sacerdote et al., 2005).

## 3. Primary aldosteronism and resistant hypertension

Primary aldosteronism (PA) is a clinical condition sustained by overproduction of the mineralocorticoid hormone aldosterone by the adrenal glands. The overproduction is relatively independent by the renin-angiotensin system (RAS) activity, and non suppressible by sodium loading. PA was considered to be a rare cause of secondary hypertension until recently. Early epidemiologic studies have claimed the prevalence of PA to be less than 1% of hypertensive patients. On the contrary, there is evidence from several recent studies that PA is a much more common cause of resistant hypertension than had been suspected before, and particularly common in patients with resistant hypertension, its prevalence being between 10 and 15% among patients with severe hypertension (Gordon et al., 1994; Fardella et al., 2000; Mosso et al., 2003). Several authors have suggested a direct role of aldosterone autonomy as a mechanism for drug resistance and have recommended the search for primary aldosteronism in cases of severe or drug resistant hypertension as primary aldosteronism was found in 20% of patients with resistant hypertension. Primary aldosteronism is, therefore, the most common cause of secondary hypertension.

Bilateral idiopathic hyperaldosteronism (IHA) and aldosterone-producing adenoma (APA) are the most common subtypes of primary aldosteronism. A rarer cause of primary aldosteronism, unilateral hyperplasia or primary adrenal hyperplasia, is generated in a single adrenal gland by hyperplasia of the zona glomerulosa. Two forms of familial hyperaldosteronism (FH) have been described: FH type I and FH type II. FH type I, or glucocorticoid-remediable aldosteronism, is autosomal dominant in inheritance and associated with variable degrees of hyperaldosteronism, high levels of hybrid steroids (e.g. 18-hydroxycortisol and 18-oxocortisol), ameliorated by exogenous glucocorticoids. FH type II refers to the familial occurrence of APA or IHA, or both (Young, 2003) .

A number of studies demonstrate that primary aldosteronism is strongly associated with target organ damage and elevated rate of cardiovascular events. Indeed, hyperaldosteronism produces oxidative stress with oxidative damage to DNA, inflammation, and nongenomic effects (with cardiovascular remodeling, hypertrophy, fibrosis, endothelial dysfunction and increased arterial stiffness). This reflects in increased cardiovascular events, such as impaired systolic and diastolic ventricular function, atrial fibrillation, microalbuminuria, increased incidence of ischemic and hemorrhagic stroke, pulmonary edema and myocardial infarction. (Takeda et al., 1995; Rocha et al., 2002; Farquharson & Struthers, 2002; Sechi et al., 2006; Rossi et al., 2008; Schupp et al., 2010).

### 3.1 Diagnosis

Diagnosis of PA is made by a three step approach: screening; confirmation / exclusion; subtype diagnosis. Serum potassium level cannot be used as an indicator of the presence of hidden primary aldosteronism due to high prevalence of normokalemic PA, and the prevalence of hypokalemia increasing with severity of hypertensive disease. These data suggest that hypokalemia is a late manifestation of the disorder following the onset of hypertension.

#### 3.1.1 Screening test

Resistant hypertension is enlisted among the subtypes of hypertension which should undergo a screening test for primary aldosteronism (Funder et al, 2008) .

There is general consensus that ARR is the most reliable available mean for primary aldosteronism screening, a validated and assured index of inappropriate aldosterone activity, and a valid screening assay even without discontinuation of antihypertensive medications (Gallay et al., 2001). ARR provides the best parting of patients with primary aldosteronism from essential hypertensive subjects. However, there is no agreement on the ARR cut-off value and on whether the absolute aldosterone level should also be taken into account. It should be noted that the optimal ARR cut-off value (as well as the aldosterone level after confirmatory test) is dependent on the assay used to measure aldosterone. Different assays, although demonstrating good overall correlation with one another, often show significant differences in absolute aldosterone concentrations (Pizzolo et al., 2006). In order to compare results from different studies and to use the same cut-offs for screening and confirmation, aldosterone assays thus need to be standardized. Moreover, ARR is strongly dependent on plasma renin activity (PRA), so that anyone with suppressed PRA will have increased ARR: this implies that ARR needs to be interpreted in light of aldosterone plasma level (>15 nd/dL) and the lowest detectable level of PRA. Another debated issue is the use of direct active renin assay instead of PRA. PRA and direct renin are closely and strongly correlated, but the correlation is weaker for the low range of values compared with the high/normal range of values (Hartman et al., 2004) .

### 3.1.2 Confirmatory testing

Because of the high prevalence of low renin hypertension, it is important to stress that increased ARR is not diagnostic of PA by itself, and a confirmatory test is most often required. This is to avoid a large number of hypertensive patients inappropriately undergoing costly and potentially harmful procedures. The choice of the test remains a matter of debate and there is currently insufficient direct evidence to recommend one in particular. The most widely used and approved by the guidelines tests are: fludrocortisone suppression test (FST), intravenous saline load test (SLT), oral sodium loading test (OLT) and captopril challenge (CC). FST, SLT and OLT include the administration of salt and thus should be considered preferable to CC for confirming PA (Mulatero et al., 2010). CC has the advantage of being relatively cheap, safe, well tolerated and easy to perform. Because of the high rate of false positive diagnoses to which it is related, it should only be used in patients at risk of volume expansion.

### 3.1.3 Subtype differentiation

All patients affected by PA should undergo an adrenal HTCT scan as the initial study for subtype differentiation in order to rule out an adrenocortical carcinoma. Magnetic resonance offers no advantage over CT, and adrenal scintiscan with [6 -131I] iodomethyl-19-norcholesterol has a low sensitivity and specificity for APA. CT scanning should be performed by an expert and motivated radiologist to diminish inadequacy of CT scanning to distinguish between APA and IHA because of small size of some adenomas. The Endocrine Society Guidelines recommend that all patients for whom the surgical treatment is practicable and desired should undergo adrenal venous sampling (AVS) as the gold standard to differentiate unilateral from bilateral disease (Young & Stanson, 2009)

### 3.1.4 ARR to identify disproportionate aldosterone production

High aldosterone secretion may play a role in the pathogenesis of increased blood pressure in resistant hypertensives even when PA cannot be diagnosed by clinical and instrumental criteria. We have shown that a mild elevation of ARR and plasma aldosterone, which are not reduced to a significant extent by oral captopril administration during CC, predict poor blood pressure response to antihypertensive agents. The clinical features and outcome of these patients with high ARR were indistinguishable from those of hypertensive patients with clinically diagnosed IHA: both reached blood pressure goal in a smaller fraction and in a longer time than patients with ARR in the normal range (Sartori et al., 2006). The cause(s) of the disproportionately high aldosterone levels which are not inhibited to a significant extent by the inhibition of Ang II production by captopril remain(s) unknown but they may be related to abnormal regulation of aldosterone production by Ang II (see below). ARR should be, therefore, performed in all patients with resistant hypertension to demonstrate a disproportionate aldosterone secretion and encourage treatment with aldosterone antagonists to achieve a more effective blood pressure reduction.

### 3.2 Treatment of primary aldosteronism

Surgical treatment should be offered to eligible patients with unilateral adrenal disease; it consists in unilateral adrenalectomy. It has been shown to improve blood pressure control. In patients who are unable or unwilling to undergo surgery, or with a bilateral adrenal disease, treatment with a mineralcorticoid receptor antagonist should be started. Treatment of aldosterone excess either with spironolactone or with unilateral adrenalectomy was found to reduce the high cardiovascular risk of this patient group (Milliez et al., 2005). The benefit of controlling PA is also demonstrated after a long period of therapy: treated patients with PA had similar rates of cardiovascular events as hypertensive patients without PA after a 12-years follow up. The best cardiovascular outcome was seen in younger patients and in those with a shorter duration of disease. These results stress the need of early recognition and treatment to reverse the adverse effects of aldosterone excess.

#### 3.2.1 Mineralocorticoid receptor antagonists

Spironolactone is a direct antagonist of the mineralcorticoid receptor and it is a powerful add-on agent to the antihypertensive regimen in patients with resistant hypertension. When added to a regimen of three drugs including a diuretic, spironolactone lowers blood pressure significantly, with achievement of blood pressure control in a high percentage of patients. This effect is similar in patients with or without evidence of aldosterone excess, with no gender or ethnic difference. Indeed, similar degrees of blood pressure reduction were achieved regardless of baseline plasma aldosterone or PRA values. This underscores the contributory role of relative aldosterone excess to treatment resistance, such that even those with presumably low levels of aldosterone benefit from mineralcorticoid receptor antagonists use. (Nishizaka et al., 2003; Sartori et al., 2006; De Souza et al., 2010) This is in contrast with other studies that showed that high ARR predicted the antihypertensive efficacy of spironolactone (Eide et al., 2004); these contrasting results may be explained by the considerably higher spironolactone dose administered in patients with demonstrated PA, generating a strong difference in the two populations.

The importance of relative aldosterone excess in promoting treatment resistance is emphasized also in another recent study: spironolactone was added either to an ACE-I or to an ARB theraphy and compared to ACE-I plus ARB combined therapy. Greater blood pressure reduction was achieved when spironolactone was added to an ACE inhibitor or an ARB versus dual RAS blockade (Alvarez-Alvarez et al., 2010). These results suggest that aldosterone excess plays a major role in the pathogenesis of treatment resistance, and that hypersecretion of aldosterone is relatively autonomous of the RAS activity, so that the amplitude of blood pressure lowering is greater in patients given the mineralcorticoid receptor antagonist compared to those on dual blockade. Furthermore, since the study excluded patients with PA, the results show that resistant hypertensive patients in general have an element of relative aldosterone excess, even if aldosterone falls within the normal range. (Acelajado & Calhoun, 2011).

Mineralcorticoid receptor antagonists are also anti-proteinuric: reduction of albuminuria was demonstrated in patients with diabetes or chronic kidney disease, nephropathy, or persistent microalbuminuria. In case of chronic kidney disease, spironolactone alone was able to reduce proteinuria and slow down renal progression (Bianchi et al., 2006).

Treatment with mineralcorticoid receptor antagonists not only controls blood pressure levels and proteinuria, but also reverses or attenuates the cardiovascular injury mediated by aldosterone excess. This is particularly true for the nongenomic effects, which lead to tissue fibrosis, arterial stiffness, and increased oxidative stress. In patients with resistant hypertension spironolactone reduces left ventricular mass index after 3 and 6 months of therapy, both in patient with PA and in those with normal renin - angiotensin- aldosterone levels (Gaddam et al., 2010) . The extent of regression of the left ventricular mass index achieved with spironolactone treatment is greater for patients with PA compared to those without.

If patients with both resistant hypertension and PA are selected, further interesting benefits of therapy with spironolactone are shown on nongenomic effects. Spironolactone significantly decreases brain natriuretic peptide (BNP), an effect that was not seen in those with normal or low aldosterone levels; this indicates a prominent diuretic effect even when administered on top of chronic thiazide diuretic treatment. In another study on resistant hypertension and PA, flow-mediated dilation of the brachial artery increased with spironolactone treatment as an indication of reduced arterial stiffness and improvement of endothelial function, and this effect was independent of the change of blood pressure (Nishizaka et al., 2004) .

### 3.2.2 Adverse effects

Adverse effects of spironolactone use are breast tenderness, gynecomastia, erectile dysfunction, and menstrual irregularities, as a result of the binding of spironolactone to androgen receptors, preventing their interaction with dihydrotestosterone. All these major adverse effects warrant monitoring (Marrs, 2010). The incidence of these effects is rare (2–9%) and they are all reversible after discontinuing treatment. If a more selective MR antagonist is used (such as eplerenone), no or less antiandrogen effects is shown, given its lower affinity for progesterone and androgen receptors. A comparison between spironolactone and eplerenone in patients with primary hypertension and bilateral adrenal hyperplasia showed that the two agents achieved similar degrees of blood pressure lowering in patients with PA (Karagiannis et al., 2008). A direct comparison of these two agents in patients with resistant hypertension has not been conducted so far. Furthermore, eplerenone has not yet been specifically evaluated for the treatment of resistant hypertension and it is not available in several countries.

Hyperkalemia can also be a side effect of treatment with mineralcorticosteroid antagonists, especially when multidrug therapy, including renin – angiotensin system blockers, is prescribed or in patients with chronic kidney diseases. This effect can be reversed by discontinuing the drug or reducing the dose.

## 4. RGS2

The above mentioned studies, showing benefits of aldosterone antagonists in patients with resistant hypertension, strongly support a role of aldosterone excess, beyond true primary aldosteronism, as a major cause of treatment resistance. Furthermore, data from our laboratory have shown that disproportionately high aldosterone levels associated to poor response to inhibition of Ang II production by captopril are prevalent in resistant hypertension (Sartori et al., 2006). Therefore, we have investigated the signal transduction pathways of Ang II to clarify whether the inappropriately high aldosterone levels are caused by abnormal regulation of aldosterone production by Ang II in the adrenals.

The pressor effects of Ang II action are mediated by stimulation of G protein-coupled receptors (GPCRs), which are mediators of the activity of several other important cardiovascular neurotransmitters and hormones, including noradrenaline, adrenaline, endothelin, thrombin, vasopressin, acetylcholine, serotonin and sphingosine-1-phosphate (S1P). G-proteins are widely expressed throughout the cardiovascular system and thus play an important role in the physiological regulation of the cardiovascular system.

Signaling by hormones and neurotransmitters that activate G protein-coupled receptors (GPCRs) maintains blood pressure within the normal range despite large changes of cardiac output that can occur within seconds. The blood pressure regulation requires, therefore, precise kinetic control of GPCR signaling. Alteration of GPCR signaling is a salient feature of hypertension and its associated cardiovascular complications and hypertension is often associated with increased activity of GPCR-mediated signaling in the heart and blood vessels. Accordingly, these pathways are common targets of inhibitors used to treat hypertension and heart disease (angiotensin-converting enzyme -ACE- inhibitors - and Ang II receptor antagonists) (Rockman et al., 2002).

### 4.1 G-Protein structure and function

The G-protein heterotrimer is composed of a GDP bound G$\alpha$ subunit and a G$\beta\gamma$ heterodimer. Different gene families consisting of 16$\alpha$, 6$\beta$ and 12$\gamma$ genes encode the three subunits that can form heterotrimeric complexes in various combinations. It is the G$\alpha$ subunit families (Gs, Gq, Gi etc.), however, that define the signaling context of the heterotrimer via its ability to couple selectively to a limited number of seven-transmembrane domain receptors and effectors. In the absence of extracellular ligand (inactive state -OFF state-), the G-protein heterotrimer is coupled to the intracellular surface of the receptor. Binding of receptor ligand induces the exchange of GTP for GDP on the G$\alpha$ subunit and the subsequent dissociation of G$\alpha$ from the G$\beta\gamma$ heterodimer. This condition marks the activated (active state -ON state-) state and during this time the G$\alpha$ and G$\beta\gamma$ subunits are free to engage the appropriate downstream effector pathways (Clapham & Neer, 1997; Hamm 1998). Effector signaling is terminated by the G$\alpha$-subunit catalyzed hydrolysis of GTP and reformation of the quiescent receptor-coupled heterotrimer. Thus G-proteins act as molecular time switches that control the onset and lifetime of cellular responses to extracellular signals.

### 4.2 RGS proteins promote rapid termination of G-protein mediated signals

G-protein signaling pathways are tightly coupled to rapid ON–OFF kinetics of the cell physiological effectors, including membrane ion channels. As the intrinsic rate of G$\alpha$-mediated GTP hydrolysis is very slow, GTPase-activating proteins (GAPs) are needed to achieve the rapid ON–OFF kinetics of G-protein signaling observed *in vivo*. Regulators of G protein signaling (RGS) proteins contain a 120 amino acid GAP domain (Berman et al., 1996) that increase the rate of G$\alpha$-mediated GTP hydrolysis by up to 2000 times (Ross & Wilkie, 2000). Accordingly, RGS proteins attenuate GPCR-mediated signaling by promoting faster signal termination kinetics following removal of a GPCR agonist and decreasing GPCR agonist sensitivity (higher agonist concentrations are needed to achieve the same degree of signaling). In addition, the RGS protein GAP domain can inhibit signaling by blocking G*a* binding to downstream effector molecules (Ceolotto et al., 2001). Three RGS proteins, RGS2, RGS4, and RGS5, are among the most highly expressed proteins in the heart and blood vessels. The genes encoding these three proteins are located within the region on chromosome 1 associated with blood pressure variation.

### 4.3 RGS2

Regulators of G-protein Signaling (RGS) proteins are a large family of important endogenous regulators of GPCR signaling: RGS proteins have an established role as inhibitors of G-protein signaling in cardiovascular tissues and, therefore, are important endogenous regulators of blood pressure.

#### 4.3.1 RGS2 inhibits G*α*q and adenylatecyclase-mediated signaling

RGS2 is unique owing to its preferential interaction with G*a*q/11 (and Gas) and its low affinity for G*a*i (Heximer et al., 1999; Cladman et al., 2002). RGS2 binds either directly (M1 muscarinic receptor, or a1A- and b2-adrenoceptors) or indirectly via interaction with a scaffold protein (a1B-adrenoceptor) to GPCRs. Through its unique G protein selectivity for G*a*q/11, RGS2 appears to play a key role in cardiovascular pathophysiology, in which deleterious processes are often initiated via G*a*q/11-coupled GPCRs; for example, in blood vessels, many contractile responses are mediated via G*a*q (Wieland et al., 2007) .

Activation of G*a*q-mediated vasoconstrictor signaling pathways in vascular smooth muscle cells (VSMCs) mediates the action of several vasoconstrictor agonists, including noradrenaline, Ang II, vasopressin and endothelin. RGS2 is a selective and potent inhibitor of G*a*q signalling that is ubiquitously expressed throughout the cardiovascular system. The biological significance of RGS2 in cardiovascular physiology is evident from blood pressure studies carried out in mice and humans. Several studies have shown that RGS2-null mice are hypertensive (Tang et al., 2003; Gross et al., 2005), with altered G-protein signaling in a number of tissues. These mice have agonist-dependent increases in G*a*q signaling in VSMCs compared with wild-type controls. Moreover, RGS2-null mice also have increased pressor responses to infusion of Ang II and *a*-adrenergic receptor agonists compared with wild-type controls. This effect may be partly explained by increased myogenic vasoreactivity to G-protein-mediated stimuli of the RGS2-null mice (Hercule et al., 2007). RGS2 has also been shown to be highly integrated within the NO mediated vasodilator pathway. Specifically, the N-terminal of RGS2 is phosphorylated by PKG (cGMP-dependent protein kinase), resulting in plasma membrane translocation and increased function as an inhibitor of vasoconstrictor signaling (Tang et al., 2003). Results from knockout animal studies also suggest that abnormal function of the autonomic nervous system contributes to the hypertensive phenotype, since they have increased urinary noradrenaline and altered baroreflex sensitivity. Moreover, through the ability of its N-terminal domain to directly inhibit specific adenylate cyclase isoforms (Gu et al., 2008b; Salim et al., 2003), RGS2 may attenuate signaling via receptors for dopamine and vasopressin in the kidney. Consistent with this suggestion, RGS2 was shown to regulate vasopressin responses in cortical collecting duct segments *in vivo* (Zuber et al., 2007).

### 4.3.2 RGS2 and Ang II action

There is increasing evidence of a reciprocal association between RGS2 activity and Ang II signaling. RGS2 has been shown to modulate signaling through the AT1 receptor (Ang II type 1 receptor) in several reports mentioned above. However, it has also been shown that RGS2 mRNA expression is increased by Ang II signaling in several cell lines, suggesting that RGS2 is an important part of a negative-feedback loop for this pathway. Indeed, the Ang II-stimulated expression of RGS2 has been shown to be able to inhibit both Ang II signaling (Li et al., 2005) and aldosterone production (Romero et al., 2006) . Although the precise mechanism for the up regulation of *Rgs2* is not fully understood, recent findings have implicated a role for PLA2 (phospholipase A2) in this process. Together, these results suggest a reciprocal relationship between RGS2 and Ang II, which is supported by *in vivo* studies showing that the *Rgs2*-null animals are more sensitive to Ang II-induced hypertension than wild-type controls (Hercule et al., 2007).

### 4.3.3 Clinical hypertension and RGS2 deficiency

The importance of RGS2 in the regulation of blood pressure homoeostasis is evident also in human studies. Recent studies have identified human genetic polymorphisms within the *RGS2* locus that are associated with hypertension in different ethnic populations (Riddle et al., 2006; Freson et al., 2007). The *RGS2* gene consists of five exons that show minimal genetic variation between subjects. No coding polymorphisms have been yet identified in Caucasian subjects; however, one single nucleotide polymorphism (SNP) was found in Black Americans (Riddle et al., 2006), and nine different SNPs in Japanese subjects (of which five are non-synonymous) (Yang et al., 2005). In the case of the Japanese population, hypomorphic *RGS2* allele function could partially explain the development of hypertension in subjects carrying missense mutations at Q2L,Q2R and R44H. For example, Q2L and Q2R variant proteins were shown to be less stable compared with normal RGS2 and, as a result, these subjects are thought to express lower steady-state levels of RGS2. By contrast, another study showed that the R44H variant of RGS2, although not compromising stability, disrupt the amphipathic *α*-helix that is crucial for proper plasma-membrane targeting and function (Gu et al., 2008a). Notably, another mutation at the Arg44 position, R44G, has also been shown to be associated with hypertension and higher than normal BMI (body mass index), suggesting a further role of RGS2 in causing obesity and metabolic syndrome. In addition, to those changes identified in the coding regions, the promoter region, introns and untranslated regions of *RGS2* also contain several SNPs and I/D (insertion/deletion) polymorphisms, of which one has been shown to result in enhanced calcium mobilization in fibroblasts in response to Ang II (Semplicini et al., 2006), and one has been linked to an increase in risk of the metabolic syndrome in white Caucasian Europeans (Freson et al., 2007). Remarkably, their allelic frequency differs markedly between ethnicity, and some are exclusively found in one ethnic group. Taken together, these studies of both non-synonymous mutations and extra-exonic polymorphisms suggest the possibility that *RGS2* variation contributes to some of the variability of blood pressure observed between different ethnic groups.

Noteworthy, too much RGS2 may also provide a pathophysiological stimulus within the cardiovascular tissues. It has been reported that the RGS2 protein is overexpressed in patients with Bartter's syndrome (B/S) and Gitelman's syndromes (G/S), and that this abnormally high expression inhibits Ang II-mediated intracellular calcium release (Calo' et al., 1998) and promotes altered vascular remodeling. Indeed, fibroblasts taken from patients with B/S and G/S have enhanced RGS2 expression and reduced signaling through the AT1 receptor (Calo' et al., 2004), the effects of which can be normalized by the knockdown of RGS2 expression (Calo' et al., 2008).

All these findings strongly suggest that the precise control of RGS2 protein level and function is extremely important for the normal regulation of vascular function and blood pressure control. This hypothesis received further support by our findings that 1) RGS2 expression is reduced in PBMs and in cultured fibroblasts from hypertensive patients in comparison with normotensive individuals (Semplicini et al., 2006), 2) low RGS2 expression predicts a poor response to antihypertensive treatment. In fact, resistant hypertensives were characterized by higher plasma aldosterone, ARR and reduced RGS2 expression in peripheral blood mononuclear cells in comparison to responder to antihypertensive drugs. (Semplicini et al., 2010).

The association between resistant hypertension and low RGS2 expression suggests increased vascular tone of the resistance vessels due to unopposed Ang II-mediated vasoconstriction, while the association with high plasma aldosterone and high ARR is an indicator of disproportionate aldosterone response to Ang II in the adrenals.

In the vasculature, chronic upregulation of Ang II activity, due to low RGS2 expression, was suggested not only by the finding of increased BP, but also of increased plasma BUN and urate levels, an indicator of increased renal efferent artery resistance, reduction of renal blood flow and increased hydraulic pressure in the glomerular capillary, with consequent increased glomerular filtration rate, and urate and sodium reabsorption along the early proximal tubule. (Perlstein et al., 2004; Johnson et al., 2005).

In the adrenals, the association between low RGS2 and high plasma aldosterone and high ARR is an indicator of disproportionate aldosterone response to Ang II (Semplicini et al., 2010).

## 5. Disproportionate aldosterone secretion and reduced RGS2 expression: a proposed link in resistant hypertension deserving further investigations

Identification and treatment of uncontrolled and resistant hypertension is a task of paramount importance in cardiovascular preventive medicine. In fact, poor blood pressure control carries unacceptably high risk of cardiovascular complications and premature death. Improving blood pressure control at individual and population level may reduce cardiovascular morbidity and mortality but this major goal can not be achieved with such a high prevalence of uncontrolled and resistant hypertension.

The data summarized so far suggest which pathways should be investigated to unravel the pathophysiology of resistant hypertension and how to improve its drug treatment. The research results of our and others' laboratories indicate that aldosterone plays a key role in the pathogenesis of resistant hypertension and suggest that aldosterone antagonists should be tested in selected patients with resistant hypertension.

Calhoun et al. (2008) and Gallay et al. (2001) reported that PA is present in 20% of individuals with resistant hypertension. High-normal levels of circulating aldosterone increase the risk of poor blood pressure control. High aldosterone with high ARR and low PRA may reflect either primary aldosterone overproduction or, more likely, increased adrenal response to Ang II.

Our working hypothesis is that the exaggerated aldosterone production in resistant hypertensives is due to low RGS2 expression. This hypothesis originates from our recent findings (Semplicini et al., 2010) showing in a cohort of resistant hypertensives that:

1. there is an inverse correlation between RGS2 expression and baseline BP,
2. low RGS2 expression is associated with resistant hypertension,
3. resistant hypertension with low RGS2 expression is associated with high plasma BUN and acid uric, indicating increased sodium and water reabsorption in the renal proximal tubules,
4. resistant hypertension with low RGS2 is associated with high plasma aldosterone and ARR,
5. the accuracy of RGS2 and ARR in predicting response to antihypertensive treatment is similar and not additive.

Aldosterone stimulates RGS2 expression, and upregulation of RGS2 by Ang II functions as a negative feedback of aldosterone production. The fact that we showed in resistant hypertensives high aldosterone with low RGS2 expression provides strong support to our hypothesis that abnormal regulation of RGS2 expression increases the duration of action of the intracellular signaling cascade, leading to persistently increased secretion of aldosterone in resistant hypertensives.

RGS2 is one of the genes involved in human essential hypertension, because it regulates the cell responses to Ang II and other vasoconstrictive agents and it controls peripheral vasoconstriction and blood pressure. Our data provide robust indication that reduced expression of RGS2 acts also as a promoter of aldosterone excess in resistant and uncontrolled hypertension.

Dysregulation of RGS2 plays a crucial role in the pathogenesis of cardiovascular diseases, making RGS2 as a potential therapeutic target or biomarker of hypertension or hypertensive heart disease. There is no firm evidence of the cause of reduced RGS2 expression in resistant hypertension, but it could be associated to a susceptible genetic polymorphism, and it is still unknown how to control the activity of its gene to up-regulate its expression.

On clinical grounds, according to our hypothesis, we propose a short course of aldosterone antagonists in resistant hypertensives. If it provides a good blood pressure response, long term treatment with aldosterone antagonists is recommended. This therapeutic approach has to be tested in long term controlled studies. In the meanwhile, further in depth studies of these mechanisms are recommended to allow a wider comprehension of resistant hypertension and to provide further support to its therapeutic approach with aldosterone antagonists.

## 6. References

Acelajado, MC & Calhoun, DA. (2011). Aldosteronism and resistant hypertension. *Int J Hypertens*. 2011 Jan 20;2011:837817]

Alvarez-Alvarez, B; Abad-Cardiel, M.; Fernandez-Cruz, A. & Martell-Claros, N. (2010). Management of resistant arterial hypertension: role of spironolactone versus double blockade of the renin-angiotensin-aldosterone system. *J. Hypertension*. 2010 Nov;28(11):2329-35.

Aqel, RA.; Zoghbi, GJ.; Baldwin, SA.; Auda, WS.; Calhoun, DA.; Coffey, CS.; Perry, GJ. & Iskandrian, AE. (2003). Prevalence of renal artery stenosis in high-risk veterans referred to cardiac catheterization. *J Hypertens*. 2003;21: 1157-1162.

Aguilera, MT.; de la Sierra, A.; Coca, A.; Estruch, R.; Fernández-Solá, J. & Urbano-Márquez, A. (1999). Effect of alcohol abstinence on blood pressure: assessment by 24-hour ambulatory blood pressure monitoring". *Hypertension*. 1999 Feb;33(2):653-7.

Bakris, GL. A practical approach to achieving recommended blood pressure goals in diabetic patients. (2001). *Arch Intern Med*. 2001 Dec 10-24;161(22):2661-7.

Berman, DM; Kozasa, T. & Gilman, A. G. (1996). The GTPase-activating protein RGS4 stabilizes the transition state for nucleotide hydrolysis. *J Biol Chem*. 1996 Nov 1;271(44):27209-12.

Bianchi, S.; Bigazzi, R. & Campese, VM. (2006). Long-term effects of spironolactone on proteinuria and kidney function in patients with chronic kidney disease. *Kidney Int*. 2006 Dec;70(12):2116-23.

Björklund, K.; Lind, L.; Zethelius, B.; Berglund, L. & Lithell, H. (2004). Prognostic significance of 24-h ambulatory blood pressure characteristics for cardiovascular morbidity in a population of elderly men. *J Hypertens*. 2004 Sep;22(9):1691-7.

Boudville, N.; Ward, S.; Benaroia , M. & House, AA. (2005). Increased sodium intake correlates with greater use of antihypertensive agents by subjects with chronic kidney disease. *Am J Hypertens*. 2005 Oct; 18(10):1300 –1305.

Bramlage, P.; Pittrow, D.; Wittchen, HU.; Kirch, W.; Boehler, S.; Lehnert, H.; Hoefler, M.; Unger, T. & Sharma, AM. (2004). Hypertension in overweight and obese primary care patients is highly prevalent and poorly controlled. *Am J Hypertens*. 2004 Oct;17(10):904-10.

Brown, MA.; Buddle, ML. & Martin, A. (2001). Is resistant hypertension really resistant?. *Am J Hypertens*. 2001 Dec;14(12):1263-9.

Buckalew, VM Jr; Berg, RL.; Wang, SR.; Porush, JG.; Rauch, S. & Schulman, G. (1996). Prevalence of hypertension in 1,795 subjects with chronic renal disease: the modification of diet in renal disease study baseline cohort. Modification of Diet in Renal Disease Study Group. *Am J Kidney Dis*. 1996 Dec;28(6):811-21.

Calhoun, DA.; Jones, D.; Textor, S.; Goff, DC.; Murphy, TP.; Toto, RD.; White, A.; Cushman, WC.; White, W.; Sica, D.; Ferdinand, K.; Giles, TD.; Falkner, B. & Carey, RM. (2008). Resistant Hypertension: Diagnosis, Evaluation, and Treatment. A Scientific Statement From the American Heart Association Professional Education Committee of the Council for High Blood Pressure Research. *Hypertension*. 2008 Jun;51(6):1403-19.

Calo', LA.; Davis, PA.; Milani, M.; Cantaro, S.; Bonfante, L.; Favaro, S. & D'Angelo A. (1998). Bartter's syndrome and Gitelman's syndrome: two entities sharing the same abnormality of vascular reactivity. *Clin Nephrol*. 1998 Jul;50(1):65-7.

Calo', L. A.; Pagnin, E.; Davis, P. A.; Sartori, M.; Ceolotto, G.; Pessina, AC. & Semplicini, A. (2004) Increased expression of regulator of G protein signaling-2 (RGS-2) in Bartter's/Gitelman's syndrome. A role in the control of vascular tone and implication for hypertension. *J Clin Endocrinol Metab.* 2004 Aug;89(8):4153-7.

Calò, L. A.; Pagnin, E.; Ceolotto, G.; Davis, PA.; Schiavo, S.; Papparella, I.; Semplicini, A. & Pessina, AC. (2008). Silencing regulator of G protein signaling-2 (RGS-2) increases angiotensin II signaling: insights into hypertension from findings in Bartter's/Gitelman's syndromes. *J Hypertens.* 2008 May;26(5):938-45.

Caro, JJ.; Speckman, JL.; Salas, M.; Raggio, G. & Jackson, JD. (1999). et al. Effect of initial drug choice on persistence with antihypertensive therapy: the importance of actual practice data. *CMAJ.* 1999 Jan 12;160(1):41-6.

Ceolotto, G.; Gallo, A.; Sartori, M.; Valente, R.; Baritono, E.; Semplicini, A. & Avogaro, A.(2001). Hyperglycemia acutely increases monocyte extracellular signal-regulated kinase activity in vivo in humans. *J Clin Endocrinol Metab.* 2001 Mar;86(3):1301-5.

Cladman, W. & Chidiac, P. (2002). Characterization and comparison of RGS2 and RGS4 as GTPase-activating proteins for M2 muscarinic receptor-timulated Gi. *Mol Pharmacol.* 2002 Sep;62(3):654-9.

Clapham, DE. & Neer, EJ. (1997) G protein $\beta\gamma$ subunits. *Annu Rev Pharmacol Toxicol.* 1997;37:167-203.

Conlin, PR.; Moore, TJ.; Swartz, SL.; Barr, E.; Gazdick, L.; Fletcher, C.; DeLucca, P. & Demopoulos, L. et al. "Effect of indomethacin on blood pressure lowering by captopril and losartan in hypertensive patients". *Hypertension.* 2000 Sep;36(3):461-5.

Cuckson AC, Moran P, Seed, P.; Reinders, A. & Shennan, AH. (2004). Clinical evaluation of an automated oscillometric blood pressure wrist device. *Blood Press Monit.* 2004 Feb;9(.1):31-7

Dedier, J.; Stampfer, MJ.; Hankinson, SE.; Willett, WC.; Speizer, FE. & Curhan, GC. (2002). "Nonnarcotic analgesic use and the risk of hypertension in US women. *Hypertension.* 2002 Nov;40(5):604-8; discussion 601-3.

De Souza, F.; Muxfeldt, E.; Fiszman, R. & Salles, G, (2010). Efficacy of spironolactone therapy in patients with true resistant hypertension. *Hypertension.* 2010 Jan;55(1):147-52.

Eide IK, Torjesen PA, Drolsum A, Babovic A, Lilledahl NP. (2004). Low-renin status in therapy-resistant hypertension: a clue to efficient treatment. *J Hypertens.* 2004 Nov;22(11):2217-26.

Fardella, CE.; Mosso, L.; Gómez-Sánchez, C.; Cortés, P.; Soto, J.; Gómez, L.; Pinto, M.; Huete, A.; Oestreicher, E.; Foradori, A. & Montero, J. (2000). Primary hyperaldosteronism in essential hypertensives: prevalence, biochemical profile, and molecular biology. *J Clin Endocrinol Metab.* 2000 May;85(5):1863-7.

Farquharson, CA. & Struthers, AD. (2002). Aldosterone induces acute endothelial dysfunction in vivo in humans: evidence for an aldosteroneinduced vasculopathy. *Clin Sci (Lond).* 2002 Oct;103(4):425-31.

Ferrari, P. (2003). Cortisol and the renal handling of electrolytes: role in glucocorticoid-induced hypertension and bone disease. *Best Pract Res Clin Endocrinol Metab.* 2003 Dec;17(4):575-89.

Forman, JP.; Stampfer, MJ. & Curhan, GC. (2005). Non-narcotic analgesic dose and risk of incident hypertension in US women. *Hypertension*. 2005 Sep;46(3):500-7.

Freson, K.; Stolarz, K.; Aerts, R.; Brand, E.; Brand-Herrmann, SM.; Kawecka-Jaszcz, K.; Kuznetsova, T.; Tikhonoff, V.; Thijs, L.; Vermylen, J.; Staessen, JA.; Van Geet, C. & European Project on Genes in Hypertension Investigators. (2007) −391 C to G substitution in the regulator of G-protein signalling-2 promoter increases susceptibility to the metabolic syndrome in white European men: consistency between molecular and epidemiological studies. *J Hypertens*. 2007 Jan;25(1):117-25.

Funder, JW.; Carey, RM.; Fardella, C.; Gomez-Sanchez, CE.; Mantero, F.; Stowasser, M.; Young, WF. Jr; Montori, VM. & Endocrine Society. (2008). Case detection, diagnosis and treatment of patients with primary aldosteronism: an endocrine society clinical practice guidelines. *J Clin Endocrinol Metab*. 2008 Sep;93(9):3266-81.

Gaddam, K.; Corros, C.; Pimenta, E.; Ahmed, M.; Denney, T.; Aban, I.; Inusah, S.; Gupta, H.; Lloyd, SG.; Oparil, S.; Husain, A.; Dell'Italia, LJ. & Calhoun DA. (2010). Rapid reversal of left ventricular hypertrophy and intracardiac volume overload in patients with resistant hypertension and hyperaldosteronism: a prospective clinical study, *Hypertension*. 2010 May;55(5):1137-42.

Gallay, BJ.; Ahmad, S.; Xu, L.; Toivola, B. & Davidson, RC. (2001). Screening for primary aldosteronism without discontinuing hypertensive medications: plasma aldosterone-renin ratio. *Am J Kidney Dis*. 2001 Apr;37(4):699-705.

Givens RC, Lin YS, et al. "CYP3A5 gentoype predicts renal CYP3A activity and blood pressure in healthy adults." *J Appl Physiol*. 2003;95: 1297–1300

Gordon RD, Stowasser M, et al. "High incidence of primary aldosteronism in 199 patients referred with hypertension". *Clin Exp Pharmacol Physiol*. 1994;21:315–318.

Grassi, G.; Facchini, A.; Trevano, FQ.; Dell'Oro, R.; Arenare, F.; Tana, F.; Bolla,G.; Monzani, A.; Robuschi, M. & Mancia, G. (2005). Obstructive sleep apnea dependent and -independent adrenergic activation in obesity. *Hypertension*. 2005 Aug;46(2):321-5.

Gross, V.; Tank, J.; Obst, M.; Plehm, R.; Blumer, KJ.; Diedrich, A.; Jordan, J. & Luft FC. (2005). Autonomic nervous system and blood pressure regulation in RGS2-deficient mice. *Am J Physiol Regul Integr Comp Physiol*. 2005 May;288(5):R1134-42.

Grote, L.; Hedner, J. &Peter JH. (2000). Sleep-related breathing disorder is an independent risk factor for uncontrolled hypertension. *J Hypertens*. 2000 Jun;18(6):679-85.

Gu, S.; Tirgari, S. and Heximer, SP. (2008a). The RGS2 gene product from a candidate hypertension allele shows decreased plasma membrane association and inhibition of Gq. *Mol Pharmacol*. 2008 Apr;73(4):1037-43.

Gu, S.; Anton, A.; Salim, S.; Blumer, KJ.; Dessauer, CW. & Heximer, SP. (2008b). Alternative translation initiation of human regulators of G-protein signaling-2 yields a set of functionally distinct proteins. *Mol Pharmacol*. 2008 Jan;73(1):1-11.

Hall, JE. (2003). The kidney, hypertension, and obesity. *Hypertension*. 2003; 41(part 2):625–633.

Hamm, H. E. (1998). The many faces of G protein signaling. *J Biol Chem*. 1998 Jan 9;273(2):669-72.

Hannila-Handelberg, T.; Kontula, K.; Tikkanen, I.; Tikkanen, T.; Fyhrquist, F.; Helin, K.; Fodstad, H.; Piippo, K.; Miettinen, HE.; Virtamo, J.; Krusius, T.; Sarna, S.; Gautschi,

I.; Schild, L. & Hiltunen, TP. (2005). Common variants of the beta and gamma subunits of the epithelial sodium channel and their relation to the plasma renin and aldosterone levels in essential hypertension. *BMC Med Genet.* 2005 Jan 20;6:4.

Hartman, D.; Sagnella, GA.; Chester, CA. & MacGragor, GA. (2004). Direct renin assay and plasma rennin activity assay compared. *Clin Chem.* 2004 Nov;50(11):2159-61.

He FJ, MacGregor GA. (2004). Effect of longer-term modest salt reduction on blood pressure. *Cochrane Database Syst Rev.* 2004;(3):CD004937.

Henningsen, NC.; Ohlsson, O.; Mattiasson, I.; Trell, E.; Kristensson, H. & Hood, B. (1980). Hypertension, levels of serum gamma glutamyl transpeptidase and degree of blood pressure control in middle-aged males. *Acta Med Scand.* 1980;207(4):245–251.

Hercule, HC.; Tank, J.; Plehm, R.; Wellner, M.; da Costa Goncalves, AC.; Gollasch, M.; Diedrich, A.; Jordan, J.; Luft, FC. & Gross, V. (2007). Regulator of G protein signalling 2 ameliorates Ang II-induced hypertension in mice. *Exp Physiol.* 2007 Nov;92(6):1014-22.

Hermida, RC.; Ayala, DE.; Calvo, C.; López, JE.; Mojón, A.; Fontao, MJ.; Soler, R. & Fernández JR. (2005). Effects of time of day of treatment on ambulatory blood pressure pattern of patients with resistant hypertension. *Hypertension.* 2005 Oct;46(4):1053-9.

Heximer, SP.; Srinivasa, SP.; Bernstein, LS.; Bernard, JL.; Linder, ME.; Hepler, JR. & Blumer. KJ. (1999). G protein selectivity is a determinant of RGS2 function. *J Biol Chem.* 1999 Nov 26;274(48):34253-9.

Ho H, Pinto A, Hall SD, Flockhart DA, Li L, Skaar TC, Cadman P, O'Connor DT, Wagner U, Fineberg NS, Weinberger MH. (2005). Association between CYP3A5 genotype and blood pressure. *Hypertension.* 2005 Feb;45(2):294-8.

Johnson, RJ.; Segal, MS.; Srinivas, T.; Ejaz, A.; Mu, W.; Roncal, C.; Sánchez-Lozada, LG.; Gersch, M.; Rodriguez-Iturbe, B.; Kang, DH. & Acosta, JH. (2005). Essential hypertension, progressive renal disease, and uric acid: a pathogenetic link?. *J Am Soc Nephrol.* 2005 Jul;16(7):1909-19.

Karagiannis, A.; Tziomalos, K.; Papageorgiou, A.; Kakafika, AI.; Pagourelias, ED.; Anagnostis, P.; Athyros, VG. & Mikhailidis, DP. (2008). Spironolactone versus eplerenone for the treatment of idiopathic hyperaldosteronism. *Expert Opin Pharmacother.* 2008 Mar;9(4):509-15

Kikuya, M.; Hozawa, A.; Ohokubo, T.; Tsuji, I.; Michimata, M.; Matsubara, M.; Ota, M.; Nagai, K.; Araki, T.; Satoh, H.; Ito, S.; Hisamichi, S. & Imai, Y. (2000). Prognostic significance of blood pressure and heart rate variabilities: the Ohasama study". *Hypertension.* 2000 Nov;36(5):901-6.

Klahr, S.; Levey, AS.; Beck, GJ.; Caggiula, AW.; Hunsicker, L.; Kusek, JW. & Striker, G. (1994). The effects of dietary protein restriction and blood-pressure control on the progression of chronic renal disease. Modification of Diet in Renal Disease Study Group. *N Engl J Med.* 1994 Mar 31;330(13):877-84.

Lavie, P. & Hoffstein, V. (2001). Sleep apnea syndrome: a possible contributing factor to resistant. *Sleep.* 2001 Sep 15;24(6):721-5.

Leiner, T.; de Haan, MW.; Nelemans, PJ.; van Engelshoven, JM. & Vasbinder GB (2005). Contemporary imaging techniques for the diagnosis of renal artery stenosis. *Eur Radiol*. 2005 Nov;15(11):2219-29.

Li, Y.; Hashim, S. & Anand-Srivastava, MB. (2005). Angiotensin II-evoked enhanced expression of RGS2 attenuates Gi-mediated adenylyl cyclase signaling in A10 cells. *Cardiovasc Res*. 2005 Jun 1;66(3):503-11.

Lloyd-Jones DM, Evans JC, Larson MG, Levy D. (2002).Treatment and control of hypertension in the community: a prospective analysis. *Hypertension*. 2002 Nov;40(5):640-6.

Luft, FC. & Weinberger, MH. (1988). Review of salt restriction and the response to antihypertensive drugs: satellite symposium on calcium antagonists. *Hypertension*. 1988 Feb;11(2 Pt 2):I229-32.

Mancia, G.; De Backer, G.; Dominiczak, A.; Cifkova, R.; Fagard, R.; Germano, G.; Grassi, G.; Heagerty, AM.; Kjeldsen, SE.; Laurent, S.; Narkiewicz, K.; Ruilope, L.; Rynkiewicz, A.; Schmieder, RE.; Boudier, HA.; Zanchetti, A.; Vahanian, A.; Camm, J.; De Caterina, R.; Dean, V.; Dickstein, K.; Filippatos, G.; Funck-Brentano, C.; Hellemans, I.; Kristensen, SD.; McGregor, K.; Sechtem, U.; Silber, S.; Tendera, M.; Widimsky, P.; Zamorano, JL.; Erdine, S.; Kiowski, W.; Agabiti-Rosei, E.; Ambrosioni, E.; Lindholm, LH.; Viigimaa, M.; Adamopoulos, S.; Bertomeu, V; Clement, D; Erdine, S.; Farsang, C.; Gaita, D.; Lip, G.; Mallion, JM.; Manolis, AJ.; Nilsson, PM.; O'Brien, E.; Ponikowski, P.; Redon, J.; Ruschitzka, F.; Tamargo, J.; van Zwieten, P.; Waeber, B. & Williams B. (2007). Management of Arterial Hypertension of the European Society of Hypertension; European Society of Cardiology. 2007 Guidelines for the Management of Arterial Hypertension: The Task Force for the Management of Arterial Hypertension of the European Society of Hypertension (ESH) and of the European Society of Cardiology (ESC). *J Hypertens*. 2007 Jun;25(6):1105-1187.

Marrs JC, (2010). Spironolactone management of resistant hypertension. *Ann Pharmacoter* 2010Nov;44(11):1762-9.

Mazzaglia, G.; Mantovani, LG.; Sturkenboom, MC.; Filippi, A.; Trifirò, G.; Cricelli, C.; Brignoli, O. & Caputi, AP. (2005). Patterns of persistence with antihypertensive medications in newly diagnosed hypertensive patients in Italy: a retrospective cohort study in primary care. *J Hypertens*. 2005 Nov;23(11):2093-100.

McFarlane, SI.; Banerji, M. & Sowers, JR. (2001). Insulin resistance and cardiovascular disease. *J Clin Endocrinol Metab*. 2001 Feb;86(2):713-8.

Milliez, P.; Girerd, X.; Plouin, PF.; Blacher, J.; Safar, ME. & Mourad, JJ. (2005). Evidence for an increased rate of cardiovascular events in patients with primary aldosteronism. *J Am Coll Cardiol*. 2005 Apr 19;45(8):1243-8.

Moneva, MH. & Gomez-Sanchez, CE. (2002). Pathophysiology of adrenal hypertension. *Semin Nephrol*. 2002 Jan;22(1):44-53.

Mosso, L.; Carvajal, C.; González, A.; Barraza, A.; Avila, F.; Montero, J.; Huete, A.; Gederlini, A. & Fardella, CE. (2003). Primary aldosteronism and hypertensive disease. *Hypertension*. 2003 Aug;42(2):161-5.

Mulatero, P.; Monticone, S.; Bertello, C.; Mengozzi, G.; Tizzani, D.; Iannaccone, A. & Veglio, F. (2010). Confirmatory tests in the diagnosis of primary aldosteronism. *Horm Metab Res*. 2010 Jun;42(6):406-10.

Muxfeldt, ES.; Bloch, KV.; Nogueira, AR. & Salles, GF. (2003). Twenty-four hour ambulatory blood pressure monitoring pattern of resistant hypertension. *Blood Press Monit*. 2003 Oct;8(5):181-5.

Nieto, FJ.; Young, TB.; Lind, BK.; Shahar, E.; Samet, JM.; Redline, S.; D'Agostino, RB.; Newman, AB.; Lebowitz, MD. & Pickering, TG. (2000). "Association of sleep-disordered breathing, sleep apnea, and hypertension in a large community-based study. Sleep Heart Health Study. *JAMA*. 2000 Apr 12;283(14):1829-36.

Nishizaka, MK.; Zaman MA. & Calhoun DA. (2003). Efficacy of low-dose spironolactone in subjects with resistant hypertension. *Am J Hypertens*. 2003 Nov;16(11 Pt 1):925-30.

Nishizaka, MK.; Zaman, MA.; Green, SA.; Renfroe, KY. & D. A. Calhoun, DA. (2004). Impaired endothelium-dependent flowmediated vasodilation in hypertensive subjects with hyperaldosteronism, *Circulation*. 2004 Jun 15;109(23):2857-61.

Nishizaka, MK.; Pratt-Ubunama, M.; Zaman, MA.; Cofield, S. & Calhoun. DA. (2005). Validity of plasma aldosterone-to-renin activity ratio in African American and white subjects with resistant hypertension. *Am J Hypertens*. 2005 Jun;18(6):805-12.

Omura, M.; Saito, J.; Yamaguchi, K.; Kakuta, Y. & Nishikawa, T. (2004). "Prospective study on the prevalence of secondary hypertension among hypertensive patients visiting a general outpatient clinic in Japan". *Hypertens Res*. 2004 Mar;27(3):193-202.

Peppard, PE.; Young, T.; Palta, M. & Skatrud, J. (2000). Prospective study of the association between sleep-disordered breathing and hypertension. *N Engl J Med*. 2000 May 11;342(19):1378-84.

Perlstein, TS.; Gumieniak, O.; Hopkins, PN.; Murphey, LJ.; Brown, NJ.; Williams, GH.; Hollenberg, NK. & Fisher, ND. (2004). Uric acid and the state of the intrarenal renin-angiotensin system in humans. *Kidney Int*. 2004 Oct;66(4):1465-70.

Pickering, TG.; Hall, JE.; Appel, LJ.; Falkner, BE.; Graves, J.; Hill, MN.; Jones, DW.; Kurtz, T.; Sheps, SG. & Roccella, EJ. (2005). Recommendations of blood pressure measurement in humans and experimental animals. Part 1: blood pressure measurement in humans. A Statement for Professionals from the Subcommittee of Professional and Public Education of the American Heart Association Council on High Blood Pressure Research. *Circulation*. 2005 Feb 8;111(5):697-716.

Pierdomenico, SD.; Lapenna, D.; Bucci, A.; Di Iorio, A.; Neri, M.; Cuccurullo, F. & Mezzetti, A. (2004). Cardiovascular outcome in treated hypertensive patients with responder, masked, false resistant, and true resistant hypertension. *Am J Hypertens*. 2004 Oct;17(10):876-81.

Pizzolo, F.; Corgnati, A.; Guarini, P.; Pavan, C.; Bassi, A.; Corrocher, R. & Olivieri, O. Plasma aldosterone assays: comparison between chemiluminescence-based and RIA methods. *Clin Chem*. 2006 Jul;52(7):1431-2.

Radack, KL.; Deck, CC. & Bloomfield, SS. (1987). Ibuprofen interferes with the efficacy of antihypertensive drugs. A randomized, double-blind, placebo-controlled trial of ibuprofen compared with acetaminophen. *Ann Intern Med*. 1987 Nov;107(5):628-35.

Redon, J.; Campos, C.; Narciso, ML.; Rodicio, JL.; Pascual, JM. & Ruilope, LM. (1998). Prognostic value of ambulatory blood pressure monitoring in refractory hypertension: a prospective study". *Hypertension*. 1998 Feb;31(2):712-8

Riddle, EL.; Rana, BK.; Murthy, KK.; Rao, F.; Eskin, E.; O'Connor, DT. & Insel, PA. (2006). Polymorphisms and haplotypes of the regulator of G protein signaling-2 gene in normotensives and hypertensives. *Hypertension*. 2006 Mar;47(3):415-20.

Rocha, R.; Rudolph, AE.; Frierdich, GE.; Nachowiak, DA.; Kekec, BK.; Blomme, EA.; McMahon, EG. & Delyani, JA. (2002). Aldosterone induces a vascular inflammatory phenotype in the rat heart. *Am J Physiol Heart Circ Physiol*. 2002 Nov;283(5):H1802-10.

Rockman, HA.; Koch, WJ. & Lefkowitz, RJ. (2002). Seven-transmembrane-spanning receptors and heart function. *Nature*. 2002 Jan 10;415(6868):206-12.

Romero, DG.; Plonczynski, MW.; Gomez-Sanchez, EP.; Yanes, LL. & Gomez-Sanchez, CE. (2006). RGS2 is regulated by angiotensin II and functions as a negative feedback of aldosterone production in H295R human adrenocortical cells. *Endocrinology*. 2006 Aug;147(8):3889-97.

Ross, EM. & Wilkie, TM. (2000). GTPase-activating proteins for heterotrimeric G proteins: regulators of G protein signaling (RGS) and RGS-like proteins. *Annu Rev Biochem*. 2000;69:795-827.

Rossi GP, Sechi LA, Giacchetti G, Ronconi V, Strazzullo P, Funder JW. (2008). Primary aldosteronism: cardiovascular, renal and metabolic implications. *Trends Endocrinol Metab*. 2008 Apr;19(3):88-90.

Sacerdote, A.; Weiss, K.; Tran, T.; Rokeya Noor, B. & McFarlane, SI. (2005). Hypertension in patients with Cushing's disease: pathophysiology, diagnosis, and management. *Curr Hypertens Rep*. 2005 Jun;7(3):212-8.

Salim, S.; Sinnarajah, S.; Kehrl, JH. & Dessauer, CW. (2003). Identification of RGS2 and type V adenylyl cyclase interaction sites. *J Biol Chem*. 2003 May 2;278(18):15842-9.

Sartori, M.; Calò, LA.; Mascagna, V.; Realdi, A.; Macchini, L.; Ciccariello, L.; De Toni, R.; Cattelan, F.; Pessina, AC. & Semplicini A. (2006). Aldosterone and Refractory Hypertension: A Prospective Cohort Study. *Am J Hypertens*. 2006 Apr;19(4):373-9; discussion 380.

Schupp, N.; Queisser, N.;Wolf, M.; Kolkhof, P.; Barfacker, L.; Schafer. S.; Heidland, A. & Stopper, H. et al. (2010). Aldosterone causes DNA strand breaks and chromosomal damage in renal cells, which are prevented by mineralocorticoid receptor antagonists. *Horm Metab Res*. 2010 Jun;42(6):458-65.

Sechi, LA.; Novello, M.; Lapenna, R.; Baroselli, S.; Nadalini, E.; Colussi GL. & Catena, C. (2006). Long-term renal outcomes in patients with primary aldosteronism. *JAMA*. 2006 Jun 14;295(22):2638-45.

Semplicini, A.; Lenzini, L.; Sartori, M.; Papparella, I.; Calò, LA.; Pagnin, E.; Strapazzon, G.; Benna, C.; Costa, R.; Avogaro, A.; Ceolotto, G. & Pessina, AC. (2006) Reduced expression of regulator of G-protein signaling 2 (RGS2) in hypertensive patients increases calcium mobilization and ERK1/2 phosphorylation induced by angiotensin II. *J Hypertens*. 2006 Jun;24(6):1115-24

Semplicini, A.; Strapazzon, G.; Papparella, I.; Sartori, M.; Realdi, A.; Macchini, L.; Calò, LA. & Ceolotto G. (2010). RGS2 expression and aldosterone : renin ratio modulate response to drug therapy in hypertensive patients. *J Hypertens.* 2010 May;28(5):1104-8.

Sinclair, AM.; Isles, CG.; Brown, I.; Cameron, H.; Murray, GD. & Robertson, JW. (1987). Secondary hypertension in a blood pressure clinic. *Arch Intern Med.* 1987 Jul;147(7):1289-93.

Takeda R, Matsubara T, Miyamori I, Hatakeyama H, Morise T. (1995). Vascular complications in patients with aldosterone producing adenoma in Japan: comparative study with essential hypertension. The Research Committee of Disorders of Adrenal Hormones in Japan. *J Endocrinol Invest.* 1995 May;18(5): 370-3.

Tang, KM.; Wang, GR.; Lu, P.; Karas, RH.; Aronovitz, M.; Heximer, SP.; Kaltenbronn, KM.; Blumer, KJ.; Siderovski, DP.; Zhu, Y. & Mendelsohn, ME. (2003). Regulator of G-protein signaling-2 mediates vascular smooth muscle relaxation and blood pressure. *Nat Med.* 2003 Dec;9(12):1506-12.

Van Wijk, BLG.; Klungel, OH.; Heerdink, ER. & de Boer, A. (2005). Rate and determinants of 10-year persistence with antihypertensive drugs. *J Hypertens.* 2005 Nov;23(11):2101-7.

Weinberger, MH.; Cohen, SJ.; Miller, JZ.; Luft, FC.; Grim, CE. & Fineberg, NS. (1988). Dietary sodium restriction as adjunctive treatment of hypertension. *JAMA.* 1988 May 6;259(17):2561-5.

Wieland, T.; Lutz, S. & Chidiac, P. (2007). Regulators of G protein signalling: a spotlight on emerging functions in the cardiovascular system. *Curr Opin Pharmacol.* 2007 Apr;7(2):201-7.

Wildman, RP; Gu, D.; Muntner, P.; Huang, G.; Chen, J.; Duan, X. & He J. (2005). Alcohol intake and hypertension subtypes in Chinese men. *J Hypertens.* 2005 Apr;23(4):737-43.

Yang, J.; Kamide, K.; Kokubo, Y.; Takiuchi, S.; Tanaka, C.; Banno, M.; Miwa, Y.; Yoshii, M.; Horio, T.; Okayama, A.; Tomoike, H.; Kawano, Y. & Miyata, T. (2005). Genetic variations of regulator of G-protein signaling 2 in hypertensive patients and in the general population. *J Hypertens.* 2005 Aug;23(8):1497-505.

Young WF Jr. (2003). Minireview: primary aldosteronism--changing concepts in diagnosis and treatment. *Endocrinology.* 2003 Jun;144(6):2208-13.

Young, WF. & Stanson, AW. (2009). What are the keys to successful adrenal venous sampling (AVS) in patients with primary aldosteronism?. *Clin Endocrinol (Oxf).* 2009 Jan;70(1):14-7.

Yiannakopoulou, ECh.; Papadopulos, JS.; Cokkinos, DV. & Mountokalakis, TD. (2005). "Adherence to antihypertensive treatment: a critical factor for blood pressure control". Eur J Cardiovasc Prev Rehabil. 2005 Jun;12(3):243-9.

Zuber, AM.; Singer, D.; Penninger, JM.; Rossier, BC. & Firsov, D. (2007). Increased renal responsiveness to vasopressin and enhanced V2 receptor signaling in RGS2−/− mice. *J Am Soc Nephrol.* 2007 Jun;18(6):1672-8.

Zelinka, T.; Strauch, B.; Petrák, O.; Holaj, R.; Vranková, A.; Weisserová, H.; Pacák, K. & Widimský, J. Jr. (2005). Increased blood pressure variability in pheochromocytoma compared to essential hypertension patients. *J Hypertens*. 2005 Nov;23(11):2033-9.

4

# Is Low Baroreflex Sensitivity only a Consequence of Essential Hypertension or also a Factor Conditioning Its Development?

Natasa Honzikova and Eva Zavodna
*Masaryk University, Faculty of Medicine, Department of Physiology*
*Czech Republic*

## 1. Introduction

Baroreflex is the most important nervous regulatory mechanism of blood pressure homeostasis. Its role in a short-time regulation of blood pressure is very well documented. On the other hand, the answer to the question whether primary low baroreflex sensitivity could also be the cause of the development of hypertension remains unresolved. This question is now topical.

Baroreflex has several branches: reflex control of the peripheral resistance, of the tone of capacitance vessels, of the heart rate and contractility. Heart rate response to blood pressure variations is studied most intensively. Heart rate changes caused by stimulation of baroreceptors are usually quantified as the index of baroreflex sensitivity (BRS), which corresponds to a prolongation of the cardiac interval due to the increase of blood pressure in ms/mmHg. This mechanism operates beat-by-beat and is evaluated from recordings of blood pressure and inter-beat intervals (IBI) lasting for several minutes or several seconds respectively, depending on the method used. Despite the fact that BRS fluctuates in healthy subjects at rest, it represents a characteristic individual feature. Baroreflex sensitivity decreases with age and in different pathological states. This is of major clinical relevance as a risk factor of sudden cardiac death in patients after myocardial infarction, which is included among complications of hypertension. Therefore, many studies have paid attention to this problem providing evidence that metabolic and sympathetic/parasympathetic changes, especially during obesity, activate mechanisms (for instance thickening of the carotid wall) causing suppression of BRS. On the other hand, some healthy children and adolescents have as low BRS as elderly patients with hypertension. Some genetic studies provided evidence for an inborn disposition to low BRS. This opened the question whether an inborn low BRS could represent an additive factor disposing to blood pressure elevation. This is important with respect to epidemic obesity and to an increased prevalence of hypertension among young people.

We have proved by our own method of a summed-weighted-fuzzified index that low BRS is an index partially independent of obesity, which is linked with blood pressure elevation in young population (Krontoradova et al., 2008).

In the methodological part of this Chapter, we describe a cross-spectral method of baroreflex sensitivity determination and the difference in the signification of this index determined in ms/mmHg (BRS) as usual, or in mHz/mmHg (BRSf). BRS is inter-beat interval-dependent and reflects best the total parasympathetic/sympathetic control of the heart rhythm. BRSf is inter-beat interval-independent and reflects preferably sensitivity of the baroreceptors. This fact is important when comparing groups of subjects with different mean inter-beat intervals, for instance, during childhood and adolescence.

## 2. Baroreflex in short-term and long-term homeostasis of blood pressure

The scientists proceeded from the observation that baroreceptors adapt to an increased blood pressure and are set to a higher level of blood pressure - the so-called resetting (Lohmeier et al., 2005). After baroreceptor denervation in experimental animals, blood pressure is increased by more than 50 mmHg, but during several days it resumes the original level due to the loss of blood volume by an increased urinary output. The result is an increase in blood pressure variability with the mean value of blood pressure corresponding to the value before the denervation. Based on the interpretation of these experiments it was concluded that the main function of baroreflex is the short-time regulation of blood pressure (Cowley et al., 1973). Only the recent experiments with chronic electrical stimulation of the carotid baroreceptor afferent nerve fibres and chronic recording of the renal sympathetic activity as well as some other experiments demonstrated the role of baroreceptors in the long-term control of blood pressure (Brooks & Sved, 2005; Cowley et al., 1992; Thrasher, 2005). The therapy of chronic hypertension resistant to antihypertensive drugs by stimulation of carotid nerves confirmed that baroreflex is likewise effective in long-term blood pressure regulation (Filippone & Bisognano, 2007).

### 2.1 Measurement of heart rate baroreflex sensitivity

The methods used to stimulate baroreceptors include administration of vasoconstrictive or vasodilative substances. The other possibility of stimulating baroreceptors is the so-called "neck suction". Another group of methods applies different mathematical procedures to the evaluation of recordings of blood pressure and inter-beat fluctuations which last several minutes. Baroreflex sensitivity calculated by different methods slightly differs (Laude et al., 2004; Persson et al., 2001).

In our laboratory, we published the first spectral analysis of blood pressure resting fluctuations in humans (Penaz et al., 1978). We have been using spectral analysis for baroreflex sensitivity determination since 1992 (Honzikova et al., 1992). Since then, we have obtained ample methodological experience and we would like to point out some of it.

#### 2.1.1 Cross-spectral method of baroreflex sensitivity determination

At first, we can shortly describe our approach to the determination of baroreflex sensitivity using one of the options, the cross-spectral method.

The recordings of continuous blood pressure and of inter-beat interval duration (IBI) are quasi-periodical. Therefore a pre-processing is essential. The recording of blood pressure is digitized (for instance by a 250 Hz sampling rate and 12-bit resolution), and then stored.

From the stored signal, the sequences of IBI, systolic blood pressure values (SBP), and diastolic blood pressure (DBP) are determined. The data acquired represent irregularly sampled values (concomitantly with variations of IBI) of a continuous time system. They are interpolated and equidistantly re-sampled.

The next step is a spectral analysis of these pre-processed data. There are two possibilities of evaluating the spectra: discrete Fourier transformation (DFT) applied directly on the signals and DFT applied to the autocorrelation function or the cross-correlation function of the signals. The latter method allows proving the legitimacy of the results by coherence. Therefore, we use this second method: the autocorrelation functions of IBI, SBP, DBP, and the cross-correlation function of IBI and SBP are calculated, and then, in the second step, the power spectra of the autocorrelation functions IBI, SBP and DBP, and the cross-spectrum of the cross-correlation function of IBI and SBP are calculated by fast Fourier transformation.

The gain factor between variations in systolic blood pressure and inter-beat intervals calculated at a frequency of 0.1 Hz is taken as a measure of baroreflex sensitivity (BRS) in ms/mmHg (Honzikova et al., 1992, 2003; Persson et al., 2001; Zavodna et al., 2006).

The frequency ranges between 0.07 and 0.012, or between 0.05 and 0.15 Hz, respectively, are used for the determination of BRS. The values of BRS are taken into account only if the coherence is higher than 0.5 (Fig. 1).

We calculate not only the BRS index in ms/mmHg, but also the BRSf index in mHz/mmHg. The reason for such approach is explained in detail in part 2.1.2 of this Chapter.

Continuous blood-pressure recordings are taken under different conditions. We use recordings at rest, in sitting position, during metronome-controlled breathing at a frequency of 0.33 Hz for about 5 minutes for the determination of the resting value of baroreflex sensitivity, or recordings at spontaneous breathing during a dynamic test, for instance workload, when controlled breathing is impossible.

During the testing of long duration, a time-frequency map of the spectra is computed. An example is given in Fig. 1, representing an experiment lasting 18 minutes: 3 minutes at rest (controlled breathing 0.33 Hz), 9 minutes of bicycling (0.5 W/kg of body weight, spontaneous breathing), and 6 min at rest after exercise (Honzikova et al., 2003).

To get such a time course of the system properties the whole signal is processed in segments step by step from the beginning to the end.

The results of the time-frequency map of spectral analysis presented in Fig. 1 revealed two characteristic features. First, all calculated parameters - the frequency at which BRS was determined (f), the maximal power of the product of IBI and SBP spectral component (P), the selected maximal spectral components in a frequency range between 0.05 and 0.15 Hz of IBI and SBP (vIBI and vSBP), the time-shift between vIBI and vSBP spectral components in a frequency range between 0.05 and 0.15 Hz, and baroreflex sensitivity fluctuate in time course. Second, for some short time intervals, coherence between variability of the signals is insignificant and so some data are omitted. Therefore, in principle, we never get identical values of these parameters during repeated measurements. Nevertheless, it was shown in several studies that there is a significantly lower intra-individual than inter-individual variability of BRS, SBP or IBI (Dietrich et al., 2010; Honzikova et al., 1990; Jira et al., 2006, 2010a; Penaz et al., 1978).

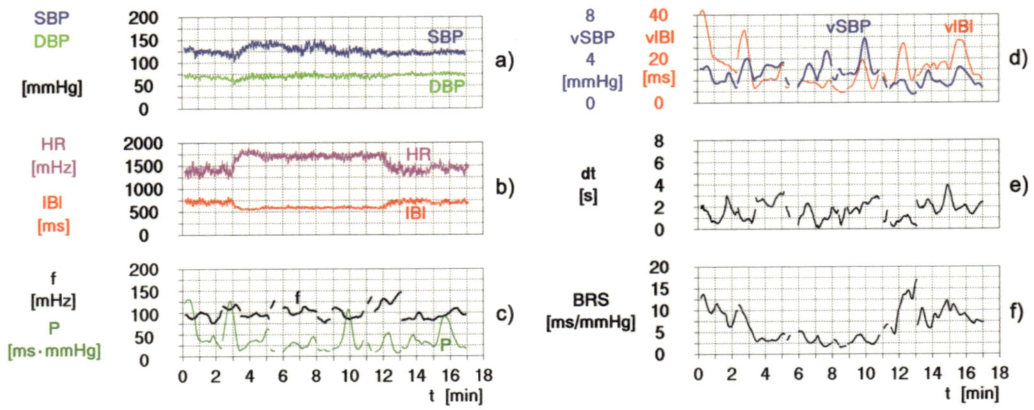


Fig. 1. An example of the time course of circulatory variables at rest (3 min, controlled breathing), during exercise (9 min, spontaneous breathing), and during recovery (6 min, controlled breathing). The individual graphs represent: a) the time course of the following parameters: systolic and diastolic blood pressure (SBP and DBP); b) inter-beat intervals and their inverse, heart rate values (IBI and HR); c) fluctuation of the frequency at which BRS was determined (f) with respect to the maximal power, i.e. the product of IBI and SBP spectral component amplitudes (P); d) the selected spectral components in the frequency range between 0.05 and 0.15 Hz of IBI and SBP (vIBI and vSBP); e) the time-shift between vIBI and vSBP spectral components in the frequency range between 0.05 and 0.15 Hz; f) baroreflex sensitivity (BRS).

### 2.1.2 Indices of baroreflex sensitivity calculated in ms/mmHg and mHz/mmHg

Baroreflex sensitivity can be expressed as the change of IBI due to a change of systolic blood pressure in ms/mmHg (BRS index) or as the change of heart rate (HR) due to a change of systolic blood pressure in bpm/mmHg (Ackermann et al., 1989) or in mHz/mmHg (Al Kubati et al., 1997). The BRS index is used in most studies, the second method is not used frequently, and there is no standard abbreviation for the indication that heart rate was used for the assessment of baroreflex sensitivity. In our laboratory, we apply calculation of baroreflex sensitivity in both units, in ms/mmHg and in mHz/mmHg, and we use the abbreviations BRS and BRSf (f in this abbreviation expresses that we use beat-to-beat values of heart rate for the calculation). To get the BRSf index (mHz/mm Hg), it is necessary to calculate the value of a modulus at a frequency of 0.1 Hz in a similar way as in case of the BRS index using spectral analysis of instantaneous values of the heart rate measured beat-by-beat and the corresponding systolic blood pressure values.

Even though in many dynamic tests or examinations of patients with severely suppressed baroreflex sensitivity the interpretation of the results is independent of the procedure (units) used, it is not so in all conditions. For example, examination of BRS and BRSf in 139 patients 7-14 days after the first signs of myocardial infarction had a similar discriminating significance between patients at risk and not at risk. Both indices were significantly decreased in patients who died within one year after examination in comparison with the survivors (Semrad et al., 1998). On the other hand, there is a difference in the age-related values of BRS and BRSf (Zavodna et al., 2006).

It seems to be useful to explain our approach. The theoretical background is in a non-linear relationship between IBI and HR (in the scheme below there are big differences in mean IBI for a better demonstration of the effect discussed). The difference in the values of BRS and BRSf calculated at a different mean value of IBI is schematically presented in Fig. 2 (left).

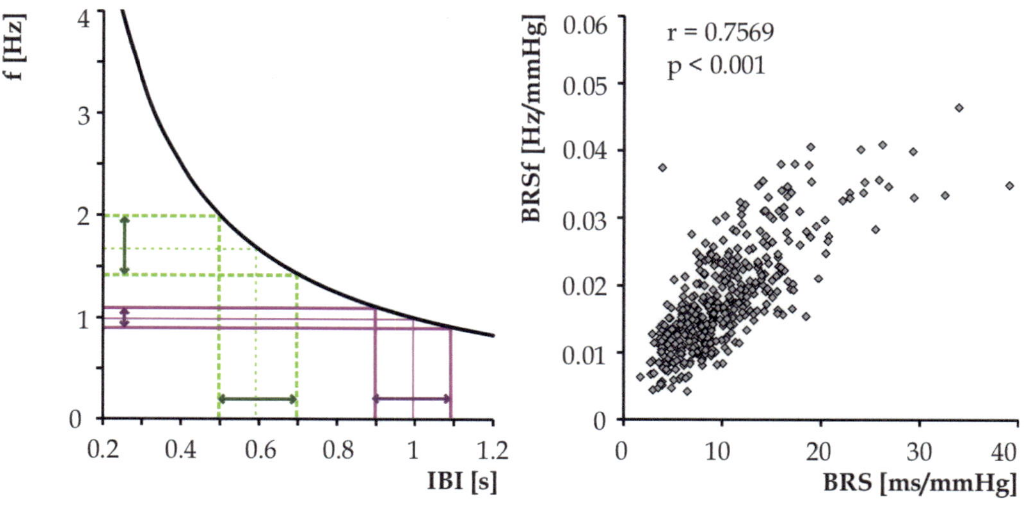


Fig. 2. Left: The non-linear relationship between IBI and HR influences BRS and BRSf indices presented by arrows. Right: The relationship between BRS and BRSf determined in 415 subjects (aged 11-20 years). The correlation coefficient calculated after normalization by a cube root.

Thus, with the same mean IBI in the two groups tested, the BRS index corresponds to the baroreflex responsiveness of the heart to blood pressure changes. Such a situation is very frequent, though mean IBI differs in individuals of such groups.

On the other hand, in a tested group with different mean IBI, the BRSf index should be preferred. For example, the effect of the development of parasympathetic control of the heart rate in childhood is manifested by prolongation of the mean IBI (Fig. 2 right). In the study of Zavodna et al. (2006), 415 healthy subjects at the age of 11-20 years were examined (under resting conditions, sitting, controlled breathing 0.33 Hz). The BRS and BRSf indices were determined by the cross-spectral method at a frequency of 0.1 Hz. BRS did not correlate with age, but BRSf significantly decreased with age. The baroreflex sensitivity determined as BRS in ms/mmHg was significantly positively dependent on the mean IBI. This relationship was found not only in the whole group of subjects, but also in the respective age subgroups. A different situation was encountered in the relationship between baroreflex sensitivity expressed in mHz/mmHg as BRSf and the mean IBI. BRSf correlated negatively with IBI in the age range between 11 to 20 years, but in the individual age subgroups the BRSf index was IBI independent. The greatest impact of IBI on baroreflex sensitivity was recorded in children aged 11-15 years in whom the mean IBI was prolonged with age. This means that the BRS index was influenced by the prolongation of mean IBI reflecting an age-dependent increased tonic vagal nerve activity. On the other hand, it could be hypothesized that BRSf better expressed the baroreceptor sensitivity.

Some other studies also examined the problem of the relationship between the heart rate and BRS in children (Allen et al., 2000). It was proposed to standardize the patients' BRS to a fixed heart rate of 60 b.p.m. by regression (Abrahamsson et al., 2003). This approach has some limitation, because the linearity between log-BRS and heart rate is guaranteed only between the heart rates of 80 and 120 b.p.m. (Wesseling, 2003).

We decided to evaluate a suppression of systolic blood pressure variability by a baroreflex regulation of the heart rhythm at a frequency of 0.1 Hz using the BRS and BRSf indices (Honzikova et al., 2007). This study was performed in 58 subjects (20–22 years of age). SBP variability (SBPv) at 0.1 Hz (LF range) was used for statistical evaluation.

To enable a comparison of the quantitative effects of BRS and BRSf on SBPv, both variables were expressed as multiples of standard deviations. A negative correlation was found between SBPv and BRSsd and between SBPv and BRSfsd.

The multiple regression equation

$$SBPv = 9.43 - 0.0052*IBI/ms + 0.15*BRSsd - 1.85*BRSfsd \; ; \quad F = 2.92, p<0.05 \qquad (1)$$

revealed a higher regression coefficient of BRSfsd than the regression coefficient of BRSsd.

In conclusion, this analysis revealed that the inter-beat interval-independent index BRSf (mHz/mmHg) is a better indicator for evaluation of the efficacy of baroreflex sensitivity to suppress the SBP variability than the inter-beat interval-dependent index BRS (ms/mmHg).

## 3. Physiology of baroreflex sensitivity

### 3.1 Resting heart rate baroreflex sensitivity as an individual characteristic feature and the influence of respiration

Baroreflex sensitivity, heart rate, and blood pressure variability are closely interrelated. This is especially so in the case that all the three variables are determined at a frequency of 0.1 Hz. This is the frequency range of a dominant role of baroreflex suppression of variations in blood pressure by heart rate changes. If the frequency range of respiration is included in a measurement or calculation, non-baroreflex factors are involved in respiratory sinus arrhythmia, such as a central component (Eckberg, 2003; Gilad et al., 2005; Eckberg & Karemaker, 2009; Tzeng et al., 2009), afferent stimuli from stretch receptors in the lungs and thoracic wall (Taha et al., 1995), and resonance (van de Vooren et al., 2007). Thus, there is a difference between BRS values determined at a respiratory frequency and a frequency of 0.1 Hz (Bothova et al., 2010; Fredericks et al., 2000). Bothova et al. (2010) have shown that on average the determination of BRS by the spectral method at the breathing frequency overestimates the real BRS. This phenomenon was present only statistically and an opposite relationship can occur in some subjects. From the point of view of clinicians it is important that this effect is also present at low BRS values. Therefore, for diagnostic purposes we recommend the evaluation of BRS at a frequency of 0.1 Hz using metronome-controlled breathing at a frequency that is substantially higher than 0.1 Hz and is not a multiple of 0.1 Hz to eliminate the respiratory baroreflex-non-related influence and a resonance effect on heart rate fluctuations.

### 3.2 Physiology of baroreflex sensitivity in children and adolescents

Relatively few studies of physiological BRS values in children and adolescents have been published. These studies indicate that BRS values are similar to those of young healthy adults and that inter-individual differences are also considerable. Quite different values of BRS were reported in 1868 children (10-13 years old) by Dietrich et al. (2006) - between 2.3 and 73 ms/mmHg. We found smaller differences in a group of 415 subjects 11-20 years old (Zavodna et al., 2006), ranging between 3.9 ms/mmHg for the 5th percentile and 18.7 ms/mmHg for the 95th percentile.

These results are surprising and change the view on the role of low BRS as a potentially primary factor involved in the early elevation of blood pressure. Low values of BRS in some children (Zavodna et al., 2006; Dietrich et al., 2006) approach the critical value for the risk of sudden cardiac death in patients after myocardial infarction and correspond to values present in hypertensive patients. BRS is usually less than 5 ms/mmHg in hypertensive patients (Labrova et al., 2005) and BRS lower than 3ms/mmHg is a marker of an increased risk of sudden cardiac death in patients after myocardial infarction (La Rovere et al., 1998; Honzikova et al., 2000).

Concerning the age-dependent BRS, a decrease was repeatedly described in adults by many authors (Gribbin et al., 1971; Kardos et al., 2001). Fewer studies on BRS in children were published (Allen et al., 2000; Lenard et al., 2004; Rudiger et al., 2001). No significant age-dependent baroreflex-sensitivity decrease was found in 400 subjects aged 10 to 19 years, as long as baroreflex sensitivity was expressed by the BRSf index in mHz/mmHg or after normalization of BRS on the cardiac interval by multiple regression analysis (Zavodna et al., 2006). This can be explained by an increase in the parasympathetic tone and a prolongation of IBI, and this special approach was explained in part 2.1.2 of this Chapter.

### 3.3 Genetics of BRS

The genetic contribution to a BRS value could involve different components of the baroreceptor reflex arc, including baroreceptors, central neuronal transmission, reflex afferent and efferent pathways. In all of these there act numerous ligands, receptors, channels, etc. A serious understanding of genetically conditioned BRS will be very complicated because of multiple interactions of these factors.

Baroreceptors are mechanosensory nerve endings that innervate the adventitia of large arteries - the carotid and aortic sinus. An explanation of the conversion of mechanical energy into the action potential is still an open question. In the last two decades, a member of the degenerin family with mechanosensitive properties was detected in baroreceptor terminals: amiloride-sensitive epithelial Na channels (ENaC) (Drummond et al., 1998). The ENaC channels are usually under the aldosterone control. We might presume that aldosterone would increase Na+ current in baroreceptor terminals and improve baroreceptor sensation of blood pressure rise. In the promotor region of the gene for enzyme 11/18-beta-hydroxylase (CYP11B2) in position -344 it is possible to find the C/T substitution which may influence the binding of regulatory factors (Lim et al., 2002). The T allele has been associated with increased plasma and urinary levels of aldosterone (Paillard et al., 1999; Davies et al., 1999), corresponding to the results of Ylitalo et al. (2000). They found, in a group of premenopausal women (41-46 years) who were TT homozygotes, increased mean and inter-individual variability of baroreflex sensitivity. The data are close to our unpublished data; however, we observed them in a group of young men (20-24 years) but not in women.

Gollasch et al. (2002) tested several mutations of the potassium large conductance calcium-activated channel (KCNMB1) and showed that individuals having SNP AA in exon 4b had greater baroreflex slopes in the high-frequency range than had CA or CC subjects. Their findings suggest that potassium channel heterogeneity could mainly influence the rapid baroreflex-mediated adjustment of heart rate by the parasympathetic nervous system. This idea is also supported by Pedarzani et al. (2000), who documented the presence of very high levels of $\alpha$-subunit potassium channel mRNA in rat dorsal vagal neurons.

The processing of the baroreceptor input is mediated in the CNS by several neurotransmitters, especially by angiotensin II. Generally, angiotensin II has a sympathoexcitatory effect. It was shown that long-term intracerebroventricular infusion of angiotensin II decreased BRS in rabbits, but therapy with the angiotensin blocker losartan resulted in BRS increase (Gaudet et al., 2000). We have found in our group of healthy young subjects (20-24 years) an association between the less frequent homozygotes CC and decreased baroreflex sensitivity (Jira et al., 2010b).

There are also other studies that were more or less successful in the association of the mutation in genes with blood pressure variability and its buffering via the baroreflex pathway, e.g. endothelin (Ormezzano et al., 2005), acid sensing ion channel (Lu et al., 2009), neuropeptide Y1 receptor (Wang et al., 2009), eNOS (Jira et al., 2011), etc.

## 4. Low baroreflex sensitivity as a risk factor

### 4.1 Significance of low baroreflex sensitivity as a risk factor

The significance of a short-time blood pressure regulation by high BRS as a protection of an ischemic myocardium from the risk of sudden cardiac death was shown about 15 years ago and BRS lower than 3ms/mmHg was determined as the critical value of BRS (Honzikova et al., 2000; La Rovere et al., 1998). At high BRS, a quick prolongation of IBI following a sudden blood pressure elevation decreases cardiac workload. This is important in an ischemic myocardium, especially after myocardial infarction, and therefore high BRS prevents sudden cardiac death.

Myocardial infarction is a frequent complication of essential hypertension. Studies of BRS in hypertensive patients are important with respect to the potential risk of hypertensive patients in a possible situation of a later myocardial infarction. BRS is usually lower than 5 ms/mmHg in hypertensive patients (Cowley, 1992; Labrova et al., 2005; Thrasher et al., 2005). Different comorbidities (diabetes mellitus or heart failure) have an additive effect either by decreasing BRS, or increasing the risk of myocardial infarction (Mortara et al., 1997).

Patients at risk of sudden cardiac death profit from implantation of an implantable cardioverter-defibrillator (ICD). Indication for ICD implantation is done invasively. It would be desirable to develop a non-invasive approach to risk stratification of patients. Many trials were carried out to find a combination of non-invasive risk-stratification techniques for identifying the patients at risk. Although the low left ventricular ejection fraction has been used effectively to select high-risk patients for the application of therapy to prevent sudden cardiac death, it has a limited sensitivity. Reviews of nearly 15 non-invasive markers of high-risk patients also include BRS (Bailey et al., 2007; Goldberger et al., 2008).

### 4.2 Logit and fuzzy models in risk-data analysis

Multiregression analysis is used for evaluation of the influence of different factors on some functional states, as well as the logistic regression analysis and calculation of the odds ratio for a group of risk factors. Such approach provides the basic information, for instance for the understanding of the pathogenesis of any process. Medical practice very often needs not only identification of risk predictors, but also determination of their critical values, sensitivity, specificity, and a positive predictive value in the diagnostics or a therapeutic decision in patients. Calculation of the receiver operating curve (ROC) is used for this purpose. The improvement of the predictive power of a group of risk factors needs to take the following physiological assumptions into account. First, the edge between a risky and a non-risky value of each predictor is not an exact value; secondly, different risk predictors have different weight.

We have developed fuzzified and weighted models for a sum of risk predictors (Honzik et al., 2003, 2010). First, ROC and the area under ROC were determined for each single predictor. The measure of the increasing risk of each single predictor was determined with one fuzzy set of data with an output range from 0 to 1. The fuzzy weighted method multiplied each individual risk of each predictor with the predictor's area under ROC. The final measure of the risk of each patient was determined as the sum of partial fuzzified weighted risks of individual predictors. These new individual predictors were also evaluated by ROC and the area under ROC. For each predictor (measured predictors and a new fuzzified-weighted-summed predictor) critical values, sensitivity, specificity, and positive predictive values were calculated. Our new fuzzified-weighted-summed predictor favourably affected the predictive power of non-invasive risk predictors in individuals. This approach can be applied in similar decision processes (Krontoradova et al., 2008).

## 5. Low baroreflex sensitivity due to factors associated with hypertension

### 5.1 Low BRS and the increased stiffness of the carotid wall

The association between BRS and intima-media thickness (IMT) in the carotid bulb, a region with high baroreceptor density, was shown as a marker of subclinical atherosclerosis and essential hypertension (Gianaros et al., 2002; Honzikova et al., 2006a; Labrova et al., 2005; Zanchetti et al. 1998). Carotid IMT also correlated with age in people who were not hypertensives (Labrova et al., 2005). Besides intimal thickening due to the atherosclerotic process, smooth muscle hypertrophy and/or hyperplasia may develop due to a pressure overload in hypertensive patients. Thus, remodelling of the carotid wall linked to high blood pressure and an increased stiffness of the carotid sinus leads to lower distensibility of the baroreceptor carotid region during blood pressure increase. BRS is also inversely associated with the relative wall thickness and the left ventricular mass index, and is significantly impaired in hypertensive patients with concentric left ventricular remodelling (Milan et al., 2007). All these findings suggest that BRS is a target in arterial hypertension.

As mentioned above, we determined baroreflex sensitivity in hypertensive patients not only by the BRS index, but also using the BRSf index. Hypertensive patients had thicker IMT and lower both indices of baroreflex sensitivity, BRS and BRSf, than healthy controls (Labrova et al., 2005). The positive correlation between age and IMT, the negative correlation between age and BRS and BRSf, and the positive correlation between IMT and BMI in healthy subjects were in agreement with the hypothesis that the age-dependent decrease of baroreflex sensitivity corresponded to the age-related structural changes of the carotid wall. A different situation appeared in hypertensive patients. We did not see any additive thickening of their IMT or any decrease of BRS with age, but BRSf decreased significantly with age. IMT in hypertensive patients was not additively influenced by age or BMI. This means that the additive influence of age on baroreflex sensitivity in hypertensive patients could be detected by the BRSf index only. Using two indices of baroreflex sensitivity, BRS and BRSf, we were able to show that baroreflex sensitivity in hypertensives is lower not only due to thickening of the carotid wall, but also due to ageing (Labrova et al., 2005; Honzikova et al., 2006).

The examination of the BRSf index implies the question whether low BRS in hypertensive patients is only a secondary effect of the mechanisms described above or whether an individually inborn low BRS could participate in the development of hypertension.

### 5.2 Obesity, sympathetic activation and hypertension

The relationship between obesity and a higher risk of high blood pressure was established for both adults and children in dozens of studies, (e.g. Krontoradova et al., 2008; Lurbe et al., 1998; Rahmouni et al., 2005). The Framingham study brought evidence of the prevalence of hypertension in obese individuals, which was twice that of individuals of normal weight, across all ages in men and women (Hubert et al., 1983). It was also reported in several studies that weight loss in hypertensive subjects lowered blood pressure (Gordon et al., 1997; Kriketos et al., 2001; Neter et al., 2003), though the results of some studies showed that blood pressure decrease related to weight loss could be only transient (Laaksonen et al., 2003). Also, white coat hypertension is more frequent in individuals with overweight (Helvaci et al., 2007; Honzikova et al., 2006).

Nowadays, the prevalence of obesity increases not only in adults, but also in adolescents. It is hypothesized that it could be linked with increased prevalence of hypertension in adolescents and young adults. The data on the epidemics of obesity are alarming. Data from 45 pairs of surveys from 11 countries were analysed in studies by Lobstein & Jackson-Leach (2006). Annual increases in the prevalence of overweight (including obesity) rose from typically below 0.5 percentage points in the 1980s to over 1.0 percentage points in the late 1990s. The variations across countries may relate to changes and differences in the key environmental factors (Wang et al., 2002).

More mechanisms leading to blood pressure increase in obese subjects have been described. Many studies have documented that sympathetic activation takes part in linking obesity to hypertension. Particularly, intra-abdominal obesity is a major risk factor for cardiovascular morbidity and mortality. It seems that leptin plays a key role. Leptin is a hormone secreted by adipocytes and its blood concentration is proportional to the fat mass content. It acts in the hypothalamus and, besides controlling the body weight by a suppression of food intake and stimulating the metabolic rate, it also increases sympathetic nervous activity. Hypertension in obesity is explained by a selective leptin resistance to the appetite reducing activity, but by preservation of the sympathetic activation and the sympathetic action on the kidney. Thus, chronic hyperleptinemia in obesity produces hypertension. Sympathetic activation is linked with an activation of the renin-angiotensin system (RAS) in obesity. Adipocyte-derived angiotensinogen can act locally to effect adipocyte growth and differentiation, and thus it can partially attribute to the increased fat mass (Rahmouni et al., 2005). It can be also secreted into the blood stream (Rahmouni et al., 2005). Rahmouni et al. (2004) found in mice with obesity induced by high-fat diet greater angiotensinogen gene expression in the intra-abdominal fat but not in other fat depots or non-adipose tissue. As regards visceral obesity and hypertension, high circulating levels of free fatty acids in obese subjects are involved in sympathetic activation. They are released into the portal vein from lipolysis in visceral fat depots, and this could explain the association between visceral obesity and sympathetic activation (Rahmouni et al., 2005).

The elevated circulating leptin is associated with impaired baroreflex function. BRS is reduced in obese children (Lazarova et al., 2009). Leptin receptors are present on vagal afferent fibres and neurons within the solitary tract nucleus, providing an anatomic distribution consistent with baroreflex modulation. It was shown in experiments in rats that leptin microinjection at sites within the solitary tract nucleus impairs the baroreflex sensitivity for bradycardia induced by increases in arterial pressure (Arnold et al., 2009).

In addition to the effects on homeostasis of body weight and sympathetic activity, leptin has a broad range of effects in different tissues. The effect on glucose homeostasis supports the development of type II diabetes mellitus, and this is an additive mechanism related to blood pressure elevation and BRS decrease.

Endothelial dysfunction such as decreased nitric oxide (NO) responsiveness is also a common abnormality in obesity. Damage to the endothelium leads to structural changes of the vessel wall such as thickening of the intima-media of the vessel wall (Rahmouni et al., 2005). Usually, this mechanism is accepted as a principal one in a decreased BRS because of a low compliance of the arterial wall where baroreceptors are present. However, it is necessary to take into account the effect of NO activity involved in low frequency variability in circulation.

There are data showing that NO is involved in the control of blood pressure variability (BPV) via release of NO by endothelial cells (Just et al., 1994; Nafz et al., 1997). The greatest difference in BPV was reported in a frequency range of 0.1 to 0.5 Hz in dogs and 0.2 to 0.6 in rats, i.e. a frequency range in which the sympathetic nervous system is most effective. NO buffers blood pressure fluctuations by opposing the sympathetic nervous activity (Stauss et al., 2000). Moreover, Hogan et al. (1999) demonstrated nitric oxide as a possible factor which causes a significant reduction in the diastolic and systolic blood pressure low-frequency power by infusion of the NO donor sodium nitroprusside in humans. In this experiment, the hypotensive action of sodium nitroprusside was prevented by phenylephrine, but a reduction in the BP low-frequency power persisted. This corresponds to the fact that in carriers of less frequent alleles enhanced BPV was observed at a frequency of 0.1 Hz, which is the frequency of sympathetic activity in humans (Jira et al., 2011).

Many genetically hypothetic mechanisms could be involved in the pathophysiology of the individual disposition for an increase of blood pressure in dependence on obesity. However, they seldom show a linkage between obesity and variability in circulation in a frequency range of 0.1 Hz or baroreflex sensitivity.

Fatso/fat mass and obesity associated gene (FTO gene) was established as contributing to obesity. It is expressed in the hypothalamus and influences energy metabolism. Since hypothalamus is also involved in blood pressure regulation, the relationship of polymorphism of the FTO gene to blood pressure control was studied (Pausova et al., 2009). It was found in this study, carried out nearly in 500 adolescents, that individuals with the FTO-risk genotype, compared with those who lacked it, demonstrated greater adiposity, including the amount of intra-abdominal fat, higher systolic blood pressure, and a higher sympathetic modulation of the vasomotor tone evaluated as a variability of diastolic blood pressure in a frequency range of 0.1 Hz by spectral analysis. It was hypothesized that sex differences and inter-individual differences in linking intra-abdominal obesity to hypertension could be explained by mechanisms of action of androgens. Voluminous intra-abdominal fat, higher blood pressure, and a prominent sympathetic modulation of the vasomotor tone (evaluated as a variability of diastolic blood pressure in a frequency range of 0.1 Hz by spectral analysis) were found in boys aged 12 to 18 years, who had a low CAG-repeat number in the androgen-receptor gene in comparison with those with a high CAG-repeat number. No such differences were seen among girls. This study documented not only that this gene represents a genetic risk factor for linkage between intra-abdominal obesity and hypertension, but also that sympathoactivation may be an underlying link between these states (Pausova et al., 2010).

## 6. Low BRS as a factor causing blood pressure elevation in adolescents

### 6.1 Prevalence of hypertension and white coat hypertension in children and adolescents

The concept of white coat hypertension is used in situations when blood pressure measured at a causal office examination is elevated, but is within the physiological range during its repeated measurement or a 24-hour blood-pressure measurement. Some authors believe that white coat hypertension does not require pharmacological therapy (Cavallini et al., 1995), but an increased risk of cardiovascular diseases was reported in other studies (Gustavsen et al., 2003; Lande et al., 2008).

Prevalence of white coat hypertension is relatively high in different countries in both adults and children. Prevalence of white coat hypertension was higher in obese children, but differences as to age or sex were insignificant (Stabouli et al., 2005). Dozens of studies have brought similar results. Elevation of blood pressure mainly concerns its systolic value. The difference measured in diastolic blood pressure could be conditioned by the technical difficulty of its measurement, especially in small children (Hornsby et al., 1991). Nowadays, ambulatory blood pressure measurement is a standard for the diagnostics of white coat hypertension.

### 6.2 Primary low baroreflex sensitivity as an additive factor of blood pressure elevation in children and adolescents

Recently, several studies have shown that an increase in the body mass index (BMI) correlates significantly with the elevation of blood pressure and a decrease of BRS.

Differences in the BMI, BRS/BRSf indices, mean IBI, and systolic blood pressure variability were compared in healthy controls, adolescents with white coat hypertension, and hypertensive adolescents (Honzikova et al., 2006b). The stepwise blood pressure elevation in these groups was associated with a stepwise increase of BMI and a stepwise decrease of both indices of baroreflex sensitivity, BRS and BRSf; the mean IBI was unchanged. Systolic blood pressure variability was increased in hypertonic adolescents only.

Such a finding may correspond with the idea that subclinical atherosclerosis and a remodelling of the vascular wall may develop very early, though the finding of a similarly lower BRS in children, adolescents and young adults with white coat hypertension suggests a contradicting interpretation. This group of young subjects with white coat hypertension has a physiological blood pressure over 24 hours and there is no reason for remodelling the vascular wall. Nevertheless, they have lower BRS than healthy controls and BRSf as well. These results suggest the only interpretation, namely that low BRS precedes blood pressure elevation (Honzikova et al., 2009).

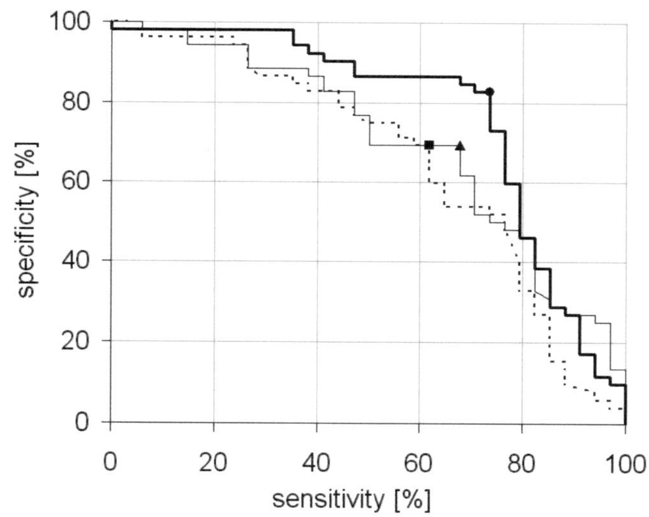


Fig. 3. Receiver operating curves of baroreflex sensitivity (BRS, thin line), body mass index (BMI, dashed line), and a combination of both factors (full line). Optimal critical values determined as values at which the maximum achievable combination of sensitivity and specificity was reached: 7.08 ms/mmHg for BRS (triangle), 22.20 kg/m$^2$ for BMI (square), and 0.439 normalized units for a combination of BMI and BRS (point). Reproduced with permission of Physiological Research.

Direct evidence that low baroreflex sensitivity is a partially independent risk factor for the development of essential hypertension was provided by Krontoradova et al. (2008). In this study hypertonic subjects had a significantly lower BRS and a significantly higher BMI (the BRSf index was not evaluated with respect to the same mean IBI in controls and hypertonics). On the other hand, no correlation was found between BMI and BRS either in the group of hypertonics or in controls. The predicting power of BMI, BRS, and a combination of both factors determined by logistic regression analysis for hypertension was evaluated by sensitivity and specificity. The optimal critical values were determined by the receiver operating curves (ROC), i.e. a plot of sensitivity versus specificity for moving critical values in steps. Also, the area under the ROC curve was calculated. The approach described in part 4.2 of this Chapter was applied for the evaluation of association of decreased BRS and increased BMI with a risk of hypertension. The sensitivity, specificity and area under ROC were increased for a combination of both factors, BRS and BMI, in predicting hypertension (see Fig. 3).

This means that low BRS may serve as an independent risk factor for the development of essential hypertension. What mechanism of blood pressure elevation due to individually low BRS could be taken into consideration? Stressing situations increase the sympathetic nervous activity as well as blood pressure. Blood pressure elevation is partially blunted by the heart rate baroreflex response. This suppression of blood pressure increase is insufficient in children with low BRS; therefore, white coat hypertension occurs and frequent vasoconstrictive reactions could lead to the development of essential hypertension after a longer time.

## 7. Conclusion

Baroreflex sensitivity is, to a certain extent, an individually characteristic index. It fluctuates spontaneously even at rest and therefore, regardless of how it is further processed mathematically, a particular value measured represents an approximate estimate of its size. On the other hand, low values of baroreflex sensitivity are highly repeatable in some individuals, and it is just the low BRS values that pose a risk for the development of hypertension and its complications. Bearing in mind the fact that essential hypertension is a disease of higher age, the majority of studies done in previous years were naturally focused on baroreflex sensitivity in older population. The increased arterial stiffness, increased IMT, and sympathetic activation in obesity represent indubitable factors which lead to hypertension and, consequently, result in a decrease of BRS. The hypothesis ensuing from these studies, which states that the drop in baroreflex sensitivity accompanies the development of hypertension as a secondary manifestation of the disease, is proved by these studies. Low baroreflex sensitivity is then a risk factor in further complications of the disease, particularly after myocardial infarction. Also, the pathophysiological mechanism of protection of the myocardium from ischemia through high baroreflex sensitivity is obvious. Quick prolongation of IBI following a sudden blood pressure elevation decreases cardiac workload.

On the other hand, measurements of BRS in children and adolescents and the first genetic studies on the inborn conditionality of BRS have provided enough evidence that some individuals possess congenitally low baroreflex sensitivity. This condition does not mean any risk for a healthy organism. Without a targeted study, we cannot even speculate on how this assumption will manifest itself in advanced age in terms of increased risk of sudden cardiac death, since in the meantime the long-term pathological influence of other mechanisms lowering baroreflex sensitivity will have presented itself in the other risky patients.

However, low baroreflex sensitivity apparently represents a risk. It is probably a further factor which disposes an individual towards blood pressure elevation. Low baroreflex sensitivity will manifest itself as blood pressure hyperreactivity. It may lead to white coat hypertension in adolescents as a step in the development of essential hypertension. Therefore, congenitally low baroreflex sensitivity may be considered as another risk factor for the development of essential hypertension. This is the reason why in the young population, including children and adolescents with low baroreflex sensitivity, increased emphasis should be put on the prevention of obesity and sufficient physical activity as on easily influenceable stimuli which additively increase blood pressure.

Measuring baroreflex sensitivity is a simple, in no way stressful, non-invasive method. It requires just a couple of minutes taking non-invasive record of blood pressure by means of a pressure cuff applied on a finger and subsequent mathematical processing. However, if a BRS determination is to provide the presumed relevant clinical information, it is not that easy. BRS evaluation in the young may only be carried out on the basis of repeated measurements. In child age and adolescence, it is appropriate to take into account the average heart rate when quantifying BRS. One of the possibilities is the BRSf index or some other adequate method. This area of research is therefore substantial from the point of view of the study of baroreflex sensitivity, prevention of hypertension and its severe complications, and may be of significance for preventative medicine.

## 8. Acknowledgement

This study was supported by grant MSM 0021622402 from the Ministry of Education, Youth and Sports of the Czech Republic. We gratefully acknowledge A. Krticka for help with the methodology part.

## 9. References

Abrahamsson, C., Ahlund, C., Nordlander, M. & Lind, L. (2003). A method for heart rate-corrected estimation of baroreflex sensitivity. *Journal of Hypertension,* Vol. 21, No. 11, (November 2003), pp. 2133-2140, ISSN 02636352

Ackermann, U., Irizawa, T.G. & Barber. B. (1989). Angiotensin restores atrial natriuretic factor-induced decrease of baroreceptor sensitivity in normotensive rats, but not in spontaneously hypertensive rats. *Canadian Journal of Physiology and Pharmacology,* Vol. 67, No. 6, (June 1989), pp. 675-81, ISSN 00084212

Al-Kubati, M.A.A., Fiser, B. & Siegelova, J. (1997). Baroreflex sensitivity during psychological stress. *Physiological Research,* Vol. 46, No. 1, (February 1997), pp. 27-33, ISSN 08628408

Allen, M.T., Matthews, K.A. & Kenyon, K.L. (2000). The relationships of resting baroreflex sensitivity, heart rate variability and measures of impulse control in children and adolescents. *International Journal of Psychophysiology,* Vol. 37, No. 2, (August 2000), pp. 185-194, ISSN 01678760

Arnold, A.C., Shaltout, H.A., Gallagher, P.E. & Diz, D.I. (2009). Leptin impairs cardiovagal baroreflex function at the level of the solitary tract nucleus. *Hypertension,* Vol. 54, No. 5, (November 2009), pp. 1001-1008, ISSN 0194911X

Bailey, J.J., Hodges, M. & Church, T.R. (2007). Decision to implant a cardioverter defibrillator after myocardial infarction: The role of ejection fraction v. other risk factor markers. *Medical Decision Making,* Vol. 27, No. 2, (March 2007), pp. 151-160, ISSN 0272989X

Bothova, P., Honzikova, N., Fiser, B., Zavodna, E., Novakova, Z., Kalina, D., Honzikova, K. & Labrova, R. (2010). Comparison of baroreflex sensitivity determined by cross-spectral analysis at respiratory and 0.1 Hz frequencies in man. *Physiological Research,* Vol. 59, Suppl. 1, (May 2010), pp. S103-111, ISSN 08628408

Brooks, V.L. & Sved, A.F. (2005). Pressure to change? Re-evaluating the role of baroreceptors in the long-term control of arterial pressure. *American Journal of Physiology - Regulatory Integrative and Comparative Physiology,* Vol. 288, No. 4 57-4, (April 2005), pp. R815-R818, ISSN 03636119

Cavallini, M.C., Roman, M.J., Pickering, T.G., Schwartz, J.E., Pini, R. & Devereux, R.B. (1995). Is white coat hypertension associated with arterial disease or left ventricular hypertrophy? *Hypertension,* Vol. 26, No. 3, (September 1995), pp. 413-419, ISSN 0194911X

Cowley Jr., A.W. (1992). Long-term control of arterial blood pressure. *Physiological Reviews,* Vol. 72, No. 1, (January 1992), pp. 231-280, ISSN 00319333

Cowley Jr., A.W., Liard, J.F. & Guyton, A.C. (1973). Role of baroreceptor reflex in daily control of arterial blood pressure and other variables in dogs. *Circulation Research,* Vol. 32, No. 5, (May 1973), pp. 564-576, ISSN 00097330

Davies, E., Holloway, C.D., Ingram, M.C., Inglis, G.C., Friel, E.C., Morrison, C., Anderson, N.H., Fraser, R. & Connell, J.M.C. (1999). Aldosterone excretion rate and blood pressure in essential hypertension are related to polymorphic differences in the aldosterone synthase gene CYP11B2. *Hypertension,* Vol. 33, No. 2, (February 1999), pp. 703-707, ISSN 0194911X

Dietrich, A., Riese, H., Van Roon, A.M., Van Engelen, K., Ormel, J., Neeleman, J. & Rosmalen, J.G.M. (2006). Spontaneous baroreflex sensitivity in (pre)adolescents. *Journal of Hypertension,* Vol. 24, No. 2, (February 2006), pp. 345-352, ISSN 02636352

Dietrich, A., Rosmalen, J.G.M., Althaus, M., van Roon, A.M., Mulder, L.J.M., Minderaa, R.B., Oldehinkel, A.J. & Riese, H. (2010). Reproducibility of heart rate variability and baroreflex sensitivity measurements in children. *Biological Psychology,* Vol. 85, No. 1, (September 2010), pp. 71-78, ISSN 03010511

Drummond, H.A., Price, M.P., Welsh, M.J. & Abboud, F.M. (1998). A molecular component of the arterial baroreceptor mechanotransducer. *Neuron,* Vol. 21, No. 6, (December 1998), pp. 1435-1441, ISSN 08966273

Eckberg, D.L. (2003). The human respiratory gate. *Journal of Physiology,* Vol. 548, No. 2, (April 2003), pp. 339-352, ISSN 00223751

Eckberg, D.L. & Karemaker, J.M. (2009). Point:Counterpoint: Respiratory sinus arrhythmia is due to a central mechanism vs. respiratory sinus arrhythmia is due to the baroreflex mechanism. *Journal of Applied Physiology,* Vol. 106, No. 5, (May 2009), pp. 1740-1744, ISSN 87507587

Filippone, J.D. & Bisognano, J.D. (2007). Baroreflex stimulation in the treatment of hypertension. *Current Opinion in Nephrology and Hypertension,* Vol. 16, No. 5, (September 2007), pp. 403-408, ISSN 10624821

Frederiks, J., Swenne, C.A., TenVoorde, B.J., Honzikova, N., Levert, J.V., Maan, A.C., Schalij, M.J. & Bruschke, A.V.G. (2000). The importance of high-frequency paced breathing in spectral baroreflex sensitivity assessment. *Journal of Hypertension,* Vol. 18, No. 11, (November 2000), pp. 1635-1644, ISSN 02636352

Gaudet, E., Godwin, S.J. & Head, G.A. (2000). Effects of central infusion of ANG II and losartan on the cardiac baroreflex in rabbits. *American Journal of Physiology - Heart and Circulatory Physiology*, Vol. 278, No. 2 47-2, (February 2000), pp. H558-H566, ISSN 03636135

Gianaros, P.J., Jennings, J.R., Olafsson, G.B., Steptoe, A., Sutton-Tyrrell, K., Muldoon, M.F. & Manuck, S.B. (2002). Greater intima-media thickness in the carotid bulb is associated with reduced baroreflex sensitivity. *American Journal of Hypertension*, Vol. 15, No. 6, (June 2002), pp. 486-491, ISSN 08957061

Gilad, O., Swenne, C.A., Davrath, L.R. & Akselrod, S. (2005). Phase-averaged characterization of respiratory sinus arrhythmia pattern. *American Journal of Physiology - Heart and Circulatory Physiology*, Vol. 288, No. 2 57-2, (February 2005), pp. H504-H510, ISSN 03636135

Goldberger, J.J., Cain, M.E., Hohnloser, S.H., Kadish, A.H., Knight, B.P., Lauer, M.S., Maron, B.J., Page, R.L., Passman, R.S., Siscovick, D., Stevenson, W.G. & Zipes, D.P. (2008). American Heart Association/American College of Cardiology Foundation/Heart rhythm society scientific statement on noninvasive risk stratification techniques for identifying patients at risk for sudden cardiac death: A scientific statement from the American heart association council on clinical cardiology committee on electrocardiography and arrhythmias and council on epidemiology and prevention. *Circulation*, Vol. 118, No. 14, (September 2008), pp. 1497-1518, ISSN 00097322

Gollasch, M., Tank, J., Luft, F.C., Jordan, J., Maass, P., Krasko, C., Sharma, A.M., Busjahn, A. & Bahring, S. (2002). The BK channel β1 subunit gene is associated with human baroreflex and blood pressure regulation. *Journal of Hypertension*, Vol. 20, No. 5, (May 2002), pp. 927-933, ISSN 02636352

Gordon, N.F., Scott, C.B. & Levine, B.D. (1997). Comparison of single versus multiple lifestyle interventions: Are the antihypertensive effects of exercise training and diet-induced weight loss additive? *American Journal of Cardiology*, Vol. 79, No. 6, (March 1997), pp. 763-767, ISSN 00029149

Gribbin, B., Pickering, T.G., Sleight, P. & Peto, R. (1971). Effect of age and high blood pressure on baroreflex sensitivity in man. *Circulation Research*, Vol. 29, No. 4, (October 1971), pp. 424-431, ISSN 00097330

Gustavsen, P.H., Hoegholm, A., Bang, L.E. & Kristensen, K.S. (2003). White coat hypertension is a cardiovascular risk factor: A 10-year follow-up study. *Journal of Human Hypertension*, Vol. 17, No. 12, (December 2003), pp. 811-817, ISSN 09509240

Helvaci, M.R., Kaya, H., Yalcin, A. & Kuvandik, G. (2007). Prevalence of white coat hypertension in underweight and overweight subjects. *International Heart Journal*, Vol. 48, No. 5, (November 2007), pp. 605-613, ISSN 13492365

Hogan, N., Kardos, A., Paterson, D.J. & Casadei, B. (1999). Effect of exogenous nitric oxide on baroreflex function in humans. *American Journal of Physiology - Heart and Circulatory Physiology*, Vol. 277, No. 1 46-1, (July 1999), pp. H221-H227, ISSN 03636135

Honzik, P., Hrabec, J., Labrova, R., Semrad, B. & Honzikova, N. (2003). Fuzzification, weight and summation of risk factors in a patient improve the prediction of risk for cardiac death. *Scripta Medica*, Vol. 76, No. 3, (June 2003), pp. 141-148, ISSN 12113395

Honzik, P., Krivan, L., Lokaj, P., Labrova, R., Novakova, Z., Fiser, B. & Honzikova, N. (2010). Logit and fuzzy models in data analysis: Estimation of risk in cardiac patients. *Physiological Research*, Vol. 59, Suppl. 1, (May 2010), pp. S89-96, ISSN 08628408

Honzikova, N., Penaz, J. & Fiser, B. (1990). Individual features of circulatory power spectra in man. *European Journal of Applied Physiology,* Vol. 59, No. 6, pp. 430-434, ISSN 03015548

Honzikova, N., Fiser, B. & Honzik, J. (1992). Noninvasive determination of baroreflex sensitivity in man by means of spectral analysis. *Physiological Research,* Vol. 41, No. 1, (February 1992), pp. 31-37, ISSN 08628408

Honzikova, N., Rybkova, I. & Honzik, J. (1996). Baroreflex sensitivity, heart rate and blood pressure during mental load and emotional activation. *Homeostasis in Health and Disease,* Vol. 37, No. 1-2, (April 1996), pp. 72-76, ISSN 09607560

Honzikova, N., Semrad, B., Fiser, B. & Labrova, R. (2000). Baroreflex sensitivity determined by spectral method and heart rate variability, and two-years mortality in patients after myocardial infarction. *Physiological Research,* Vol. 49, No. 6, (November 2000), pp. 643-650, ISSN 08628408

Honzikova, N., Krticka, A., Novakova, Z. & Zavodna, E. (2003). A dampening effect of pulse interval variability on blood pressure variations with respect to primary variability in blood pressure during exercise. *Physiological Research,* Vol. 52, No. 3, (June 2003), pp. 299-309, ISSN 08628408

Honzikova, N., Labrova, R., Fiser, B., Maderova, E., Novakova, Z., Zavodna, E. & Semrad, B. (2006a). Influence of age, body mass index, and blood pressure on the carotid intima-media thickness in normotensive and hypertensive patients. *Biomedizinische Technik,* Vol. 51, No. 4, (October 2006), pp. 159-162, ISSN 00135585

Honzikova, N., Novakova, Z., Zavodna, E., Paderova, J., Lokaj, P., Fiser, B., Balcarkova, P. & Hrstkova, H. (2006b). Baroreflex sensitivity in children, adolescents, and young adults with essential and white-coat hypertension. *Klinische Padiatrie,* Vol. 218, No. 4, (July-August 2006), pp. 237-242, ISSN 03008630

Honzikova, N., Fiser, B., Zavodna, E., Novakova, Z. & Krticka, A. (2007). Effectiveness of suppression of systolic blood pressure variability by baroreflex. *Clinical Autonomic Research,* Vol. 17, No. 5, (October 2007), pp. 281, ISSN 0959-9851

Honzikova, N. & Fiser, B. (2009). Baroreflex sensitivity and essential hypertension in adolescents. *Physiological Research,* Vol. 58, No. 5, (October 2009), pp. 605-612, ISSN 08628408

Hornsby, J.L., Mongan, P.F., Taylor, A.T. & Treiber, F.A. (1991). 'White coat' hypertension in children. *Journal of Family Practice,* Vol. 33, No. 6, (June 1991), pp. 617-623, ISSN 00943509

Hubert, H.B., Feinleib, M., McNamara, P.M. & Castelli, W.P. (1983). Obesity as an independent risk factor for cardiovascular disease: A 26-year follow-up of participants in the Framingham heart study. *Circulation,* Vol. 67, No. 5, (May 1983), pp. 968-977, ISSN 00097322

Jackson-Leach, R. & Lobstein, T. (2006). Estimated burden of paediatric obesity and co-morbidities in Europe. Part 1. The increase in the prevalence of child obesity in Europe is itself increasing. *International Journal of Pediatric Obesity, Vol.* 1, No. 1, (January 2006), pp. 26-32, ISSN 17477166

Jira, M., Zavodna, E., Honzikova, N., Novakova, Z. & Fiser, B. (2006). Baroreflex sensitivity as an individual characteristic feature. *Physiological Research,* Vol. 55, No. 3, (June 2006), pp. 349-351, ISSN 08628408

Jira, M., Zavodna, E., Novakova, Z., Fiser, B. & Honzikova, N. (2010a). Reproducibility of blood pressure and inter-beat interval variability in man. *Physiological Research,* Vol. 59, Suppl. 1, (May 2010), pp. S113-121, ISSN 08628408

Jira, M., Zavodna, E., Honzikova, N., Novakova, Z., Vasku, A., Izakovicova Holla, L. & Fiser, B. (2010b). Association of A1166C polymorphism in AT1 receptor gene with baroreflex sensitivity. *Physiological Research,* Vol. 59, No. 4, (August 2010), pp. 517-528, ISSN 08628408

Jira, M., Zavodna, E., Honzikova, N., Novakova, Z., Vasku, A., Holla, L.I. & Fiser, B. (2011). Association of eNOS gene polymorphisms T-786C and G894T with blood pressure variability in man. *Physiological Research,* Vol. 60, No. 1, (February 2011), pp. 193-197, ISSN 08628408

Just, A., Wittmann, U., Nafz, B., Wagner, C.D., Ehmke, H., Kirchheim, H.R. & Persson, P.B. (1994). The blood pressure buffering capacity of nitric oxide by comparison to the baroreceptor reflex. *American Journal of Physiology - Heart and Circulatory Physiology,* Vol. 267, No. 2 36-2, (August 1994), pp. H521-H527, ISSN 03636135

Kardos, A., Rudas, L., Gingl, Z., Szabados, S. & Simon, J. (1995). The mechanism of blood pressure variability. Study in patients with fixed ventricular pacemaker rhythm. *European Heart Journal,* Vol. 16, No. 4, (April 1995), pp. 545-552, ISSN 0195668X

Kardos, A., Watterich, G., De Menezes, R., Csanady, M., Casadei, B. & Rudas, L. (2001). Determinants of spontaneous baroreflex sensitivity in a healthy working population. *Hypertension,* Vol. 37, No. 3, (March 2001), pp. 911-916, ISSN 0194911X

Kriketos, A.D., Robertson, R.M., Sharp, T.A., Drougas, H., Reed, G.W., Storlien, L.H. & Hill, J.O. (2001). Role of weight loss and polyunsaturated fatty acids in improving metabolic fitness in moderately obese, moderately hypertensive subjects. *Journal of Hypertension,* Vol. 19, No. 10, (October 2001), pp. 1745-1754, ISSN 02636352

Krontoradova, K., Honzikova, N., Fiser, B., Novakova, Z., Zavodna, E., Hrstkova, H. & Honzik, P. (2008). Overweight and decreased baroreflex sensitivity as independent risk factors for hypertension in children, adolescents, and young adults. *Physiological Research,* Vol. 57, No. 3, (June 2008), pp. 385-391, ISSN 08628408

La Rovere, M.T., Bigger Jr., J.T., Marcus, F.I., Mortara, A. & Schwartz, P.J. (1998). Baroreflex sensitivity and heart-rate variability in prediction of total cardiac mortality after myocardial infarction. *Lancet,* Vol. 351, No. 9101, (February 1998), pp. 478-484, ISSN 01406736

Laaksonen, D.E., Laitinen, T., Schönberg, J., Rissanen, A. & Niskanen, L.K. (2003). Weight loss and weight maintenance, ambulatory blood pressure and cardiac autonomic tone in obese persons with the metabolic syndrome. *Journal of Hypertension,* Vol. 21, No. 2, (February 2003), pp. 371-378, ISSN 02636352

Labrova, R., Honzikova, N., Maderova, E., Vysocanova, P., Novakova, Z., Zavodna, E., Fiser, B. & Semrad, B. (2005). Age-dependent relationship between the carotid intima-media thickness, baroreflex sensitivity, and the inter-beat interval in normotensive and hypertensive subjects. *Physiological Research,* Vol. 54, No. 6, (December 2005), pp. 593-600, ISSN 08628408

Lande, M.B., Meagher, C.C., Fisher, S.G., Belani, P., Wang, H. & Rashid, M. (2008). Left ventricular mass index in children with white coat hypertension. *Journal of Pediatrics,* Vol. 153, No. 1, (July 2008), pp. 50-54, ISSN 00223476

Laude, D., Elghozi, J.-L., Girard,A., Bellard, E., Bouhaddi, M., Castiglioni, P., Cerutti, C., Cividjian, A., Di Rienzo, M., Fortrat, J.O., Janssen, B., Karemaker, J.M., Leftheriotis,

G., Parati, G., Persson, P.B., Porta, A., Quintin, L., Regnard, J., Rudiger, H., Stauss, H.M. (2004). Comparison of various techniques used to estimate spontaneous baroreflex sensitivity (the EUROBAVAR study). *American Journal of Physiology. Regulatory, Integrative and Comparative Physiology,* Vol. 286, No. 1, (January 2004), pp. R226–R231, ISSN 0363-6119

Lazarova, Z., Tonhajzerova, I., Trunkvalterova, Z., Brozmanova, A., Honzikova, N., Javorka, K., Baumert, M. & Javorka, M. (2009). Baroreflex sensitivity is reduced in obese normotensive children and adolescents. *Canadian Journal of Physiology and Pharmacology,* Vol. 87, No. 7, (July 2009), pp. 565-571, ISSN 00084212

Lenard, Z., Studinger, P., Mersich, B., Kocsis, L. & Kollai, M. (2004). Maturation of cardiovagal autonomic function from childhood to young adult age. *Circulation,* Vol. 110, No. 16, (October 2004), pp. 2307-2312, ISSN 00097322

Lim, P.O., Macdonald, T.M., Holloway, C., Friel, E., Anderson, N.H., Dow, E., Jung, R.T., Davies, E., Fraser, R. & Connell, J.M.C. (2002). Variation at the aldosterone synthase (CYP11B2) locus contributes to hypertension in subjects with a raised aldosterone-to-renin ratio. *Journal of Clinical Endocrinology and Metabolism,* Vol. 87, No. 9, (September 2002), pp. 4398-4402, ISSN 0021972X

Lobstein, T. & Jackson-Leach, R. (2006). Estimated burden of paediatric obesity and co-morbidities in Europe. Part 2. Numbers of children with indicators of obesity-related disease. *International Journal of Pediatric Obesity,* Vol. 1, No. 1, (January 2006), pp. 33-41, ISSN 17477166

Lohmeier, T.E., Hildebrandt, D.A., Warren, S., May, P.J. & Cunningham, J.T. (2005). Recent insights into the interactions between the baroreflex and the kidneys in hypertension. *American Journal of Physiology - Regulatory Integrative and Comparative Physiology,* Vol. 288, No. 4, (April 2005), pp. R828-R836, ISSN 03636119

Lu, Y., Ma, X., Sabharwal, R., Snitsarev, V., Morgan, D., Rahmouni, K., Drummond, H.A., Whiteis, C.A., Costa, V., Price, M., Benson, C., Welsh, M.J., Chapleau, M.W. & Abboud, F.M. (2009). The ion channel ASIC2 is required for baroreceptor and autonomic control of the circulation. *Neuron,* Vol. 64, No. 6, (December 2009), pp. 885-897, ISSN 08966273

Lurbe, E., Alvarez, V., Liao, Y., Tacons, J., Cooper, R., Cremades, B., Torro, I. & Redon, J. (1998). The impact of obesity and body fat distribution on ambulatory blood pressure in children and adolescents. *American Journal of Hypertension,* Vol. 11, No. 4 I, (April 1998), pp. 418-424, ISSN 08957061

Milan, A., Caserta, M.A., Del Colle, S., Dematteis, A., Morello, F., Rabbia, F., Mulatero, P., Pandian, N.G. & Veglio, F. (2007). Baroreflex sensitivity correlates with left ventricular morphology and diastolic function in essential hypertension. *Journal of Hypertension,* Vol. 25, No. 8, (August 2007), pp. 1655-1664, ISSN 02636352

Mortara, A., La Rovere, M.T., Pinna, G.D., Prpa, A., Maestri, R., Febo, O., Pozzoli, M., Opasich, C. & Tavazzi, L. (1997). Arterial baroreflex modulation of heart rate in chronic heart failure: clinical and hemodynamic correlates and prognostic implications. *Circulation,* Vol. 96, No. 10, (November 1997), pp. 3450-3458, ISSN 0009-7322

Nafz, B., Wagner, C.D. & Persson, P.B. (1997). Endogenous nitric oxide buffers blood pressure variability between 0.2 and 0.6 hz in the conscious rat. *American Journal of Physiology - Heart and Circulatory Physiology,* (February 1997), pp. H632-H637, ISSN 03636135

Neter, J.E., Stam, B.E., Kok, F.J., Grobbee, D.E. & Geleijnse, J.M. (2003). Influence of weight reduction on blood pressure: A meta-analysis of randomized controlled trials. *Hypertension,* Vol. 42, No. 5, (November 2003), pp. 878-884, ISSN 0194911X

Ormezzano, O., Poirier, O., Mallion, J., Nicaud, V., Amar, J., Chamontin, B., Mounier-Vehier, C., François, P., Cambien, F. & Baguet, J.P. (2005). A polymorphism in the endothelin-A receptor gene is linked to baroreflex sensitivity. *Journal of Hypertension,* Vol. 23, No. 11, (November 2005), pp. 2019-2026, ISSN 02636352

Paillard, F., Chansel, D., Brand, E., Benetos, A., Thomas, F., Czekalski, S., Ardaillou, R. & Soubrier, F. (1999). Genotype-phenotype relationships for the renin-angiotensin-aldosterone system in a normal population. *Hypertension,* Vol. 34, No. 3, (September 1999), pp. 423-429, ISSN 0194911X

Pausova, Z., Syme, C., Abrahamowicz, M., Xiao, Y., Leonard, G.T., Perron, M., Richer, L., Veillette, S., Smith, G.D., Seda, O., Tremblay, J., Hamet, P., Gaudet, D. & Paus, T. (2009). A common variant of the FTO gene is associated with not only increased adiposity but also elevated blood pressure in French Canadians. *Circulation: Cardiovascular Genetics,* Vol. 2, No. 3, (May 2009), pp. 260-269, ISSN 1942325X

Pausova, Z., Abrahamowicz, M., Mahboubi, A., Syme, C., Leonard, G.T., Perron, M., Richer, L., Veillette, S., Gaudet, D. & Paus, T. (2010). Functional variation in the androgen-receptor gene is associated with visceral adiposity and blood pressure in male adolescents. *Hypertension,* Vol. 55, No. 3, (March 2010), pp. 706-714, ISSN 0194911X

Pedarzani, P., Kulik, A., Muller, M., Ballanyi, K. & Stocker, M. (2000). Molecular determinants of Ca2+ -dependent K+ channel function in rat dorsal vagal neurones. *Journal of Physiology,* Vol. 527, No. 2, (September 2000), pp. 283-290, ISSN 00223751

Penaz, J., Honzikova, N. & Fiser, B. (1978). Spectral analysis of resting variability of some circulatory parameters in man. *Physiologia Bohemoslovaca,* Vol. 27, No. 4, (August 1978), pp. 349-357, ISSN 03699463

Persson, P.B., DiRienzo, M., Castiglioni, P., Cerutti, C., Pagani, M., Honzikova, N., Akselrod, S. & Parati, G. (2001). Time versus frequency domain techniques for assessing baroreflex sensitivity. *Journal of Hypertension,* Vol. 19, No. 10, (October 2001), pp. 1699-1705, ISSN 02636352

Rahmouni, K., Correia, M.L.G., Haynes, W.G. & Mark, A.L. (2005). Obesity-associated hypertension: New insights into mechanisms. *Hypertension,* Vol. 45, No. 1, (January 2005), pp. 9-14, ISSN 0194911X

Rahmouni, K., Mark, A.L., Haynes, W.G. & Sigmund, C.D. (2004). Adipose depot-specific modulation of angiotensinogen gene expression in diet-induced obesity. *American Journal of Physiology - Endocrinology and Metabolism,* Vol. 286, No. 6 49-6, (June 2004), pp. E891-E895, ISSN 01931849

Rudiger, H. & Bald, M. (2001). Spontaneous baroreflex sensitivity in children and young adults calculated in the time and frequency domain. *Autonomic Neuroscience: Basic and Clinical,* Vol. 93, No. 1-2, (October 2001), pp. 71-78, ISSN 15660702

Semrad, B., Fiser, B. & Honzikova, N. (1998). Aging and cardiac autonomic status, In: *Clinical guide to cardiac autonomic tests*, Malik, M., (Ed.), pp. (285-300), Kluwer Academic Publishers, ISBN 0-7923-5178-9, The Netherlands.

Stabouli, S., Kotsis, V., Toumanidis, S., Papamichael, C., Constantopoulos, A. & Zakopoulos, N. (2005). White-coat and masked hypertension in children: Association with target-organ damage. *Pediatric Nephrology,* Vol. 20, No. 8, (August 2005), pp. 1151-1155, ISSN 0931041X

Stauss, H.M. & Persson, P.B. (2000). Role of nitric oxide in buffering short-term blood pressure fluctuations. *News in Physiological Sciences,* Vol. 15, No. 5, (October 2000), pp. 229-233, ISSN 08861714

Taha, B.H., Simon, P.M., Dempsey, J.A., Skatrud, J.B. & Iber, C. (1995). Respiratory sinus arrhythmia in humans: An obligatory role for vagal feedback from the lungs. *Journal of Applied Physiology,* Vol. 78, No. 2, (February 1995), pp. 638-645, ISSN 87507587

Thrasher, T.N. (2005). Effects of chronic baroreceptor unloading on blood pressure in the dog. *American Journal of Physiology - Regulatory Integrative and Comparative Physiology,* Vol. 288, No. 4 57-4, (April 2005), pp. R863-R871, ISSN 03636119

Tzeng, Y.C., Sin, P.Y.W., Lucas, S.J.E. & Ainslie, P.N. (2009). Respiratory modulation of cardiovagal baroreflex sensitivity. *Journal of Applied Physiology,* Vol. 107, No. 3, (September 2009), pp. 718-724, ISSN 87507587

Van De Vooren, H., Gademan, M.G.J., Swenne, C.A., TenVoorde, B.J., Schalij, M.J. & Van der Wall, E.E. (2007). Baroreflex sensitivity, blood pressure buffering, and resonance: What are the links? Computer simulation of healthy subjects and heart failure patients. *Journal of Applied Physiology,* Vol. 102, No. 4, (April 2007), pp. 1348-1356, ISSN 87507587

Wang, L., Rao, F., Zhang, K., Mahata, M., Rodriguez-Flores, J.L., Fung, M.M., Waalen, J., Cockburn, M.G., Hamilton, B.A., Mahata, S.K. & O'Connor, D.T. (2009). Neuropeptide Y1 receptor NPY1R discovery of naturally occurring human genetic variants governing gene expression in cells as well as pleiotropic effects on autonomic activity and blood pressure in vivo. *Journal of the American College of Cardiology,* Vol. 54, No. 10, (September 2009), pp. 944-954, ISSN 07351097

Wesseling, K.H. (2003). Should baroreflex sensitivity be corrected for heart rate? *Journal of Hypertension,* Vol. 21, No. 11, (November 2003), pp. 2015-2018, ISSN 02636352

Ylitalo, A., Juhani Airaksinen, K.E., Hautanen, A., Kupari, M., Carson, M., Virolainen, J., Savolainen, M., Kauma, H., Antero Kesaniemi, Y., White, P.C. & Huikuri, H.V. (2000). Baroreflex sensitivity and variants of the renin angiotensin system genes. *Journal of the American College of Cardiology,* Vol. 35, No. 1, (January 2000), pp. 194-200, ISSN 07351097

Zanchetti, A., Bond, M.G., Hennig, M., Neiss, A., Mancia, G., Dal Palu, C., Hansson, L., Magnani, B., Rahn, K., Reid, J., Rodicio, J., Safar, M., Eckes, L. & Ravinetto, R. (1998). Risk factors associated with alterations in carotid intima-media thickness in hypertension: Baseline data from the European lacidipine study on atherosclerosis. *Journal of Hypertension,* Vol. 16, No. 7, (July 1998), pp. 949-961, ISSN 02636352

Zavodna, E., Honzikova, N., Hrstkova, H., Novakova, Z., Moudr, J., Jira, M. & Fiser, B. (2006). Can we detect the development of baroreflex sensitivity in humans between 11 and 20 years of age? *Canadian Journal of Physiology and Pharmacology,* Vol. 84, No. 12, (December 2006), pp. 1275-1283, ISSN 00084212

# 5

# Does Music Therapy Reduce Blood Pressure in Patients with Essential Hypertension in Nigeria?

Michael Ezenwa
*Department of Psychology, Faculty of Social Sciences, Nnamdi Azikiwe University, Awka. Anambra State, Nigeria*

## 1. Introduction

Hypertension is a cardiovascular pathological condition characterized by relatively sustained elevated arterial blood pressure above normal tolerable limit. It refers to the condition wherein arterial blood pressure level is greater than the limit of normal range of 90 millimeter mercury, (Ezenwa, 2009). In fact hypertension occurs when the diastolic blood pressure {*period of relaxation of the heart*} is sustainably greater than 90 millimeter mercury (Mm Hg) and the systolic blood pressure (*period of contraction of the heart*) is greater than 135 mmHg {Guyton & Hall, 2000} However, other experts {Akinkugbe,1997, Boon & Fox,1998, Onwubere,2004} suggest a slightly higher systolic blood pressure of 140 mm Hg and diastolic of 90 mm Hg (140/90 mm Hg) for a diagnosis of the disorder. By blood pressure is meant the force exerted by the blood against the unit area of the vessel wall {Guyton & Hall, 2000} often measured in millimeter mercury {mm Hg}. It is that pressure against which the heart pumps.

The need to maintain acceptable blood pressure level is a basic condition for balance and maintenance of human life. At very high blood pressure, there is the risk of over-loading the heart compounded by possibility of bursting of minute blood vessels that supply the brain cells and other vital organs with possibility of endohemorrhegic complications and death. On the other hand, at low blood pressure level, inadequate supply could short-circuit the activities and life of vital organs including the liver, kidney and brain which will obviously lead to organ-system fatigue, collapse and eventual death. Therefore, just as an electronic device depends on adequate supply of electric current for optimal performance, the human body system requires regulated blood pressure level to maintain its homeostasis. This is assured through combined activities particularly of the heart, the kidney, the brain and the endocrine system.

Unfortunately, due to many systemic, hereditary, metabolic, dietary, environmental and/or Psychological factors that continuously impact on the capacity of these systems to maintain normal blood pressure, they occasionally become overwhelmed leading to development of hypertension.

## 2. Classification of hypertenssion

Hypertension can be classified in different forms depending on what is emphasized at a point in time. It could be categorized in terms of severity into borderline, mild, moderate or severe hypertension. Hypertension may also be collapsed in terms of pathological and clinical phases into benign, accelerated and malignant hypertension. Furthermore, it could be grouped by cardiac cycle into systolic and diastolic hypertension. Most importantly, hypertension could be understood in terms of etiology into primary or essential and secondary hypertension.

Primary or essential hypertension is the commonest type of hypertension accounting for 90-95% of all cases of hypertension in humankind {Guyton &Hall, 2000}, and is of interest to the present study. Secondary hypertension as the name implies, is hypertension secondary to some other conditions such as pregnancy and accounts for about 5-10% of all hypertension cases.

Essential hypertension is believed to run in families and is of unknown origin {Guyton & Hall, 2000}. However, it has been observed{Guyton & Hall, 2000} that patients with this disorder show characteristic inability of the kidney to excrete adequate quantities of salt and water at high extra cellular fluid levels when arterial blood pressure is high. The reason for this retention of salt and water until blood pressure becomes quite high in these patients is not known, although basic abnormalities in vascular changes in the kidneys are suspected {Guyton & Hall, 2000}.

Symptomatologically, Hypertension has no signs at its early stage{Guyton& Hall, 2000, Ezenwa,2009} but can be detected following routine medical examination that shows stably elevated arterial blood pressure level beyond acceptable normal limit. This asymptomatology of essential hypertension at the early stage makes its diagnosis often delayed thereby increasing possibility of complications and death from the disorder. Complicated hypertension may present with clinical features as headache, occasional confusional state, restlessness, easy fatigability, sweating, palpitations, recurrent backache, chest pain that disappears with rest among others.

## 3. Epidemiology of hypertension in Nigeria

Hypertension is a life long non-communicable disease (NCD) and the commonest cardiovascular disorder, Box & Fox (1998). Cardiovascular disease accounts for 30% of total global mortality rate from NCD-attributable disorders followed by cancers (13%) Chronic respiratory disease (7%) and diabetes (2%), (Peltzer, 2009). Globally, Chronic and non-communicable diseases are responsible for about 60% of all death cases, (Unwin and Alberti, 2006).

In addition, NCD impact negatively on the families, quality of life and productivity. The burden of the disease results in loss of income and opportunities with implications for low economic development (Peltzer, 2009).

In Nigeria, exact epidemiology of hypertension may be quite high, (Ezenwa, 2006) than possibly reported. This is because Hypertension related data may be inconclusive or at least under reported in Nigeria since usually only formal health sector may be reported. This stems from the fact that different paths to care exit in Nigeria whose activities are different and not coordinated centrifugally. These include orthodox (allopathic) medicine which is the formal sector, homeopathic and similar-type medicine, traditional / indigenous knowledge system medicine and prayer healing homes. These different approaches operate independently, not only in their understanding of etiology, diagnosis and treatment of physical and mental disorders, but in other areas as procedure and practice, record keeping, charges, training and certification. For instance, while The Medical and Dental Council of Nigeria regulates orthodox medical training and practice, there is no board in Nigeria for regulation of the activities of the prayer house healers, despite the fact that these healers receive, admit(both on in-patient and out-patient bases) and offer intervention to people with different physical and mental disorders. On the other hand, while Allopathic Medicine has its arms separated into different professions such as investigation (Medical Laboratory Sciences), treatment (pharmacognosis, physiotherapy, psychology, surgery etc), the traditional healer has all these professions fussed into one person. He /she is a physician, laboratory scientist, pharmacologist, nurse etc). Beyond the forgoing, there is no meeting point between these different approaches making health data collation always inconclusive. Given the forgoing, available statistics on epidemiology of hypertension in Nigeria derive from the formal (orthodox) sector only especially since these different paths to care differ in their diagnostic patterns.

Summarizing the Federal Government expert committee report on non-communicable diseases ,Onwubere (2004) observed that not less than 4.33million Nigerians over 15 years of age have hypertension of various degrees or severity (mild 2.8 million, moderate 0.85 million and severe hypertension, 0.64 million). He noted a national hypertension prevalence rate of 25 -30% with high incidence in people at the two extremes of economic spectrum and in urban than in rural communities. According to Box & Fox (1998), hypertension is the commonest cause of death in industrialized societies, occurring more in men than in women, and is of increasing importance in developing countries.

In an epidemiological study of the disorder in three communities in South West Nigeria, Copper, Rotimi, Kaufman, Muna and Mensah (1998; see also Copper Puras, Tracy, Kaufman, Ordunez and Mufunda, 1997) noted 7% prevalence rate among rural (Igboora-pa community) as against 17% rate in urban (Ibadan) settlers especially urban poor and salaried working class. They also noted almost 100% higher mortality rate in patients with hypertension when compared with those with normal blood pressure. Specifically, the authors reported 5.1% mortality rate among hypertension patients in comparison with 2.8% among people with normal blood pressure. Copper et al also (1998) observed that blood pressure rose moderately with age among participants resident in the rural communities studied unlike those that lived in the urban (Ibadan) center.

## 4. Challenges associated with contemporary management of essential hypertension in Nigeria; The problem

The major approach to the management of hypertension in Nigeria (and perhaps elsewhere) is the use of anti-hypertensive medications, (in addition to complimentary dietary control that ensures reduction of salt intake and consumption of green leafy vegetables). These drugs are basically either vasodilators that tend to widen the blood vessels in order to reduce resistance or diuretics that inhabit tabular re-absorption of salt and water with consequent reduction in blood pressure. However, the pharmacological actions of these drugs are fraught with numerous side effects (A.D.A.M.2002).

The table below shows some instances of different groups of antihypertensive medications and their known side effects (A.D.A.M., 2002)

| Serial number | Drug group | Side effects |
|---|---|---|
| 1 | Loop and Thiazide diuretics | Depletion of body's supply of potassium with consequences for development of arrhythmias and other pathological conditions |
| 2 | Beta-blockers | Increase in incidence of type 2 diabetes, depression, fatigue, lethargy, nightmares. |
| 3 | Calcium-Channel Blockers | Flushing, constipation, accumulation of fluid in the feet (Pedal edema), impotence. |
| 4 | Angiotensin converting enzyme (ACE) inhibitors | Allergic reaction, irritating cough, low blood pressure, potassium retention in kidney which increases the risk of cardiac arrest when at high level. |
| 5 | Angiotensin receptor blockers | Fatigue, nasal congestion, elevated potassium blood levels and abnormal kidney function |

Table 1.

In addition to the foregoing, antihypertensive drugs are associated with sexual dysfunction (Philips, 2000). Beyond side effects, drug treatment of hypertension may nearly be contraindicated in complicated hypertension co-morbidity with tertiary stage nephritis, diabetes mellitus, liver function disease etc.

More importantly, the use of chemotherapy in the management of hypertension harbors the possible risk of death from over dose, under dose, fake and expired medication especially in developing countries where regulation of product standards may be weak.

Finally, the economic burden imposed by prolong use of antihypertensive medication may be very challenging to indigent patients and families, the unemployed and/ or the elderly. All these factors have obvious negative outcomes for occupational, social and family adjustments as well as overall quality of life of the essential hypertension patients.

It is against the foregoing serious demands associated with pharmacological management of essential hypertension that the present study sought to examine the possible therapeutic roles of music in the management of the disorder.

## 5. Non-pharmacological agents and essential hypertension

A number of studies have suggested that non-drug based methods of intervention( including music therapy ) have therapeutic effects on vital signs of patients with different disorders such as anxiety or essential hypertension, (Stoudenmire, 1975, Kim and Lee, 1989, Rasid and Parish, 1998,). Recently, Ezenwa, (2009) investigated the effect of relaxation therapy on arterial blood pressure of patients with essential hypertension and found significant reduction in their systolic and diastolic blood pressure following 30minutes exposure. The result of the study and similar others formed the main basis to investigate the possible contributions of music therapy in the management of essential hypertension.

Music is a set of organized sound that pleases the ears and sense of balance. The use of music in different settings is as old as man. In times past and today, music is used to entertain and motivate people in competitive activities such as during games (football, wrestling, running etc). It is also used in religious contexts for worship and meditation purposes as well as during solemn moments such as funerals, festivals, marriages and similar special events.

However, of great importance to the present paper is the use of music as a therapeutic agent. In the Bible, (1st Samuel, 19:9-10) it was reported that when evil spirit came upon Saul, David would play the Lyre and evil spirit would depart from him. Campbell (1998) articulated the effects of music therapy( in particular classical music by Wolfgang Amadeus Mozart) to include restoration of learning disorders, vocal and auditory handicaps, listening disabilities as well as alteration of mood, enhancement of creativity and health.

Conversely, Burns, Labbe, Williams and McCall (1999) assigned subjects to four different groups of classical, hard rock, self- selected relaxing music and no music group. Using subjects' relaxation level, skin temperature, muscle tension and heart rate as measures, they found that skin temperature decreased for all the conditions while classical, self selected relaxing music and no music group reported significant increases in feelings of relaxation. However, in a study on the effect of music intervention on anxiety patients awaiting cardiac catheterization, Hamel (2001) found a statistically significant reduction in anxiety in the test group unlike in the control, reflected in significant reduction in heart rate and systolic blood pressure. Cardigan, Caruso, Haldeman, McMamara, Noyes, Spadofora, and Carrol (2001), found music therapy to have significantly reduced blood pressure, respiratory rate and psychological distress among cardiac patients on bed rest. However, result from patients on bed rest may differ from hypertensive patients that are active occupationally. In addition, the study was done ten years ago and in a different country from the present one.

In another instance, Smolen,Topp and Singer (2002) studied the effect of self selected music on anxiety ,heart rate and blood pressure among ambulatory patients undergoing colonoscopy. They assigned thirty two subjects randomly to either an experimental group who listened to music during the colonoscopy or standard procedure no music group. Furthermore, physiological signs of anxiety including blood pressure and heart rate were measured at four points during the procedure. The researchers reported a significant group by time interaction on the physiological signs of anxiety as well as significant decreases in heart, systolic and diastolic blood pressure among the patients. However, the participants of the study were not known hypertensive patients and they chose their music of choice unlike in the presents study.

## 6. Music therapy and human physiology

Music varies a great deal. The differences in characteristics of music play out in the different uses to which music can be put. It may also reflect cultural, historical, personality and the unique promptings and the circumstances of the particular artist/composer. These differences can form a basis for distinction of classes of music. Thus, based on rhythm, it can be divided into high and low rhythmic music. It can also be distinguished into geographical and social-cultural backgrounds thus; African traditional music, Asian / Oriental traditional music, European traditional music etc. In general, music can be classified using broad characteristics into Classical, Rock, Reggae, Disco, Blues, and Country. Despite the types of music, it has one effect or the other on its listener.

Music therapy is the employment of organized sound in a purposeful therapeutic manner, (Ezenwa , 2006). Due the characteristics, sequential, logical, and predictable nature of music, it tends to generate a sense of harmony . This harmony so generated tends to mobilize the individual towards activation (arousal) in the case of high rhythmic music, or demobilization or relaxation in case of low rhythmic music (Ezenwa 2006). In this sense, through appealing to the cognitive domain, music can activate the stimulation of the appropriate hormonal system to either increase the basal metabolic rate or decrease the physiological system depending on the tonal or rhythmic pattern of the music and the listener's perception of it.

In order to provide some empirical evidence to demonstrate the critical contribution of music therapy in the management of essential hypertension, the present author conducted a clinical trial as presented below.

For the purpose of the study, interest was limited to the comparative effects of a classical music by Ludwig Von Beethoven; violin concerto in D, op. 61, second movement entitled Larghetto, on patients with essential hypertension.

## 7. Justification for the present study

As can be deduced from the foregoing the current dominant pharmacological method of managing hypertension is associated with severe side effects that affect patients in various ways. These may include medical complications, disruption in family, social and occupational adjustments, in addition to economic burden of illness, all of which predict negative outcomes for the patient and generally poor quality of life.

In order to address these short comings and to provide an alternative or at least a complimentary therapeutic approach that is comparatively inexpensive, devoid of side effects, is not prone to overdose, faking or adulteration, the present study sought to explore the effects of classical music, larghetto, on arterial blood pressure of patients with essential hypertension.

## 8. Objectives of the study

This paper sought to answer the following research questions;

1. Will music therapy be effective in significantly reducing the systolic blood pressure of essential hypertension patients?
2. Will music therapy be effective in significantly reducing the diastolic blood pressure of essential hypertension patients?

To test the validity of the foregoing questions, 10 (5 male and 5 female) known essential hypertension patients attending Ebonyi State University Teaching Hospital Abakaliki, Ebonyi State Nigeria, (now Federal University Teaching Hospital Abakaliki following its take over by the Federal Government of Nigeria in may 2011) who met the eligibility conditions for participation in the study formed the participants. Their ages ranged from 40 to 65 with a mean age of 54 and standard deviation of 9.2. Marital status showed that they were all married.

Inclusion into the study was by cumulative addition in which all candidates who met the selection criteria were included. These criteria included that patient was interested in the study on voluntary basis , had the time to participate , had hypertension as his/her main diagnosis ,did not have laboratory or other investigations to do following consultation and had no obvious medical/ family/occupational emergency that needed his/her immediate attention and that patient must be an out-patient.

The instruments used in the study included a DVD player (Thompson Ampli DVD DTH2150A) measuring 485x108x345mm manufactured by Thompson India private limited in May 2004, with serial number 0329. Other instruments were compact disc plate containing Ludwig Van Beethoven's violin concerto in D.OP. 61 entitled second movement (Larghetto), plain sheets of paper, stethoscopes and mercury sphygmomanometer for measuring and recording systolic and diastolic blood pressure of the participants. There were also human facilitators (physicians and nurses) who assisted the researcher with selection, measurement and recording of the blood pressure of the patients before and after the exposure to the independent variable.

Execution of the research was done using the following procedure. Approval for the study was got from ethics and research committee of Ebonyi State University Teaching Hospital Abakaliki. Two consultant physicians were contacted for their assistance in releasing their patients for the study .The Head Resident Doctor in Internal Medicine Department was also contacted for his co-operation and logistic support in patient enrollment. The co-operation of the Nurses on duty was also sought. Effort was however made **not** to disclose the actual purpose of the study to the assisting doctors and nurses in order to prevent experimenter-related bias.

After recruitment of the participants, they were taken to the conference hall of the Hospital which was located in a relatively quiet area of the institution. As they all came into the hall, they were addressed thus: *You are please required to sit down .The doctors will simply take your blood pressure after which you will listen to a piece of music for 30mins. Your blood pressure may be taken from time to time. Thank you for your time with us.*

To ensure relaxation of the participants, they were encouraged to introduce themselves to the group. The facilitators (the doctors and nurses) were already known to the patients.

Matched subjects design was used in the work, while matched T- test statistics was employed for data analysis since baseline and post test blood pressure readings of same group were compared.

The result of the study was presented thus:

| Type of blood pressure(BP) | Baseline | Post test | Cal. T value | Table T value | DF | P<_.01 | 10 minutes post test BP |
|---|---|---|---|---|---|---|---|
| Systolic | 144 | 133 | 3.97 | 2.26 | 9 | 3.25 | 128 |
| Diastolic | 96 | 82.5 | 5.71 | 2.26 | 9 | 3.25 | 80 |

Based on values in table 1 above, a statistically significant mean difference (p<.01) was noted between pre-treatment systolic blood pressure reading (M=144) and post treatment value (M=133) indicating that the classical music decreased systolic blood pressure level of essential hypertension patients. This reduction was found to have decreased further (M=128) when the BP was taken 10 minutes post test period.

Table 2. Summary table of means of systolic and diastolic blood pressure of essential hypertension patients.

The table above also showed that the diastolic blood pressure of the participants manifested a statistically significant mean difference between baseline BP value (M = 96) and post test BP value (M= 82.5) at P< .01. This showed that the treatment reduced diastolic blood pressure of essential hypertension patients. This reduction was also progressive (M= 80) as noted when the BP was taken 10 minutes post treatment period.

The key findings of this study included that the classical music significantly reduced both systolic and diastolic blood pressure of the essential hypertension patients that participated in the study.

These findings are consistent with other studies. Salmore & Welson (2000 found music therapy to have significantly reduced the vital signs (including the blood pressure) of patients in gastrointestinal laboratory endoscopy. In addition, the therapy has been found to reduce state anxiety in patients with myocardial infarction( white, 1992), reduced systolic and diastolic blood pressure, respiratory rate and psychological distress in cardiac patients on bed rest, Cardigan, Caruso, Haldeman, McNamara, Noyes, Spadafora and Caroll, 2001). Campbell (1998) observed that 10 minutes exposure to Mozart's Sonata for two pianos in D major, K448, (a type of classical music) resulted in eight to nine scores higher on spatial intelligence test by 36 undergraduates at the University of California. He explained that vibrating sound formed patterns and created energy fields of resonance and movement in surrounding space. As human beings absorb these energies, '*they subtly alter breath, pulse, blood pressure, muscle tension, skin temperature and other internal rhythms*'.

One possible explanation of this effect of music therapy is the fact that music as an auditory stimulus, is a form of sound energy that reverberates in balance, logic and harmony. These characteristics of music tend to have a strong irresistible appeal to the ear which compels attention from the listener to the music. By consciously or unconsciously surrendering to the sound of music, the listener is automatically tuned to the rhythm, the driving force of music which gradually changes the mood, feeling, physiology and consequently the vital signs of the individual listener. In low rhythmic music, these vital signs reduce significantly.

A major implication of this study is the fact that music therapy, a non-pharmacological agent, significantly reduced systolic and diastolic blood pressure of the participants and as such could be useful in the management of essential hypertension. This is very important against the background that chemotherapeutic management of essential hypertension is associated with side effects that affect treatment outcome and overall quality of life of the patients. Music therapy is inexpensive, accessible, and is not associated with side effects.

It is important to observe that small sample size is a common difficulty in clinical studies and this tends to limit the extent to which the study can be generalized. This work is not an exception to this limitation. Many patients who could have participated in the study did not meet the eligibility criteria. Future studies in this area may target large sample size and perhaps record possible changes in the blood pressure over longer length of time. This may determine the half life of the therapy and as such the dose.

However, it is interesting to note that only 30minutes exposure to music therapy could significantly reduce the blood pressure of known essential hypertension patients and this reduction did not only remain stable but reduced further as shown by blood pressure readings taken 10 minutes post treatment. There is therefore the need for physicians to consider the use of music therapy independently or at least as a complimentary therapeutic option. When used as a complimentary therapy, it may reduce the amount of antihypertensive drugs patients require thus contributing to reduced side effects and better treatment outcome

## 9. Conclusion

A look at the foregoing suggests that music therapy could be an important factor in the management of essential hypertension. This finding agrees with other literature in the area and therefore justifies the need for a paradigm shift from the present dominant and often exclusive use of chemotherapy in the management of essential hypertension. Music therapy is inexpensive, accessible, convenient and devoid of known side effects. The integration of music therapy, even as an adjunct therapy in the management of essential hypertension, is expected to improve access to treatment, eliminate adverse drug interactions or reactions and consequently improve overall treatment outcome with great implication for better quality of life for the essential hypertension patients.

## 10. References

A.D.A.M Inc (2002) Retrieved from: http://www.enh.org/welconnected/articles/000014.asp

Akinkugbe, O. O. (1997) (ed.) Non-communicable diseases in Nigeria; final report of national survey. Lagos. Federal Ministry of Health and Social Services.

Beethoven, L. (1770-1827). Second movement, larghetto in the album, Beethoven Violin Concertos-Romance in F. London. Academy sound and vision limited.

Boon, N. A. & Fox, A. A( 1998) Diseases of cardiovascular system. In C. R. W. Edwards, I. A. D. Bouchie, C. Haslett, & E. Davidsons's principle and practice of medicine (7th ed.).Edinburgh: Harcourt Brace and Company Limited.

Cardigan, M. E.; Caruso, N. A.; McNamara, N. E.; Noyes, D. A.; Spadafora, M. A. and Carroll, D. L. (2001). The effect of music on cardiac patients on bed rest. Prog. Cardiovas Nurs. Winter; 16(1); 5-13.

Cambell, D, (1998) The riddle of the Mozart effect ( music theray for care and prevention) Natural Health. Jan-Feb. http://www.findarticles.com

Cooper, R. S.; Osotimehin, B.; Kaufman, J. S.; Ordunez, P. o.; Mufunda, J.(1997). Evaluation of electronic blood pressure device for epidemiological studies. Blood pressure monitoring; 2: 35-40

Cooper, R.S.; Rotimi, C. N.; Kaufman, J. S.;Muna, W. F. T.; and Mensah, G.A.(1998) Hypertension treatment and control in Sub- Saharan Africa: The epidemiological basis for policy. British Medical Journal. Feb. 21

Ezenwa, M. O. (2006). Effects of music and relaxation therapies on patients with essential hypertension.( Unpublished doctoral thesis). Nnamdi Azikiwe University, Awka, Anambra State, Nigeria.

Ezenwa, M. O. ( 2009). Effect of relaxation therapy in reducing blood pressure of essential hypertension patients. Journal of psychology in Africa, 19(3); 401-404

Guyton, A. C., & Hall. J. E. (2000). A textbook of medical physiology. New Delhi: Harcourt India Private Limited.

Hamel, W. J. (2001). The effect of music intervention on anxiety in patients waiting for cardiac catheterization. Intensive Crit. Care Nurs. Oct; 17(5); 279-85

Kim, D. S. & Lee, G. J. (1989). The effect of music relaxation training on patients with insomnia complaints. Kanho Hakhoe Chi. Aug; 19(2): 191-202

Onwubere, B. J. (2004). Hypertension as it affects the heart. A paper presented to a two day seminar organized by the cardiothoracic/intensive care nurses and students of post basic nursing School of Nursing, University of Nigeria Teaching Hospital Enugu on the theme: Cardiopulmonary resuscitation (challenges and prospects in the tropics) held on 30th & 31st March, at Rotary Lecture Hall, College of Medicine, University of Nigeria Teaching Hospital Enugu.

Perltzer, k. (2009) Self reported diabetes prevalence and risk factors in South Africa: Results from world health survey .Journal of Psychology in Africa.19 (3); 365- 370.

Philips, N. A. (2000). Female sexual dysfunction: Evaluation and Treatment. American Family physician, 62, 127-136

Rasid, Z. M. & Parish, T. S. (1998).The effect of two types of relaxation training on stdents' level of anxiety. Adolescence. Spring; 33(129);99-101

Robb, S. L. (2000). Music assisted progressive muscle relaxation, progressive muscle relaxation, and music listening and silence: A comparism of relaxation techniques. Journal of Music Therapy, 37(1), 2-21

Salmore, R. G.; & Welson, J. P. (2000).The effect of pre-procedure teaching, relaxation instruction, and music on anxiety as measured by blood pressures in an outpatient gastro-intestinal endoscopy laboratory. Gastroenterol. Nurs; 23(3)102-10

Smolen, D. Top, R. and Singer, L. (2002).The effect of selected music during colonoscopy on anxiety, heart rate and blood pressure. Appl. Nurs. Res. Aug; 15(3): 126-136

Stoudenmire, J. (1975). A comparism of muscle relaxation training and music in reduction of state and trait anxiety. J. Clin. Psychol. July; 31(3): 490-2

Unwin, N. E; & Albert, K. G. (2006). Chronic non-communicates diseases. Annals of Tropical Medicine and Parasitology, 100(5-6), 455-64.

White, J. M. (1992). Music therapy: An intervention to reduce anxiety in the myocardial infarction patients. Clin. Nurs.Spec. Summer; 6 (2): 58-63

# Part 2

## Genetics and Genomics of Hypertension

6

# Recent Trends in Hypertension Genetics Research

Padma Tirunilai and Padma Gunda
*Dept. of Genetics,*
*Osmania University,*
*Hyderabad,*
*India*

## 1. Introduction

Human genome encompasses several thousands of genes which when fail to function normally lead to a defective phenotype expressed sometimes as a disease or disorder. These diseases or disorders may be simple or complex depending upon the nature and number of genes controlling the phenotypes and also their interaction with several other confounding demographic and environmental factors leading to a mosaic pattern of aetiology. Essential hypertension is one such common complex condition prevalent in most of the world populations and stands as a major risk factor for cardio-, cerebro and renovascular diseases (Kearney et al., 2005) adding to the mortality rate when the patients are not treated promptly and managed with proper surveillance. It also causes enormous financial burden to the patients and also nation's economy. This necessitates the need to establish the causes with possible measures for prevention and cure of the condition especially in view of its high prevalence in several developed and developing countries. Research conducted especially in the past two decades were focused more on understanding the etiological factors including genetic components and their interaction with several other factors with a thrust to look for more appropriate therapeutic measures for essential hypertension (EHT).

Regulation of blood pressure is important to maintain adequate blood flow in the body. By definition, blood pressure is the pressure of the blood flowing through the arteries. It depends on the flow of the blood pumped by the heart and the resistance exerted by the blood vessels against the flow. If the pressure is high, heart is forced to work harder. Based on the aetiology, hypertension is further grouped into two major groups viz., a) **Essential or Primary Hypertension** which is caused due to unknown etiology and has no specific origin but is strongly associated with life style habits representing 90-95 % of the diagnosed cases and **b) Secondary Hypertension** which arises due to preexisting medical conditions such as congestive heart failure, arteriosclerosis and disorders of kidney, liver, adrenal and thyroid glands. It accounts to 5 to 10 % of the hypertensive cases and diagnosed by various clinical laboratory and other tests. Apart from these two types, other types of hypertension are also diagnosed based on their characteristic manifestations (*Table -1*)

| | | |
|---|---|---|
| White coat Hypertension | - | BP high in doctor's office |
| Systolic Hypertension | - | High SBP but normal DBP (age related) |
| Malignant Hypertension | - | Acute uncontrolled Blood Pressure |
| Labile Hypertension | - | Variable Blood Pressure |
| Accelerated Hypertension | - | Severe Blood Pressure of recent origin |
| Borderline Hypertension | - | Blood Pressure in the grey zone |
| Pseudo Hypertension | - | Due to rigidity of the artery (seen in elders) |
| Pulmonary Hypertension | - | High Blood Pressure in pulmonary circulation |
| Renovascular Hypertension | - | Due to narrowed renal artery |
| Pre-eclampsia | - | Pregnancy induced |
| Secondary Hypertension | - | Arising from a identifiable disorder |

Table 1. Types of blood pressure disorders.

The rhythmic contraction and relaxation of heart creates pressure which is recorded as Systolic blood pressure (SBP) when the heart contracts and Diastolic Blood Pressure (DBP) when the heart relaxes. BP levels are traditionally expressed in millimetres of mercury (1 mmHg = 133 Pascal) in the mercury column of sphygmomanometer and is usually around 120mmHg systolic and 80mmHg diastolic (120/80mmHg) in a normal individual. As per JNC VII (2003) report, based on SBP and DBP levels, individuals are grouped into four classes as given in *Table-2*. An adult with consistent systolic pressure of 140mmHg or higher and/ or a consistent diastolic pressure of 90mmHg or higher is considered to be hypertensive.

| | **Systolic BP (mm/ Hg)** | **Diastolic BP (mm /Hg)** |
|---|---|---|
| Optimal | <120 | and <80 |
| Normal | < 130 | and < 85 |
| Prehypertension | 130-139 | or 85-89 |
| Hypertension | | |
| Stage 1 (mild) | 140 - 159 | or 90 – 99 |
| Stage 2 (moderate) | 160 -179 | or 100 – 109 |
| Stage 3 (severe) | ≥180 | and ≥ 110 |
| Isolated Systolic hypertension | ≥140 | and <90 |

Table 2. Classification of blood pressure levels.

## 2. Factors influencing hypertension

Essential Hypertension is a common complex condition displaying substantial public health problem. As a multifactorial condition it involves action of several genes in conjecture with epidemiologic (environmental and demographic) factors manifesting finally into a defined phenotype Hypertension. Hypertension is found to affect 25-35% of adult and 60-70% of elderly population above the age of 70yrs both among the population of developed and developing countries (Staessen et al, 2003). Variation in the prevalence of EHT depends on the ethnicity of the population like being higher in American Blacks (32.4%) as compared to Whites (23.3%) and Mexican Americans (22.6%) (Oscar et al., 2000). Among American Blacks the condition occurs with greater severity and is associated with high rate of morbidity and mortality due to stroke, cardiac failure, left ventricular hypertrophy and end stage renal disease. While much is known about demographic and environmental factors that predispose an individual to the development of essential hypertension, the nature of the genetic factors that increase susceptibility to the condition remain virtually unknown.

Studies on the epidemiology of hypertension revealed substantial effect of age, gender, body mass index, smoking, high alcohol intake, insulin resistance and also diet with high intake of salt, and low intake of potassium and calcium (Stanton et al., 1982; Appel et al, 1997, Oscar et al., 2000). Some of these factors like obesity and alcohol consumption are additive and modifiable and thus influence variations in blood pressure and expression of hypertension phenotype. Other factors which are non-modifiable like age, gender, genetic factors etc., do not influence the variations in blood pressure and hence the associated risk levels (Fig - 1). In fact the factors like obesity, cholesterol levels etc., remain in an individual more or less stable over time while blood pressure levels keep changing several times even in a day due to the action of multiple physiological pathways to maintain the appropriate levels. Interaction between the hypertensinogenic factors and susceptibility causing genetic factors that have small effects poses a great challenge in unravelling the links, causes and management of hypertension.

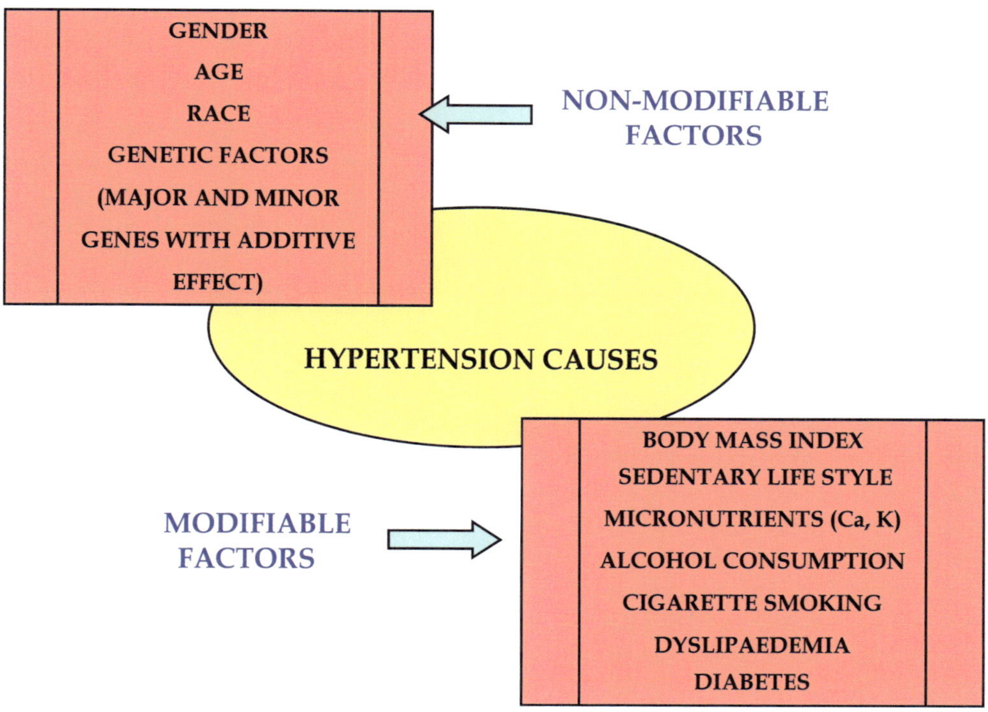


Fig. 1. Modifiable and Non-Modifiable factors influencing onset of essential hypertension.

Age is recognized as a non-modifiable risk factor for high blood pressure with continuous increase in SBP and decrease in DBP levels with ageing throughout ones life. Onset of elevated DBP is usually observed from 35-40yrs due to multiple metabolic, physiologic or genetic reasons while increase in SBP among the aged is observed due to arteriosclerosis or hardening of arteries, decrease in kidney function and physical activity. In many populations men show higher prevalence of hypertension with early onset than women. It has been suggested that estrogen levels have lowering effect on blood pressure in young women but a dramatic increase in the incidence of hypertension is observed in the postmenopausal women. Obesity and overweight also pose a major risk for chronic diseases including hypertension. Obesity induces a high secretion of insulin which brings in many modifications in the body like i) Thickening of the vessels which is responsible for an increase in the rigidity of arteries and in turn the blood pressure, ii) Increase in the cardiac output due to the secretion of increased adrenalin, iii) Induction of reabsorption of water and salt by the kidney which increases the blood volume and consequently the blood pressure iv) Over-sensitiveness to sodium which is known to increase the rigidity of the peripheral arteries.

Body Mass Index (BMI) is a simple index of weight-for-height that is commonly used to classify underweight, overweight and obesity in adults. It is defined as the weight in kilograms divided by the square of the height in meters ($kg/m^2$).

$$BMI = Mass\ (Kg) / Height\ (m)^2$$

BMI of <18.5 - Underweight; 18.5-24.9 - Normal; 25.0 - 29.9 - Overweight; >30 - Obese; >40 - Morbid obesity

Among the addictions, cigarette smoking has been investigated world wide as a risk factor for coronary heart disease (CHD), along with high blood pressure and cholesterol disorders. The nicotine in cigarettes and other tobacco products cause blood vessels to constrict and heart to beat faster, which temporarily raises the blood pressure. Drinking alcohol excessively also is found to increase the frequency of high blood pressure by one and half to two times. Alcohol when present in the blood stream it covers the blood vessels and arterial walls increasing the tension and subsequently the blood pressure. In the recent past emphasis is laid on the use of balanced high blood pressure diet with sparse amounts of saturated and trans-fats and moderate amounts of other fats. Micronutrients are also as important since intake of increased amount of sodium and low levels of potassium and calcium in the diet lead to increases in blood pressure. Increase of potassium in diet helps to balance the amount of sodium in cell fluids and rids cells of excess sodium through kidneys, which filters out extra amount of sodium while inadequate potassium can allow excess sodium to accumulate and thus increases the blood pressure. High levels of intracellular calcium increases vascular smooth muscle tone, peripheral vascular resistance, and responsiveness to the sympathetic and RAS systems that elevate blood pressure. Paradoxically it is low not high calcium intake that stimulates an increase in parathyroid hormone which leads to calcium mobilization from the bone, increased intestinal calcium absorption, decreased renal calcium excretion, increased intracellular calcium concentration with increase in blood pressure. In general, life style factors like lack of exercise and physical activity, sedentary jobs, habit of smoking and consuming alcohol all are also associated with enhancement in blood pressure and more so when the individuals are genetically predisposed to the condition.

## 2.2 Genetic factors

### 2.2.1 Inheritance of hypertension

Inter individual variations in BP levels are known to be inherited with 30% of contribution although the exact genetic factors that contribute to the variations are not clearly established The concept of genetic basis for hypertension originated 50yrs back itself with the proposal of Platt (1967) who stated that essential hypertension arises due to a single dominant gene. He observed that blood pressure values among the sibs followed a bimodal distribution with two peaks corresponding to systolic blood pressure of 130 mm mercury inherited by the normal gene and those with 160 mm mercury inherited by the gene for hypertension. At the same time Pickering (1967) proposed his view that blood pressure is inherited as a multifactorial condition since the frequency distribution curves (bell shaped) for blood pressure in the relatives of patients were observed to be similar in shape to the distribution observed in the population based sample. The distribution however showed a shift upwards to one extreme or skewed by about the same amount at all ages. Further evidences for the possible involvement of genes for hypertension comes from the population studies exhibiting greater similarity in the measurement of blood pressure within families than between families (Longini et al, 1984). This familial resemblance appears to be present at all levels of blood pressure and hence same genes can be predicted to influence blood pressure over all values- the hypothesis proposed by Pickering. Given an affected first-degree relative, the risk of hypertension is found to be increased 2-5 fold in family members as compared to the population risk. Studies conducted on familial aggregation of hypertension demonstrated correlation in the blood pressure levels between sibs and between parents and children (ranging from 0.14-0.18) and between monozygotic twins (ranging from 0.55-0.58) as opposed to dizygotic twins (ranging from 0.25-0.27) supporting the genetic basis for the condition. This observation is strengthened further by the presence of higher concordance rate among biological sibs as opposed to adopted siblings living in the same household (Mimura, 1973; Biron et al, 1976; Feinleib et al., 1977; Rice et al., 1989; Williams et al, 1991; Oscar et al., 2000). As family members share genes and environment, the correlations regarding blood pressure levels between them may also result due to interaction with shared environment. However, relatively low blood pressure correlations observed between pairs of spouse (0.06-0.08) implicate a substantial influence of genetic factors when family blood pressure correlations are considered. Furthermore, adoption studies indicated higher correlation in the levels of blood pressure between the parents and their biological children than between parents and their adopted children (Biron et al, 1976) emphasising genetic basis for blood pressure.

The strength of a genetic component for a multifactorial condition like hypertension is estimated as heritability, which is defined as the proportion of phenotypic variance due to genetic factors over the total phenotypic variance observed. Heritability encompasses two genetic components causing effects that are a) Additive and b) Dominant effects. Narrow-sense heritability, denoted as $h^2$ reflects the additive genetic effects and is considered as a measure of predictability of offspring trait values based on parental trait values whereas broad-sense heritability estimates denoted as $H^2$ include dominant gene effects which explain part of the heritability resulting due to the effects of major genes. However, these major genes do not generally contribute substantially to the heritability of complex quantitative traits like blood pressure in the general population. Large family-based studies conducted have estimated 20-40% narrow-sense heritabilities for DBP and SBP (North et al, 2003) and around 60% in twin studies (Williams et al, 1991).

Effect of age was also demonstrated on the heritability estimates for blood pressure by the studies on adult twins which was higher than in case of infant twins (Scott et al, 2010). This suggests that blood pressure heritability increases with age. In general heritability of blood pressure attributed to all the genetic factors varies from 25% in pedigree studies to 65% in twin studies.

### 2.2.2 Genetic determinants

Genes responsible for hypertension in reality may be the ones that are meant to regulate blood pressure levels in an individual. Such genes are not likely to be the causative mutations, but they may be akin to "oncogenes" which are essential to life but may be getting abnormal in function at a given time. So the genes for hypertension are normal but impacted by the confounders raising the blood pressure level leading to clinical expression of the condition. Neel et al. (1998) rightly used the term "Syndromes of impaired genetic homeostasis" to diseases arising due to mismatching of previously adaptive genotypes and modern environmental conditions. In populations without any hypertensinogenic factors blood pressure measurements follow a normal distribution but will be skewed towards right of the curve with narrow base or less variance. With the addition of hypertensinogenic factors like insulin resistance, obesity, high sodium intake, circulating angiotensin levels etc., the distribution may be skewed further to the right, with flatter curve and more variance indicating increase in the frequency of subjects with hypertension who get plotted under the tail end of the distribution (Oscar et al., 2000, Fig-2) The hypertensinogenic factors themselves may possibly have important genetic component and may act as intermediary phenotypes enhancing or decreasing the blood pressure levels like in case of obesity which is observed to be a risk factor for enhancing blood pressure. Severe the obesity greater is the risk observed for developing hypertension. Concerning the molecular basis of essential hypertension, the focused view is that in populations blood pressure has a quasi-unimodal distribution and in a person with higher blood pressure values, higher are the chances of him possessing the disease-type variant alleles of the susceptibility causing gene. Thus greater number of susceptibility genes are likely to be impaired in hypertensives as compared to normotensives (Kato, 2002) (Fig-3).

The advanced molecular biological technologies developed in the recent past helped in identifying as many as 17 independent mutations in genes associated with hypertension (8 genes) or hypotension (9 genes) (Lifton et al., 2001; *Table- 3*). These monogenic Mendelian forms of hypertension are rare and arise mostly due to the errors in different metabolic pathways. Mechanism underlying these genes does not explain the blood pressure variability observed in populations (Staessen et al., 2003). Hence efforts were focused more on the gene(s) and interacting confounding factors that influence the blood pressure variations leading to the clinical expression of essential hypertension. Several strategies were applied to meet this end which led to the consensus that hypertension is more likely a

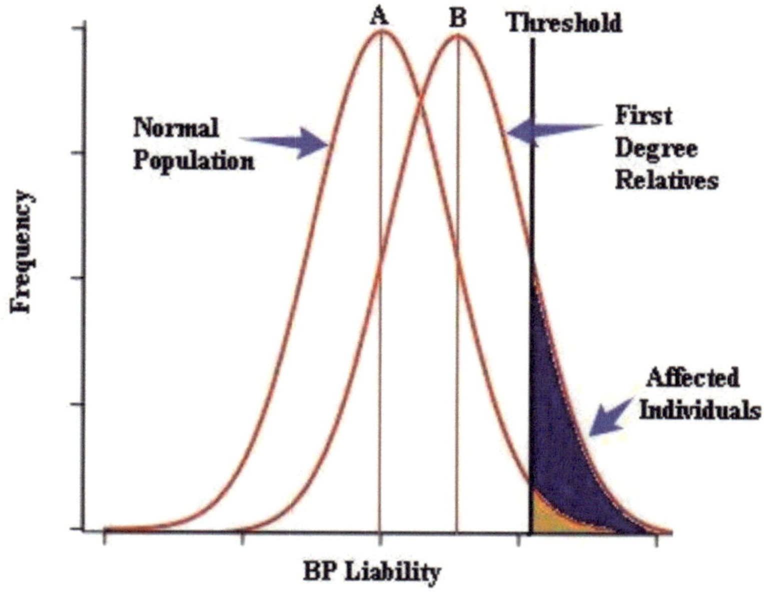


Fig. 2. Hypothetical Curves of liability for BP in general population and relatives of Probands. A- Mean BP levels in population; B-Mean BP levels in relatives of probands.

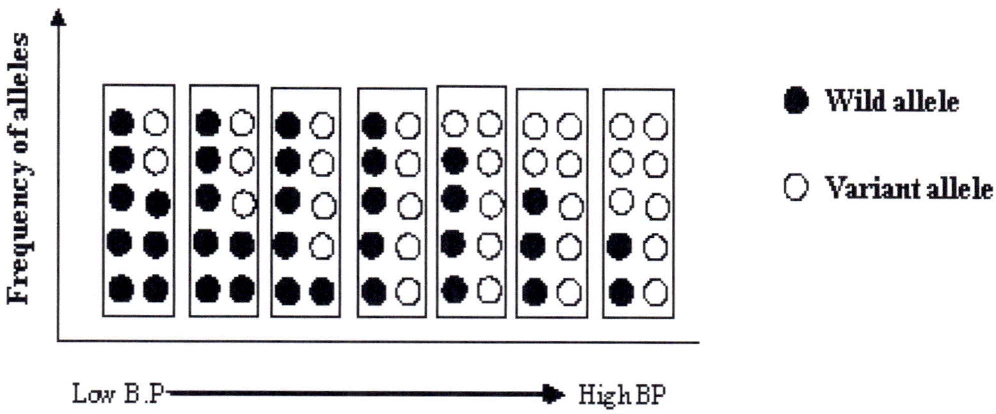


Fig. 3. Linear increase of BP levels with increasing variant alleles.

cumulative burden of many genes with small effects. It is now accepted that hypertension is a multifactorial condition with the interplay of several genes with small effects. The search proved to be tough due to the realities like a) Lack of standardisation and arbitrary dichotomisation of a continuous variable into hypertensive and normotensive groups b) Requirement of very large sample sizes to obtain good statistical power c) Inappropriate selection of controls d) Population admixture and stratification e) Failure to account for confounders like environmental and epigenetic factors which themselves may be associated with independent genetic variants (like obesity, salt and potassium intake etc.), f) Assessment of the effects of environmental factors on genetic variants which develops over time at different levels in different individuals and finally g) Presence of genetic heterogeneity where inter-individual variations in blood pressure levels are observed with reference to the associated genetic variants and also environmental factors which adds to the reduction in the power of the study considerably. Against all the odds, research on hypertension genetics has made remarkable progress in the last two decades towards better understanding of the condition mainly due to the development of wet lab technologies, biostatistical approaches for data analysis and bioinformatics tools.

| **Syndrome** | **Mutations In** | **Mode of Inheritance** |
|---|---|---|
| Glucocorticoid remediable aidosteron ism (GRA) | Chimerical gene containing promoter area of AS and coding region of 11βH | Dominant |
| Apparent mineralocorticoid excess (AME) | Absence of 11βHSD | Recessive |
| Liddle syndrome | β or γ subunit of ENaC | Dominant |
| Pseudohypoaldosteronism type 2 | One of the Genes mapped to 1q31-42, 12p13 and 17p11-q21 | Dominant |
| Hypertension induced by pregnancy | Mineralocorticoid receptor | Dominant |
| Hypertension with brachydactyly | Gene mapped to 12p11.2-12.2 | Dominant |
| Defective aldosterone | Aldosterone Synthase or 21 hydroxylase | Recessive |
| Dominant Pseudohypoaldosteronism type 1 (PHA1) | Mineralocorticoid receptor | Dominant |
| Recessive Pseudohypoaldosteronism type 1 (PHA1) | α,β or γ subunit of ENac | Recessive |
| Peroxisome proliferators activated receptor gamma (PPARγ) | PPARγ | Dominant |
| Gitelman's syndrome | Thiazide sensitive Nacl cotrans -porter | Recessive |
| Bartter's syndrome | Ion transporters | Recessive |

Table 3. Mendelian forms of blood pressure dysregulation.

## 3. Methods for identifying genetic determinants

Presently two major approaches viz., a) Association studies b) Linkage analysis are being adopted to identify the genetic components underlying complex diseases including essential hypertension.

### 3.1 Association studies

This approach is based on comparison of cases with controls to examine whether an allele or genotype of particular **polymorphism** (*Table- 4*) at candidate gene loci are seen more frequently in disease populations than in a control population. This approach requires careful selection of controls with adequate sample size that has statistical power to validate the results. The controls planned should match with the disease population for parameters like sex, age, ethnicity, socioeconomic status, accurate diagnosis etc. The controls should also be screened for the presence of hypertension and history of associated conditions like diabetes, thyroid disorders, cardiac disorder, stroke etc., (which may have genes overlapping with genes for hypertension) and should be drawn at random from the same population/ethnic group from where the patient group is selected. The controls drawn from the population are unrelated and thus expected to have random distribution of the marker alleles selected. For age related condition like hypertension which increases in frequency with age, one should be certain that the control subjects are not likely to be the carriers for the hypertension susceptible genes. It is rather difficult to achieve this requirement and one way of reducing the bias in selecting the controls will be to include such of the individuals who are older than the mean age of onset reported for the patient group and also subjects who do not have the family history of the condition. A better alternative choice of controls would be the unaffected normal sibs who are elder to the patients so that they would have crossed the age at expression of the condition in that family at the time of investigation. Further sibs share common environment and hence it would be possible to sort out the genetic component underlying the condition from the environmental factors. The careful selection of the controls can avoid the spurious conclusion on the associations found between the disease and the polymorphic loci.

| Type of Marker | No. of Loci | Features |
|---|---|---|
| Blood Group antigens | >25 | Genotype cannot always be inferred from the phenotypes. Difficult for physical localization |
| Serum Proteins | 30 | Often limited polymorphism. Difficult for physical localization |
| Leaucocyte antigens (HLA) | 1 | HLA system with A, B, C, D and DR loci each harboring hundreds of alleles thus resulting extensive polymorphism. Is highly informative |
| Restriction Fragment Length Polymorphisms (RFLPs) | $>10^5$ | Two allele markers, maximum heterozygosity 0.5, genotyped using Southern blotting and PCR techniques. Easy for physical localization |
| Variable number of tandemn repeats (VNTRs) | $>10^4$ | Many alleles and highly informative. Easy for physical localization. Tend to cluster near the ends of chromosomes |
| Microsatellites | $>10^5$ | Many alleles and highly informative.Easy for physical localization. Distributed throughout the genome |
| Single Nucleotide Polymorp-hisms (SNPs) | $>4x10^5$ | Less informative than microsatellites. Can be genotyped on a very large scale using automated equipment |

Table 4. Polymorphic genetic markers used in genetic analysis and identification of disease genes.

Association studies rely on the phenomenon of **linkage disequilibrium (LD)** and are conducted to evaluate the risk for developing the disease by the individuals carrying a specific genotype or allele of polymorphic candidate loci. These loci when co-dominant have three genotypes (AA, Aa and aa) determined by the combination of two alleles (A and a). In normal population the distribution of genotypes and the alleles are expected to be in **"Hardy-Weinberg equilibrium" (HWE)** and there may be deviations from the equilibrium when events of migration, genetic drift, selection etc., operate in a given population. Deviations in genotypic and allele frequencies of a marker gene from HWE in a patient population indicate possible association of the disease susceptible gene with the marker allele that may cause risk to the carrier individual of that allele for developing the condition.

Linkage disequilibrium (LD) results when the frequency of one or more gametic combinations of alleles at two loci A and B does not coincide with the combined individual frequencies of the two alleles i.e. $P_{A1B1} \neq p_{A1}p_{B1}$.

In this context the term linkage does not refer exclusively to loci on the same chromosome, but it also includes loci on other chromosomes. Linkage disequilibrium (D) is measured as the product of frequency of gametes with the same type of alleles minus the product of the frequencies of gametes with different types of alleles

$$D = P_{A1B1}\,P_{A2B2} - P_{A1B2}\,P_{A2B1}$$

When D = +0.25, only gametes with same type of alleles *A1B1* and *A2B2* occur in a population. When D = 0, the two loci are considered to be in genetic equilibrium

Lower the frequency of recombination between the loci, longer the time it takes for the genes to reach equilibrium. After several generations, the two genes do not reach equilibrium because of absence of crossing over due to absolute linkage between them.

The significance of associations is judged by the values of **"Odds Ratios" (ORs)** computed by comparing patient and control groups for the frequencies of marker alleles/genotypes as a ratio. The ORs obtained for any allele/genotype is compared against a reference value of 1.0, the ratio obtained when the distribution of genotypes of a polymorphism remains more or less similar n both patient and control groups. OR's can deviate significantly from 1.0 and when the OR is significantly >1.0, then the locus tested is considered to be in positive association with the disease, causing risk to the individuals carrying the particular genotype/allele; when it is significantly <1.0, it is interpreted that the marker allele is negatively associated and offers protection to the carrier individual against the disease. The ORs are computed for alleles (A vs. a) or for one genotype against any of the other two genotypes (AA vs. Aa; AA vs. aa and Aa vs. aa) and also for one genotype against the pooled frequencies of other two genotypes (AA vs. Aa + aa; Aa vs. AA + aa and aa vs. AA + Aa). These values are also represented as those obtained under **"Dominant Model"** [(which specifically tests the association of having at least one minor allele say 'a' (i.e. in Aa or aa individuals) versus not having it at all (AA individuals)] and **"Recessive Model"** [(which specifically tests the association of having the minor allele "a" in homozygous state (aa) versus having at least one major allele A (Aa or AA individuals)].

Odds Ratios are also computed to predict risk of alleles of individual markers and/or multiple markers. When multiple marker alleles are used to test associations, Bonferroni corrections is applied to validate the significance of risk obtained for the individual markers studied. In addition, ORs can also be computed for **haplotypes/haploblocks** formed by a set of alleles of marker genes on the same chromosome along with the disease gene. Haplotype associations provide information on the combinations of certain alleles present on the same chromosome as the disease gene. Associations of the disease gene found with certain haplotypes may enhance or circumvent the risk estimates obtained for single marker allele.

The association detected can be positive or negative and the criteria required for high quality positive and negative case control studies are described by Sharma and Jeunemaitre (2000). The criteria suggested for Positive case-control study are - large sample size; well matched controls; accurate definition of the phenotype; a priori estimation of the power of the study; small p-values adjusted to the number of SNPs tested; biological plausibility and functional significance; independent replication in several populations; confirmation in family based studies; high ORs/attributable risk and for a Negative case-control study these criteria are - large sample size; well matched controls; accurate definition of the phenotype; biological plausibility and functional significance; a priori estimation of the power of the study; testing at least three polymorphisms at the same locus; independent replication in at least one other populations; haplotype analysis.

The positive associations of the marker alleles tested with the disease may result due to a) Functional relationship between the marker allele and the disease susceptibility genes b) Pleiotropic effect of the disease causing genes c) Epistatic (Non-allelic) interaction between marker alleles and disease causing genes d) Linkage disequilibrium between marker loci and disease causing loci e) Effect of natural selection. Absence of association may indicate no role of the markers studied in the causation of the disease. The finding could be a false negative resulting obviously due to lack of power and does not refute the hypothesis of association. It should be noted that there is strong inverse relationship between the frequency of a given allele in a population and the number of probands needed to test its contribution to the phenotype particularly with those with low heritability expected like in hypertension (Sharma and Jeunemaitre, 2000). Contribution of rare alleles cannot be ruled out because of lack of power. By increasing the sample size the contribution of rare alleles can be brought to light. Negative results found in a population/ethnic group need not replicate in other populations/ ethnic groups since in different populations different genetic variants may either cause risk or protection to the condition. It is possible that in populations there may be more number of alleles causing susceptibility and less number of alleles counteracting the onset of hypertension. The analysis of intermediate demographic, biological or clinical phenotypes associated with hypertension also may help to subdivide the patient population into homogeneous groups and help in further analysis to achieve more precise results.

Association studies in general are widely pursued because i) The study is easy to conduct based on cases and controls since there is feasibility of collecting large number of samples from unrelated individuals without much difficulty, ii) It does no require any assumption about inheritance pattern, iii) Statistical power of the study is relatively large with the requirement of 1,000 samples to detect the relative risk of 1.5 for a given genotype iv) Candidate genes can be selected for conducting the study based on the physiology and biochemistry related to the disease process v) Small chromosomal region ranging between 3kb - 50kb in size is enough to detect linkage between the putative gene for the condition and marker genes vi) About 100,000 SNPs are enough to conduct genome wide association scans (GWAS). The only disadvantage in the study is the possibility of obtaining false positives because of population stratification and heterogeneity of the condition. Population stratification can be resolved by studying additional polymorphic loci located on different chromosomal regions and verifying for differences in the allele frequencies in the population. Unaffected family members can be used as controls to avoid the contribution of associated confounding factors. Other limitations of an association study are, it cannot detect genetic linkage of loosely linked loci. Since the approach can detect linkage only when the polymorphism and the disease susceptible gene loci are in linkage disequilibrium, the study can be conducted only by using candidate genes rather than the anonymous DNA markers. It should be remembered that lack of linkage disequilibrium between the loci studied does not necessarily imply absence of linkage. When the marker and disease causing mutation loci are located several million base pairs away, the linkage can still be detected using more powerful techniques to analyse the data.

### 3.2 Linkage analysis

Linkage is a phenomenon that deals with the tendency of any two traits (phenotypes, marker alleles etc.) to co-segregate among family members of extended pedigrees because the loci that harbor these genes are physically located on the same chromosome with defined distance. The strength of the linkage depends on the distance between the two loci which is represented as Centi Morgan (cM). cM is a unit that indicates the probability of recombination, consequence to the crossing over occurring between the two loci present on the same chromosome and is expressed as percentage. Greater the distance between the two loci, higher will be the frequency of crossing over leading to recombination occurring between the loci being tested. The analysis of linkage is carried out as **a) Two point analysis** where the distance between two loci i.e. disease causing locus and marker locus are assessed and **b) Multipoint analysis** where several loci presumably including the disease causing locus are tested for the distance between them. Multipoint linkage analysis helps to resolve the order of location of the candidate loci and the position of the disease causing locus in relation to them. It also identifies the candidate loci flanking the disease gene locus. Linkage between any two loci is computed as lod score based on which distance between any two loci can be determined that is expressed in terms of Centi Morgans or cM. Lod Score analysis can be **i) parametric or ii) non-parametric**. For parametric estimations a precise genetic model or inheritance pattern for the condition under study should be known along with the gene frequencies and penetrance of the genotype of the markers studied. With valid model it stands as a powerful method to scan and localize Mendelian disease genes within 20-Mb segment of the chromosome. In contrast, nonparametric method is applicable for conditions for which precise inheritance pattern can not be assigned like in hypertension. It is also referred as "model free" method and depends on identifying the alleles or chromosomal segments that are shared by affected individuals in a given family or population, resulting in resemblance/concordance for the two traits being studied.

#### 3.2.1 Parametric method

Parametric method is applied for localizing/mapping genes for the condition with definite model of inheritance. For the mapping of gene(s) for an autosomal dominant condition, conventional method of Linkage analysis is carried out based on the estimation of likelihood of the genetic marker loci (Table -4) which are polymorphic with high heterozygosity that co-segregate along with disease among the family members through generations. It is based on the estimation of Lod score (L) that is defined as the likelihood of obtaining a family/pedigree with the segregation of marker and disease loci together in the presence of certain amount of recombination between them (depicted as θ or x or r) and which varies from 0.0-0.5) compared to the likelihood of obtaining the same family/pedigree when there is no recombination between the marker and disease loci ( i.e. θ or x or r = 0.5) i.e. when the recombination frequency between the two loci is maximum which means that there is absence of linkage

Maximum likelihood estimate (mle) of recombination fraction (referred as θ or x or r) is used for determining linkage between two loci on a chromosome based on the relative probability ($P_R$) of having obtained the family. The $P_R$ is determined by calculating the probability of having obtained the various combinations of the particular trait under consideration on the assumption of there being no measurable linkage ($H_0$= No linkage; θ = 0.5) and comparing this with the probabilities based on a range of recombination fractions θ varying from 0.00 to 0.05, i.e.

$$P_R = \frac{P\left(\text{FAMILY, GIVEN } \theta = 0.0 \text{ to } 0.5\right)}{P\left(\text{FAMILY, GIVEN } \theta = 0.0 \text{ to } 0.5\right)}$$

$P_R$ is expressed as its logarithm. The $\log_{10}$ of PR is called as log of the odds or lod score. Lod score value of ≥ 3.0 indicates that the two loci tested are linked, value of 2.0 as evidence of strong linkage, value of 1.0 as evidence for tentative linkage and that of -2.0 absence of linkage. The Lod score of 2.0 that is suggestive of linkage can be further evaluated by analyzing more candidate/marker loci and by screening additional members of the family.

Large extended pedigrees with valid power are required for linkage estimations and gene mapping of an autosomal dominant condition. Extent of penetrance and population frequency of the gene in question and information on phase of linkage are required while using this method.

For an autosomal recessive condition where the parents of the affected individual are invariably blood relatives and heterozygous, different approach is adopted. It is ascertained whether both the alleles in the homozygous affected inbred individual are demonstrably transmitted representing copies of an allele present in a common recent ancestor. Such alleles in the homozygotes are referred as **"Identical by descent" or as IBD**. When the alleles carried by an individual are identical, but are not demonstrably inherited from the common ancestor implying that they have two different origins, then they are referred as **"Identical by state" or as IBS** (Fig- 4). Hence IBS analysis is based on population frequencies and not on Mendelian probabilities. The inbred individual is expected to be homozygous for the segment of the chromosome with some loci flanking to the disease causing locus. By examining the segregation of such flanking loci (haplotypes) from the phenotypically normal but heterozygous parents to the affected offspring, one can estimate whether the disease causing locus and the candidate loci are linked based on the extent of recombination occurring between the loci studied. For linkage analysis of an autosomal recessive condition less than 10 pedigrees with the affected offspring and parents are considered adequate. There is no need to have information on the extended pedigrees. This method is useful for identifying genes for rare autosomal recessive conditions where the parents are invariably blood relatives/cousins and hence have higher chance of inheriting same mutant allele from the common ancestor. Also the method is suitable to study the small families with affected children but phenotypically normal parents who could be the founder members in small communities. For very rare alleles, two independent origins of alleles in the homozygotes are unlikely and hence IBS will become similar to IBD. This is unlikely with common alleles where there is possibility of having identical genes in the homozygote individual that are not IBD in origin. For IBD analysis multiple loci with multiple alleles logically will yield better results. Both IBD and IBS methods can be used to estimate linkage by examining the shared chromosomal segments or alleles for nuclear families (sib-pair studies for concordance/resemblance for the two loci) or in the whole population descending from FOUNDER population. IBD method of analysis is more powerful but the study has to be conducted using large number of affected relatives specially the parents.

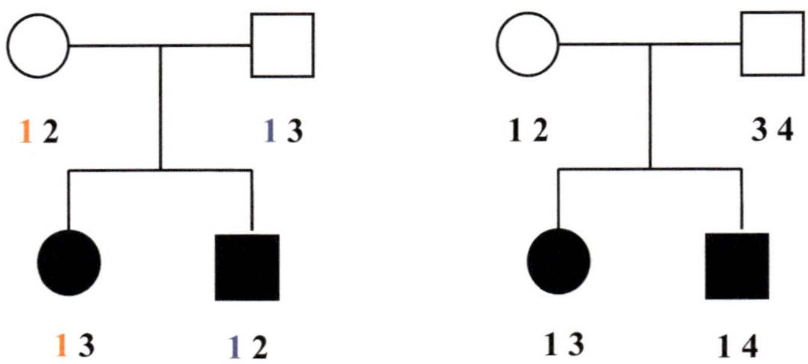


a. Identity by State for allele 1 b. Identity by Descent for allele 1

Fig. 4. Pedigrees showing transmission of alleles that are identical by state (IBS) and identical by descent (IBD).

### 3.2.2 Non-parametric or model free method

#### 3.2.2.1 Linkage disequilibrium (LD) mapping

Linkage disequilibrium may result due to a mutation in individual/individuals in the world population at some point in human history. These mutations would have segregated in the following generations along with the neighboring loci on the affected chromosome. In successive generations the recombination events scramble the alleles of the loci surrounding the disease causing gene. After several generations, the disease genes and the loci that are closely linked with it from the original chromosome remain together with no chances of further recombination between them. As a result the frequency of the two linked genes exceeds or will be in disequilibrium with that predicted by multiplying together their individual frequencies. This phenomenon referred as linkage disequilibrium (LD) is defined as non-random association of alleles at two or more loci present on the same or different chromosomes. The region of the chromosome with disease and linked neighbouring loci form a part of the unique haplotype on the ancestral chromosomal fragment and such segments help in mapping the genes more precisely for monogenic or multifactorial conditions. The distance between the loci mapped through LD estimations is often less than 1-2 cM, lower limit that can be resolved by conventional genetic linkage studies. Now several free soft wares like Haploview, PLINK, Gene hunter etc., are available to evaluate the level of LD, haplotype associations with disease causing genes, LD mapping, etc.,

LD mapping can be extended to nuclear families by performing **"Transmission Disequilibrium Test" (TDT).**

Transmission disequilibrium Test (TDT), is a family-based study to test whether a marker is associated with the disease. Families with parents and one or more children are used for the test. It is irrelevant if either parent is affected. or not. For this test parents who are heterozygotes for the marker allele are selected and number of offspring with the allele transmitted are compared with those without the transmission. The test is not affected by opulation stratification. An extended TDT test, ETDT is developed to handle data from multiallelic markers like microsatellites. The test can be applied when only one parent is available but the results may be biased. When both the parents are not available, sib-TDT can be applied. The test involves genotyping of the probands and their parents and selection of heterozygous parents (they may or may not be affected). If "a" is the frequency with which a heterozygous parent transmits the marker X1 to the affected offspring and "b" is the frequency with which the other allele X2 is transmitted, then TDT is tested by the statistic which follows chi-square distribution with 1 degree of freedom

$$\chi^2 = (a-b)^2 / (a+b)$$

### 3.2.3 Sib pair method

Identifying disease genes for hypertension following conventional Lod Score method is not possible because recombination events cannot be detected and mode of inheritance can not be easily modeled. Further the condition is age dependent and often parents of the patients will not be available for evaluation. Information on the offspring of the patients is also not useful as they would not have reached the mean age of expression of the condition in a given family and also the population from where the patients are drawn. Hence the family studies will have to be horizontal since reliable information about the disease can be obtained only from the sibs of the affected who will also be available for clinical and laboratory investigations.

Sib-pair analysis which is based on concordance or co-occurrence of marker alleles and disease susceptibility gene among pairs of sibs in multiple families is considered to be a more powerful method when compared to association studies as it does not depend on phenomenon of LD as is the case in the latter. It is a robust test for linkage analysis particularly when the inheritance model cannot be predicted. For any given locus parents carry four distinguishable alleles whose transmittance to the offspring can be traced. The sib pairs can be grouped into four categories where pairs may inherit both, one or none (2, 1, 0) of the alleles from the parents with the probability of 25%, 50% and 25% (expected ratio of 1:2:1, Fig-5).

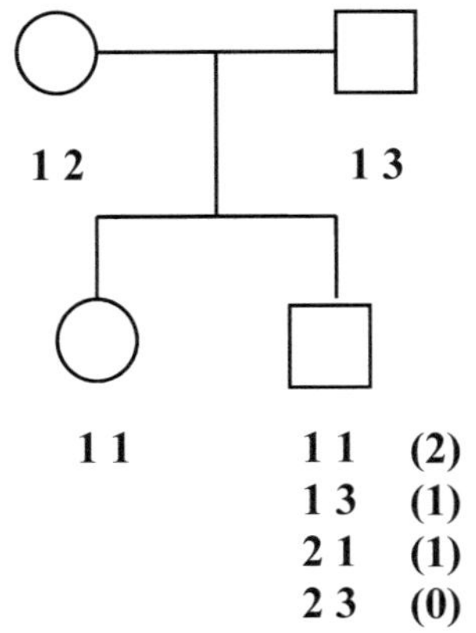


Fig. 5. Pedigree showing allele sharing between the sib pairs. Numbers in parenthesis denote the expected number of alleles shared by the sibs under Mendelian segregation.

If both the sibs in a pair are affected with a genetic disease then they are expected to share segment of the chromosome carrying disease locus. Affected sib pairs (**ASP**) are genotyped for the selected markers, and chromosomal region is searched where sharing by the sibs is above the expected 1:2:1 ratios of sharing 2, 1, and 0 alleles that are IBD. If the sib pairs are tested for IBS, the deviation from expected 1:2:1 ratio should be based on population frequencies. ASP analysis is a preferred method for studying conditions like hypertension since it is easy to identify and collect the sib pairs than the affected families and the analysis is model free. Multipoint analysis rather than the single point analysis is preferred since it offers opportunity to extract IBD information about alleles on the shared chromosomal segment **(haplotypes)** more efficiently. The lod scores computed in ASP analysis is indicated as NPL scores. The chromosomal segment identified by ASP analysis is usually large and not feasible for positional cloning. Yet the method stands as a main tool to search for the susceptibility genes for common non-Mendelian diseases like hypertension in view of its simple approach and robustness.

### 3.3 Epistatic interaction

Identification of interaction between genes and genes and environmental factors in explaining complexity of human diseases has been challenging. There is increasing evidence that epistasis or gene-gene (non-allelic) interactions play an important role in determining an individual's risk for developing complex diseases like hypertension (Williams teal, 2000; Tsai et al., 2003). New tools are developed to detect such synergistic interaction between alleles/genes arising due to epistatic phenomenon and modification of phenotypes like gradation in severity etc., due to additive effects or simple correlations between them. One such tool that is being used in interpreting the results for conditions like hypertension is **"multifactor dimensionality reduction (MDR) analysis"** - a nonparametric, model-free test alternative to logistic regression for detecting and characterizing nonlinear interactions among discrete genetic and environmental attributes.

MDR method combines attribute selection, attribute construction, classification, cross-validation and visualization to provide a comprehensive and powerful data mining approach to detect, characterize and interpret nonlinear interactions. The method is effective in detecting multilocus interactions among different polymorphisms of many different genes. It is a data reduction strategy (Ritchie et al, 2001) and in this model multilocus genotypes are pooled into high risk and low risk groups, effectively reducing the dimensionality of the genotype predictors from *N* dimensions to one dimension. The new one-dimensional multilocus genotype variable is evaluated for its ability to classify and predict disease status using cross-validation and permutation testing. MDR is advantageous program as it identifies evidence for high-order gene–gene interactions in the absence of any statistically significant independent main effects in simulated data (Ritchie et al, 2003).

## 4. Strategies

Several strategies are being used while searching for the genes causing susceptibility to essential hypertension such as i) Candidate gene approach, ii) Use of intermediary phenotypes, iii) Genome wide Association scans (GWAS) ,.iv) Animal models. Combination of two or more of these methods is also used.

### 4.1 Candidate gene approach

Candidate genes are defined as the genes that might be responsible for the onset of an inherited disorder. They are identified without reference to their chromosomal location. First a candidate chromosomal region is identified by linkage studies etc., and then the candidate genes from within the chromosomal region by verifying from the list of human genes available on the websites (NCBI; HuGe Literature Finder). From among the possible candidate genes thus identified, the one that is likely to be involved in biochemical, cellular or physiological functions contributing to the disease process are screened for mutation(s) that are likely to affect the structure, expression or function of the protein(s) associated with the disease development. The potential role of the candidate genes can be examined by using the methodologies adopted for linkage and association studies.

Now more than 350 candidate genes have been implicated for hypertension that involves several different biochemical pathways (HuGE Literature Finder). Candidate genes for hypertension are selected logically based on already established effect on cardiovascular and renal function and on the basis of known pathophysiology of hypertension. Genes for monogenic forms of hypertension identified by molecular pathology for cases mentioned in Table-3 also act as candidates to study essential hypertension. A variety of candidate genes have been identified for essential hypertension that are related to the RAAS pathway, sodium epithelial channel, adrenergic function, renal kallikrein-kinin system, alpha adducin, endothelial dysfunction, lipoprotein metabolism, hormone receptors, growth factors and many more (Table - 5).

Several studies from different ethnic groups demonstrated association of the potent candidate genes with essential hypertension that showed positive and negative results. These studies could not be replicated in different populations and the reason for the inconsistency in the results is mainly attributed to the heterogeneity in the samples studied leading to type 1 (false positive) and type 2 (false negative) errors. Lack of statistical power due to small samples screened and use of improper controls are among the other reasons.

| Genes | Chromosomal Location/Exons/ Introns | OMIM ID | SNP Associated with EHT | Population | Reference |
|---|---|---|---|---|---|
| **RENIN ANGIOTENSIN ALDOSTERONE SYSTEM** | | | | | |
| Angiotensinogen (*AGT*) | 1q42-q43; 5; 4 | 106150 | M235T | Caucasian | Jeunemaitre et al, 1992 Caulfield et al, 1994 |
| | | | | Japanese | Kamitani et al, 1994 |
| | | | | African Carribean | Caulfield et al, 1995 |
| | | | | Taiwanese | Chiang et al, 1997 |
| | | | | Chinese | Fang et al., 2010 |
| | | | T174M | Caucasian | Jeunemaitre et al (1992) |
| | | | | Canadian | Hegele et al (1994) |
| | | | -217G>A | African-Americans | Sudhir et al., 2002; Kumar et al., 2005 |
| | | | | Taiwanese | Wu et al., 2003; 2004; |
| | | | | Chinese | Liu et al., 2004 |
| | | | -20A>C | Taiwanese | Tsai et al (2003) |
| | | | -6G>A | -- | Jeunemaitre et al (1997), Wang et al (2002) Li et al (2004) |
| Renin (*REN*) | 1q32; 10; 9 | 179820 | 18-83>A | Japanese | Okura et al, 1993 |
| | | | | UAE Gulf | Frossard et al, 1998 |
| | | | -4021C>T & -3212C>T | US population of African origin | Frossord et al, 1999 |
| | | | -5312C>T | Whites | Niamh et al, 2007 |
| Angiotensin Converting Enzyme (*ACE*) | 7q23.3; 26; 25 | 106180 | Insertion/Deletion | African Americans | Duru et al, 1994 |
| | | | Polymorphism in intron 16 | Chinese | Jeng et al, 1997 ; Chiang et al , 1996 |
| | | | | Japanese | Nakno et al, 1998 |
| | | | | Malaysians | Vasudhevan et al, 2008 |
| | | | | South Indian | Bhavani et al, 2004 |
| Angiotensin II AT1 Receptor (*AGTR1*) | 3q21-25; 5; 4 | 106165 | 1166A>C | Whites | Bonnardeux et al , 1994 |

Table 5.

| | | | | | |
|---|---|---|---|---|---|
| Aldosterone Synthase (*CYP11B2*) | 8q21-22; 9; 8 | 124080 | -344C>T | French<br>Scottish<br>Japanese<br>South Indian Tamil | Brand et al, 1998<br>Davies et al, 1999<br>Matsubara et al, 2004<br>Rajan et al, 2010 |
| **SYMPATHETIC NERVOUS SYSTEM** | | | | | |
| β2 Adrenergic Receptor (*ADRA2B*) | 5q31-32; 1; 0 | 109690 | nine bp insertion/ deletion (I/D) in third intracellular loop | | Lockette et al, 1995<br>Wowern et al, 2004 |
| **ENDOTHELIAL DYFUNCTION** | | | | | |
| Endothelial Nitric Oxide Synthase (*NOS3*) | 7q36; 27; 26 | 163729 | CA repeat in intron 13 (33 repeat allele)<br>786T>C in 5′ flanking region<br>27 bp VNTR in intron 4 | Japanese<br>Canadian<br>South Indians<br>Chinese<br>South Indians | Nakayama et al, 1999<br>Hyndmann et al, 2002<br>Sushma et al, 2011<br>Wang et al, 2010<br>Sushma et al, 2009 |
| **ION TRANSPORT** | | | | | |
| β 3 subunits of G-protein (*GNβ3*) | 12p13; 11; 10 | 139130 | 825C>T | Caucasian | Schunkert et al 1998; Hengstenberg et al 2001 |
| **RENAL KALLIKREIN KININ SYSTEM** | | | | | |
| Kallikrein (*KLK1*) | 19q13.3; 5; 4 | 147910 | -58C>T<br>poly-guanine length polymorphism | African Americans<br>Chinese Han | Gainer et al, 2000<br>Hua et al, 2005 |
| **LIPID METABOLISM** | | | | | |
| Lipoprotein lipase (*LPL*) | 8p22; 10; 9 | 609708 | Intron 8 polymorphism<br>S447X | Chinese Han | Xin et al, 2005<br>Salah et al,2009 |
| **HARMONE RECEPTORS** | | | | | |
| Prostacyclin Synthase (*PNMT1*) | 17q; 10; 9 | 171190 | 9bp(CCGCCAGCC) repeat in promoter | Japanese | Naoharu et al, 1999 |

Table 5. (contd.) Some of the candidate genes reported with positive association for essential hypertension.

Selection of wrong candidate genes, location of the causative genes upstream or downstream from the candidate genes studied and discovery of new pathways for which candidates are not yet identified also contribute to the lack of success in some of the studies conducted.

### 4.1.1 Candidate genes associated with essential hypertension

*Table -5* depicts some of the positive associations reported between essential hypertension and polymorphic candidate genes related to various pathways.

**RAAS Pathway**: The RAAS is an important regulator of cardiovascular function and blood pressure (Soldner et al, 1996; Ferrario et al, 2006). It consists mainly of 4 genes including renin (*REN*) that converts angiotensinogen (*AGT*) to angiotensin I which is metabolized by angiotensin-converting enzyme (*ACE*) to form angiotensin II, which can act on angiotensin II type 1 receptors (*AGTR1*) to mediate blood pressure elevations by mechanisms including direct effects on vascular tone and indirect effects via alterations of renal function. Thus *REN, AGT, ACE* and *AGTR1* act synergistically on the phenotype of blood pressure. Each of the corresponding genes has several polymorphisms that can be associated with altered expression or function of the corresponding gene product. While each of these polymorphisms may potentially affect the regulation of blood pressure, most studies have focused on only few polymorphisms in each of these genes i.e., M235T, -217G>A, T174M, -20A>C of the *AGT* gene, an insertion deletion polymorphism involving 287bp in intron 16 of the *ACE* gene and the 1166A>G in the 3′ untranslated part of the *AGTR1* gene.

The 235T allele of the *AGT* gene is associated with a step wise increasing level of circulating angiotensinogen (gene dose response; Sethi et al, 2003). The positive correlation between polymorphism M235T and *AGT* plasma concentration has been observed in different populations (Mettimano et al, 2001; Agachan et al, 2003; Yan et al, 2006). Allele *AGT**235T shows linkage disequilibrium with a variant in the *AGT*-gene promoting area – a replacement of adenine by guanine in nucleotide 6 (-6A>G). It has been suggested that such mutation -6A>G interferes in the interaction of transcriptor factors with *AGT* promoter, thus influencing the gene transcription baseline rate. An increase in *AGT* gene expression may increase the production of angiotensin II by RAAS, thus resulting in the expansion of blood volume, which in turn would increase blood pressure. *AGT* gene is primarily expressed in the liver and adipose tissue, and C/EBPs family transcription factors play a crucial role in regulating expression of a number of genes in these tissues. A study conducted by Sudhir et al (2002) showed that recombinant glucocorticoid receptor (GR) and C/EBP family transcription factors bind strongly to nucleoside A compared with nucleoside G at -217 position of *AGT* promoter region resulting in increased transcriptional activity of -217A allele which may be involved in essential hypertension. Further, -20A>C located between the TATA box and the transcription initiation site is thought to modulate gene expression in a gender specific manner (Zhao et al, 1999). Tomoaki et al (1997) demonstrated that plasma angiotensinogen levels increase linearly with the number of -20C allele and that the subjects with the CC genotype are associated with the highest plasma levels of *AGT*. In in-vitro studies by Zhao et al (1999) the A-20C polymorphism has been found to influence basal transcription of angiotensinogen as well as stimulate transcription in response to receptor binding.

*ACE* insertion/deletion polymorphism was characterized in 1990 and studies have suggested that this polymorphism interferes in *ACE* serum concentration. DD Genotype individuals would have the highest *ACE* serum concentrations (Sayed et al, 2004; Mondry et al, 2005) and it is estimated that allele D would contribute with approximately half the variation of *ACE* plasma levels (O'Donnell et al, 1998). Significant gender differences were also reported in *ACE* I/D polymorphism. Compared with the II genotype, DD homozygosity was associated with higher risk of hypertension in studies conducted on women (Gu et al, 1994; Kiema et al, 1996; Sipahi et al, 2006) whereas two other population studies (O'Donnell et al, 1998, Higaki et al, 2000) found that the D allele was significantly associated with hypertension in men but not in women.

1166A>C at position 1166 in the 3' untranslated (UTR) region of the *AGTR1* gene was identified and was significantly shown to be associated with hypertension by Bonnardeux et al (1994). However it is not clear whether this polymorphism alters mRNA polyadenylation or destabilization signal. It is possible that this polymorphism may be in LD with a functional variant located elsewhere in the *AGTR1* gene or within a nearby gene that could explain the observed associations of this variant with cardio vascular phenotypes (Abdollahi et al, 2005). Therefore, this suppression may lead to the loss of cellular capabilities which protect against an excessive angiotensin II action (Grzegorz et al, 2002).

The renin-angiotensin system thus plays an important role in the inter-related hormonal mechanisms that regulate blood pressure and electrolyte/blood volume homeostasis. The RAS is activated when there is loss of blood volume or drop in blood pressure (such as in a hemorrhage) or low concentration of sodium in plasma, whereas factors that increase these parameters tend to suppress its function.

**Sympathetic Nervous System:** The sympathetic nervous system has also been implicated in the cardiovascular physiology and hypertension. The sympathetic nervous system primarily regulates the cardiovascular physiology by the release of catecholamines and activation of adrenergic receptors (AR). The human $\alpha_{2B}$-adrenoceptor is encoded by the *ADRA2B* gene located on chromosome 2q12 (Regan et al. 1988). A common variant form of the this gene which encodes a receptor protein with a insertion/deletion (I/D) of three glutamate residues located in the third intracellular loop of the receptor has been associated with EHT (Lockette et al.1995; Wowern et al. 2004).

**Endothelial Dysfunction:** Of the substances exerting their effect on vascular endothelium, Endothelial Nitric Oxide Synthase (*NOS3*) and Endothelin 1 (*END-1*) play an important role in regulating vascular tone. *NOS3* gene synthesizes Nitric Oxide (NO), which is a potent vasodilator and the *END-1* gene product acts as a strong vasoconstrictor called endothelin. Endothelin exerts its physiological functions via its receptors on the vascular smooth muscle cells (VSMC), by activating cascade of intracellular molecules that increase the calcium ion concentration, resulting in vasoconstriction. However, NO lowers these calcium ions to basal level, to relax the constricted VSMC, resulting in vasodilation. Thus, the delicate balance between the NO and endothelin is required for smooth functioning of vascular tone. Generation of reactive oxygen species (ROS), from various metabolic pathways, scavenge the NO, reducing the NO bioavailability leading to endothelial dysfunction. Polymorphisms in *NOS3* and *END-1* genes have been associated with hypertension in some populations.

**Lipid Metabolism:** Essential Hypertension has been frequently associated with serum lipid abnormalities. This suggests that there may be common underlying genetic determinants between blood pressure regulation and lipid metabolism. Membrane ion transport, which has been related to hypertension can be altered by lipid abnormalities and could have some involvement in the mechanisms that link high triglyceride concentrations and hypertension. *LPL* is thought to function as a "gate keeper" for fatty acid (FA) uptake into organs (Greenwood, 1985); however, patients with *LPL* deficiency have no obvious defect in adipose tissue. To date, only a few studies have explored the relation between the genetic variants near or in the *LPL* gene and blood pressure variation. Positive linkage or association has been described in some studies, which indicate that the *LPL* gene may be an important candidate for affecting the risk of Essential Hypertension or BP variation (Sass et al 2000; Pan et al 2000; Wu et al 1996; Chu et al, 2001).

**Ion Transporters:** G-Proteins are expressed in all cells of the human body and their main role is to translate signals from the cell surface into a cellular response. Polymorphisms in gene coding for G-protein subunits are expected to have a significant effect on the cardiovascular system. Hence, studying the genetic polymorphisms of the components of this system might give a new insight into the genetics of hypertension and may suggest novel downstream targets for therapy.

In addition to the above, a number of other candidate genes have been investigated as contributing to hypertension in case control studies including those involved in renal kallikrein-kinin system, growth factors (TGF-β), cytoskeletal proteins (alpha adducin), harmone receptors (*PNMT1*) etc.,

### 4.2 Intermediate phenotypes

Difficulties were observed in conducting linkage studies for hypertension using multigeneration families mainly due to the heterogeneity factor, lack of clear cut inheritance model and substantial environmental influence. It is now understood that "intermediate phenotypes" may help resolving this problem to certain extent (Dudley et al, 1992). It is based on the view that the individual genetic determinants having specific biochemical, physiological, demographic phenotype may contribute to the increase in blood pressure levels leading to hypertensive state. These phenotypes determined by single genetic loci, segregate in families following Mendelian inheritance. Such families showing intermediate phenotypes can be identified and the locus causing the phenotype may be detected. Since intermediate phenotypes are directly determined by the action of a particular gene, the influence of environment will also be less as compared to complex conditions like hypertension. Use of such phenotypes with greater heritability and early penetrance, have several advantages over the use of blood pressure phenotype as such. It helps, in identifying homogeneous group among the heterogeneous patient population like in hypertension. It also enables selection of large samples because even younger patients who are still normotensive can be identified with genetic risk for hypertension in the preclinical stage itself and this information will be useful for genetic analyses and at arriving better conclusions. In addition, it enables mapping of quantitative traits loci (QTL) in sibling pairs simultaneously testing for intermediate phenotypes. This approach is expanded to accommodate nuclear families of any size and also Transmission Disequilibrium Test (TDT; Timberlake et al., 2001). Ideal intermediate phenotype is

would be the best overall GWAS strategy. Alternate approach would be to use stringent LD threshold in genic regions to overcapture these regions.

The major limitation of GWAS study is the high expenditure involved to screen very large sample sizes, for getting small effects. A new approach to reduce the cost of GWAS is to conduct the study in stages/phases. In phase I a proportion of samples are genotyped for all the markers and then in phase II a proportion of these markers are genotyped in the remaining samples (Skol et al., 2007; Hastie et al., 2010).

The major issue in the study design of GWAS strategy is about the significance threshold. The conventional statistical significance determined using P-value threshold of 0.05 is not appropriate for GWAS because large number of tests performed increases the chance of type I error. Risch and Merikanga (1996) proposed new threshold levels now widely adopted which states that $P < 5 \times 10^{8}$ which corresponds to equivalent false positive rate of 5% for 1000 000 independent tests of association. The significance of the results can be tested using Bonferroni correction i.e. by dividing 0.05 threshold by the number of tests performed. Other issues are concerned to the evaluation of statistical power of the samples to obtain valid conclusion and resolution of problems related to population stratifications.

Initial studies of GWAS have reported positive results with identification of chromosomal regions harboring disease susceptible genes but they failed to replicate in other studies because of overestimate of effective size. Other reasons were technical errors, small sample sizes, poor choice of controls and population stratification leading to type I error or false positives. These defects are rectified to certain extent using relevant corrections. National Cancer Institute and National Human Genome Research Institute Working Group on Replication in Association Studies recommended the criteria for replication. More number of GWAS are performed in the past decade identifying susceptible regions on the human chromosomes for essential hypertension.

GWAS case-control study designs may not detect the rare variants causing blood pressure variations. From 1000 genome project - an open resource catalogue of human genetic variation run by international consortium intensely genotyped samples that can be obtained to study low frequency or rare variants for fine mapping of the regions of interest. The project aims to describe over 90% of genetic variation down to 1% minor allele frequency (MAF). Next generation deep sequencing technology also facilitates the detection of rare variants needed for fine mapping.

### 4.3.1 Genome wide scans for hypertension

Attempts to map the genes for hypertension picked in 1990s, initially based on the study of sib-pairs, affected families and by genome wide scanning for identifying the susceptible regions. One of the earliest studies by Lifton et al. (1991) reported that mean allele sharing at the locus of sodium-hydrogen antiporter (APNH) was not greater than expected from random assortment in 93 hypertensive sib pairs.

Wellcome Trust Case Control Consortium (WTCCC), Control for Heart and Aging Research in Genome Epidemiology (CHARGE), Family Blood Pressure Programme (FBPP), British Genetics of Hypertension (BRIGHT), Global Blood Pressure Genetics (Global BPgen), Amish Family Diabetes Study (AFDS) all have reported genome wide scans results on variants associated with variations in blood pressure and development of hypertension. Many of the initial studies could not meet the significance threshold criteria and in some chromosomal regions linkage were suggested. WTCCC reported the first genome-wide association scan results that captured 65 variants on 2000 hypertensives from unrelated participants of BRIGHT study (Caulfield et al., 2003). However the study did not reach the required statistical significance ($5 \times 10^{7}$) for hypertension and it was thought to be due to use of improper controls and inclusion of less number of tagged variants with large size effect (Barret et al., 2006; Padmanabhan et al., 2008). FBPP comprising four multi-centre network (GENOA, GenNet, HyperGen, SAPPHIRe) conducted studies on different ethnic groups with different selection criteria. None of the four centers reported significant results of the genome scan and the maximum lod score obtained was 2.96 showing linkage to diastolic blood pressure on the region of chromosome 1 in Caucasians (Thiel et al., 2003). BRIGHT study (Caulfield et al., 2003) with largest homogeneous Caucasian resource with 2010 sibling pairs in 1599 families found by locus counting method a principle locus for hypertension on 6q with lod score of 3.21 that attained genome wide significance and also evidence of linkage for three other loci located on 2q, 5q an 9q. These regions did not overlap with that reported in FBPP study. Xu et al, (1999) using 367 polymorphic markers studied 200,000 Chinese adults comprising sib-pairs (207 concordant, 258 high concordant and low concordant and parents) and showed that though no regions achieved 5% genome wide significance level, regions of chromosomes 3, 11, 15, 16 and 17 were linked with lod scores of >2.0. In their study on systolic blood pressure of 427 sibling pairs Krushkal et al., (1999) identified four regions on chromosome 2, 5, 6 and 15 with significant linkage. These regions include many potential candidate genes like phospholamban, dopamine receptor Type1A, Estrogen receptor calmodulin, sodium calcium exchanger etc. Pankaj Sharma et al, (2000) from a genome wide study identified the region on chromosome 11 to carry a new candidate gene for hypertension and suggested the need for replication of these results before attempting for positional cloning. Genome scan for blood pressure in Dutch dyslipidemic families (Hooman Allayee et al, 2001) showed suggestive evidence for linkage of diastolic BP to lipoprotein lipase gene locus on chromosome 8p. They also found evidence for linkage of systolic blood pressure to plasma apolipoprotein B levels to a locus on proximal chromosome 19p. Using 904 microsatellite markers, Kristjansson et al., (2002) reported linkage to chromosme18q with an allele sharing lod score of 4.60 in 490 hypertensive patients belonging to 120 extended Icelandic families. Rice et al., in the same year performed genome GWS using 509 markers on 317 black individuals from 114 families and 519 white individuals from 99 families that revealed evidence for linkage ($p<0.0023$) with base line blood pressure that replicated with other studies that located putative regions on 2p, 3p.3 and 12q.33. Von Woweren et al., (2003) from their study on genome scan of 91 Scandinavian families reported one region on chromosome 14 that reached significance threshold and 2 more regions that were suggestive of linkage with early onset hypertension. In 26 Utah pedigrees linkage of pulse pressure was suggested with loci on 8p and 12q regions by Camp et al., (2003). In a Large Chinese hypertensive kindred with 387 individuals Gong et al., (2003) found a locus on chromosome 12p that overlapped with the region containing the gene for autosomal dominant hypertension with type E brachydactyly that was mapped in large Turkish kindred (Schuster et al., 1996). This condition is now discovered as due to deletion, a reinsertion and inversion by Bahring et al., (2004). Charles et al., (2004) in their review of the GWS studies conducted earlier to 2004 summarized that all human chromosomes except for 13 and 20 have loci for blood pressure, hypertension or pre-eclampsia. Regions on chromosomes 1,2,8,11,12,15,16,18 and 19 were replicated in more than one study and there were 3 cytogenetic intervals on chromosome 2 (2p25.3-p16.3; 2p16.1-p12; 2q23.3-q24.3) harboring loci for blood pressure that was also replicated in more than one study. Caulfield et al, (2003) associated with British Genetics of hypertension (BRIGHT) programme, phenotyped 2010 affected sibling pairs drawn from 1599 severely hypertensive families completed 10 Centi Morgan genome wide scan. Their conclusion was that human essential hypertension has an oligogenic element (with a few genes involved in the determination of the trait) possibly superimposed on more genetic effects, and that several genes may be tractable to a positional cloning strategy. In a large sample of 2959 individuals from 500 families from NHLBI, Hunt et al., (2002) identified five regions with lod score suggestive of linkage of hypertension with loci on chromosomes 1,7,12 and 15 and evidence of best linkage with a locus on chromosome 6 with systolic blood pressure. In a study of 177 Australian Caucasian hypertensive sib-pairs, Rutherford et al, (2004) showed significant excess allele sharing of D18S61 marker. At this region adenylate cyclase-activating polypeptide gene-1 (ADCYAP1) involved in vasodilation shows association with hypertension. As a complement to linkage and association studies Zhu et al, (2005) carried out admixture mapping using genome scan micro satellite markers among African Americans participating in the Lung, and Blood Institute's Family Blood Pressure Programme. Using 269 microsatellite markers the authors concluded that chromosome 6q24 and chromosome 21q21 may contain genes influencing risk for hypertension in African Americans. Kamide et al, (2005) genotyped (796 hypertensives and 1084 normotensives) 47 polymorphisms in 14 genes lying between nucleotide 8,845,292 and 11,946,689 which includes D2S2278 and D2S168 loci on chromosome 2 and concluded that GREB1 and HPCAL1 are the candidates for hypertension susceptibility. Chen et al, (2005) conducted autosomal genome scan in 775 white siblings and found suggestive linkage for total area of systolic and diastolic blood pressure on chromosome 4 and diastolic blood pressure incremental area on chromosome 18. In these regions candidate genes for hypertension like alpha and beta adducin, sodium bicarbonate co-transporter and G-protein coupled receptor kinase 4 are located.

In the recent past novel regions in the genome are localized for blood pressure and hypertension employing large number of samples and SNP markers. Org et al. (2009) studied 395,102 SNPs in 1,644 individuals from the KORA S3 cohort study, but could not find the results reaching significance level of $p \leq 10^{-8}$ for blood pressure or hypertension. The authors replicated 80 strongest associations with blood pressure and hypertension in two other European cohorts and identified a variant *CDH13* (cadherin 13 preprotein) locus (rs11646213) to be associated with hypertension and blood pressure. Newton-Chech et al., (2009) in the GBP consortium performed largest GWAS study considering blood pressure as continuous trait. They identified association of SBP with three loci (*MTHFR, CYP17A1 and PLCD)*, DBP with 5 loci (*FGF5, C10orf107, SH2B3, CYP1A2 and ZNF 652)* at genome wide significance levels ($p<5 \times 10^{-8}$). They also found association of 8 variants with hypertension in the same direction as blood pressure. Levy et al., (2009) performed for the CHARGE group consortium a metanalysis of in 29,136 participants from six different cohort studies and with the population of 34,443 from GBP-gen. Their attempt revealed many novel variants for DBP and SBP with genome wide level of significance. Use of meta-analysis in the GWAS studies helps in achieving near complete genetic coverage. Meta-analysis studies by Global BPgen and CHARGE consortia have taken the number of loci to a total of 8 for systolic, 11 for diastolic pressure and 6 for hypertension (Sajjad Rafiq et al., 2010). Yet more attempts world wide are needed to fix the genes responsible for the pathogenesis of elevated blood pressure in terms of the role played by the genes, epidemiology factors and interaction between them.

### 4.4 Comparative genomics

The approach of analyzing genetic basis of any disease is through comparative genomics where data from animal studies are used to extrapolate the interpretations about the mechanisms to human conditions. For human hypertension animal models offer advantages because mating and environment can be controlled. Crossing of inbred strains resolves the problem of heterogeneity. Differences in many genes like renin, $Na+/K+$ ATPase α subunit have been reported between hypertensive and normotensive strains of rats. Genetic polymorphisms in renin gene of Dahl rats are found to co-segregate with blood pressure in a dose dependent way supporting the involvement of the genes in the regulation of blood pressure. Similar results on co-segregation was not found for the alleles of $Na+/K+$ ATPase α subunit. Data from the studies on hypertensive rodent strains indicated that genes on human chromosome 17 are responsible for human hypertension. Two closely linked microsatellite markers D17S183 and D17S934 which are close to *ACE* gene locus were significantly associated with essential hypertension (Julier et al., 1997). The region on human chromosome 17 is syntenic to rat chromosome 10. There were also studies refuting significant linkage of hypertension to chromosome 17. Study on the translation of QTLs between rats and humans predicted 26 chromosomal regions in the human genome that are likely to contain genes controlling hypertension (Stoll et al., 2000). Many other studies on animal models helped in furthering the knowledge of conserved genomic region involved in the regulation of blood pressure and progress in this direction will improve the status of knowledge of mechanisms underlying human hypertension.

## 5. Future scope for hypertension management

Despite the fact that effective drugs are available, only about one out of three people has their blood pressure successfully controlled, and the blame is attributed to the undesirable side effects and the poor oral drug compliance. Keeping in mind the increasing incidence of hypertension and the patients inconsistency for the polypharmacy, immunization against renin and the angiotensins, although with less success, are being attempted. More recently, immunization against angiotensin-I with PMD-3117 vaccine, angiotensin-II with CYT006-AngQb vaccine and targeting angiotensin-II type 1A receptor with ATR12181 vaccine have provided optimism in the development of a hypertension vaccine (Pandey et al., 2009). Ang Qb vaccine has proved to become the first vaccine ever to lower (-9/-4 mm Hg) blood pressure in human beings (Pandey et al., 2009). Vaccine could induce long lasting effects with a dosing interval of months, increasing patient acceptability and compliance and thus a better control of high blood pressure. This approach has a major advantage as it can reduce the usage of medication by the patients. The results of this new biotherapy for hypertension are intriguing and promising, and vaccination for hypertension may turn out to be very useful in many patients. The impact of this treatment can revolutionarise the management of essential hypertension- a disease that poses public health problems.

## 6. Glossary

**Bonferroni correction**: is a multiple-comparison correction used when several dependent or independent statistical tests are performed simultaneously

**Candidate gene study**: A study of specifically selected (candidate) genes in which variation is hypothesized to influence the risk of a disease.

**Diastolic blood Pressure**: represents the minimum pressure in the arteries when the heart is at rest.

**Dominant Model**: This model specifically tests the association of having at least one minor allele say 'a' (either Aa or aa) versus not having it at all (AA).

**Epistatic Interaction**: An epistatic interaction between two genes (non allelic) occurs when the phenotypic impact of one gene depends on another gene, often exposing a functional association between them.

**Hardy-Weinburg equilibrium**: An idealised state in which gene and genotypic frequencies in populatioin do not change from generation to generation in the absence of migration, genetic drift, selection

**Haplotype**: is a set of closely linked genetic markers present on one chromosome of the homologous pair which tend to be inherited together and not easily separable by recombination.

**Heretability**: Heritability is the proportion of variation in a phenotype (trait, characteristic or physical feature) that is thought to be caused by genetic variation among individuals. It is a measure of the degree to which the variance in the distribution of a phenotype is due to genetic causes. In the broad sense it is measured by the total genetic variance divided by the total phenotypic variance. In the narrow sense it is measured by the genetic variance due to additive genes divided by the total phenotypic variance.

**Hypertension (HTN)**: or high blood pressure is a cardiac chronic medical condition in which the systemic arterial blood pressure is elevated above the normal levels

**Linkage**: Linkage is the tendency of phenotypes marker alleles etc., to co-segregate in a pedigree because their determinants lie close together on a given chromosome.

**Linkage Disequilibrium**: Non random association of the gens present on the same or any other chromosome.

**Odds Ratio:** is one of a range of statistics used to assess the risk of a particular outcome (or disease) if a certain factor (or exposure) is present.

**Pleiotropy:** Pleiotropy is the phenomenon whereby a single gene has multiple consequences in numerous tissues. Pleiotropic effects stem from both normal and mutated genes, but those caused by mutations are often more noticeable and easier to study.

**Polymorphism**: Genetic Polymorphism is the presence of more than two allelic forms at a given locus in such frequencies that the rarest of them is not just due to recurring mutations but is due to a phenomenon called "polymorphisms". The frequency of the rarest allele/form as a rule is taken as > 1.0%

**Recessive Model**: This model specifically tests the association of having the minor allele "a" as both alleles (aa) versus having at least one major allele d (Aa or AA).

**Systolic Blood Pressure**: represents the maximum pressure exerted in the arteries when the heart contracts.

**Tagged SNPs**: are representative single nucleotide polymorphisms (SNP) in a region of the genome with high linkage disequilibrium

**Transmission disequilibrium test (TDT)**: A family-based study to compare the proportion of alleles transmitted (or inherited) from a heterozygous parent to an affected child. Any significant deviation from 0.50 in transmission ratio implies an association.

## 7. References

Abdollahi MR, Gaunt TR, Syddall HE, Cooper C, Phillips DI, Ye S, Day IN.. Angiotensin II type I receptor gene polymorphism: anthropometric and metabolic syndrome traits. J Med Genet. 2005; 42(5):396-401.

Agachan B, Isbir T, Yilmaz H, Akoglu E. Angiotensin converting enzyme I/D, angiotensinogen T174M-M235T and angiotensin II type 1 receptor A1166C gene polymorphism in Turkish hypertensive patients. Exp Mol Med. 2003; 35 (6): 545-9.

Appel U, Moore TJ, Obarzanek E, Vollmer WM, Svetkey LP, Sacks FM et al. A Clinical Trial of the Effects of Dietary Patterns on Blood Pressure. N Engl J Med. 1997; 336: 1117-1124.

Bahring, S., Rauch, A., Toka, O., Schroeder, C., Hesse, C., Siedler, H., Fesus, G., Haefeli, W.E., Busjahn, A., Aydin, A. et al. Autosomal-dominant hypertension with type E brachydactyly is caused by rearrangement on the short arm of chromosome 12.Hypertension, 2004; 43, 471–476.

Barrett, J. C., & Cardon, L. R. Evaluating coverage of genome-wide association studies. Nature Genetics, 2006; 38(6), 659–662.

Bhavani B A, Padma T., Sastry B.K.S. and Krishna Reddy N. Gender specific association of Insertional/Deletion Polymorphisms of the Human Angiotensin Converting Enzyme Gene with Essential hypertension Int J Hum Genet, 2004 4:207-213.

Biron P, Mongeau JG, Bertrand D: Familial aggregation of blood pressure in 588 adopted children. *Can Med Assoc J. 1976;* 115:773–774.

Biron, P., Mongeau, J. G. and Bertrand, D. Familial aggregation of blood pressure in 558 adopted children. Can. Med. Assoc. J. 1976; 115, 773–774.

Bonnardeaux, A., Davies, E., Jeunemaitre, X., Fe´ry, I., Charru, A., Clauser, E., Tiret, L., Cambien, F., Corvol, P., Soubrier, F. Angiotensin II type-1 receptor gene polymorphisms in human essential hypertension. Hypertension. 1994; 24:63–69.

Brand E, Chatelain N, Mulatero P, Féry I, Curnow K, Jeunemaitre X, et al. Structural analysis and evaluation of the aldosterone synthase gene in hypertension. Hypertension 1998; 32 : 198-204.

Camp, N.J., Hopkins, P.N., Hasstedt, S.J., Coon, H., Malhotra, A.,Cawthon, R.M. and Hunt, S.C. Genome-wide multipoint parametric linkage analysis of pulse pressure in large, extended utah pedigrees. Hypertension, 2003; 42, 322–328.

Charles A. Mein, Mark J Caulfield, Richard J Dobson, Patricia B Munroe Genetics of essential hypertension Hum Mol Genet 2004; 13(1) 169-175.

Caulfield M, Lavender P, Farral M, Munroe P, Lawson M, Turner P, Clark AJ. Linkage of the angiotensinogen gene to essential hypertension. N Engl J Med. 1994; 330:1629-1633.

Caulfield M, Lavender P, Newell-Price J, Farral M, Kamdar S, Daniel H, Lawson M, De Freitas P, Fogarty P, Clark AJ. Linkage of the angiotensinogen gene locus to human essential hypertension in African Caribbeans. J Clin Inves.1995; 96:687-692.

Caulfield M, Munroe P, Pembroke J, et al. Genome-wide mapping of human loci for essential hypertension. Lancet 2003; 361:2118–2123.

Chen W., Shengxu Li., Sathanur R. Srinivasan ., Eric Boerwinkle and Gerald S. Berenson. Autosomal genome scan for loci linked to blood pressure levels and trends since childhood: The Bogalusa Heart Study. Hypertension 2005; 45:954-959

Chiang FT, Chern TH, Lai ZP, Tseng CD, Hsu KL, Lo HM, Tseng YZ. Age and Gender Dependent Association of the Angiotensin-Converting Enzyme Gene with the Essential Hypertension in a Chinese Population. J Hum Hypertens. 1996; 10:823-826.

Chiang FT, Hsu KL, Tseng CD, Hsiao WH, Lo HM, Chern TH, Tseng YZ. Molecular variant M235T of the angiotensinogen gene is associated with essential hypertension in Taiwanese. J Hypertens.1997; 15:607-611.

Chu S, Zhu D, Xiong M, Wang GL, Jin L: Linkage analysis of candidate genes for glucose and lipid metabolism with essential hypertension. Natl Med J China 2001; 81: 20–22.

David B. Goldstein and Michael E. Weale. Population genomics: Linkage disequilibrium holds the key. Cell Biology.2001; 11:R576-R579.

Davies E, Holloway CD, Ingram MC, Inglis GC, Friel EC, Morrison C, et al. Aldosterone excretion rate and blood pressure in essential hypertension are related to polymorphic differences in the aldosterone synthase gene CYP11B2. Hypertension 1999; 33 : 703-7.

Doris A Peter Hypertension Genetics, Single nucleotide polymorphisms and the common disease: Common variant hypothesis Hypertension 2002; 39:323

Dudley C.R.K, Luis A Giuffra, Stephen T. Reeders Identifying genetic determinants in human essential hypertension J Am Soc Nephrol 1992; 3:S2-S8.

Duru K, Farrow S, Wang J, Lockbetteb W, Kurtz T. Frequency of Deletion Polymorphism in the Gene for Angiotensin Converting Enzyme is Increased in African-Americans with Hypertension. Am J Hypertens. 1994; 7:759-762.

Fang, Yu-Jing; Deng, Han-Bing; Thomas, G Neil; Tzang, Chi H; Li, Cai-Xia; Xu, Zong-Li; Yang, Mengsu; Tomlinson, Brian. Linkage of angiotensinogen gene polymorphisms with hypertension in a sibling study of Hong Kong Chinese. Journal of Hypertension. 2010; 28:1203-1209.

Feinleib m, Garrison RJ, Fabsitz R, Christian JC, Hrubec Z, Borhani NO, et al The NHLBI twin study of cardiovascular disease risk factors: methodology and summary of results Am J Epidemiol 1977; 106 284-95.

Ferrario CM, Strawn WB: Role of the renin-angiotensin-aldosterone system and proinflammatory mediators in cardiovascular disease. Am J Cardiol 2006, 98:121-128.

Frossard PM, Kane JP, Malloy MJ, Bener A. Renin gene Mbo I dimorphism is a discriminator for hypertension in hyperlipidaemic subjects. Hypertens Res. 1999; 22:285-289.

Frossard PM, Lestringant GG, Elshahat YI, John A, Obineche EN. An MboI two-allele polymorphism may implicate the human renin gene in primary hypertension. Hypertens Res. 1998; 21:221-225.

Gainer JV, Brown NJ, Bachvarova M, Bastien L, Maltais I, Marceau F, Bachvarov DR Altered frequency of a promoter polymorphism of the kinin B2 receptor gene in hypertensive African-Americans. Am J Hypertens. 2000 Dec;13(12):1268-73.

Gong M., Zhang H., Schulz H., Lee Y.A., Sun K., Baharing S., Luft F.C., Nurnberg P., Reis A., Rohde K., Genome-wide linkage reveals a locus for human essential (primary) hypertension on chromosome 12p. Human Molecular genetics, 12: 1273-1277

Greenwood, M. R. C. The relationship of enzyme activity to feeding behavior in rats: Lipoprotein lipase as the metabolic gatekeeper. Int. J. Obes. 1985; 9: 67–70.

Grzegorz Dzida, Michał Gałęziok, Tomasz Kraczkowski, Jacek Sobstyl, Patrycja Golon-Siekierska, Andrzej Puźniak, Andrzej Biłan, Jerzy Mosiewicz, Janusz Hanzlik C1166 variant of the angiotensin II receptor type 1 gene and myocardial infarction - risk factor or a chance of survival? Cardiol Pol. 2002; 56(2):138-146.

Gu X, Spaepen M, Guo C, Fagard R, Amery A, Lijnen P, Cassiman J.J. Lack of association between the ID polymorphism of the angiotensin-converting enzyme gene and essential hypertension in a Belgian population. J. Hum. Hypertens. 1994; 8:683–685.

Hastie C E, Padmanabhan S, Dominiczak A F Genome-Wide Association Studies of Hypertension:Light at the End of the Tunnel International Journal of Hypertension 2010, Article ID 509581, 10 pages

Hegele RA, Brunt JH, Connelly PW. A polymorphism of the angiotensinogen gene associated with variation in blood pressure in a genetic isolate. Circulation. 1994; 90: 2207–2212.

Hengstenberg C, Schunkert H, Mayer B, Doring A, Lowel H, Hense HW,Fischer M, Riegger GA, Holmer SR. Association between a polymorphism in the G protein _3 subunit gene (GNB3) with arterial hypertension but not with myocardial infarction. Cardiovasc Res. 2001;49: 820–827.

Higaki J, Baba S, Katsuya T, Sato N, Ishikawa K, Mannami T, Ogata J, Ogihara T. Deletion allele of angiotensin-converting enzyme gene increases risk of essential hypertension in Japanese men. Circulation. 2000; 101:2060–2065.

Hooman Allayee, Tjerk W.A. deBruin, K.Michelle Dominguez, Li S.-C. Cheng, Eli Ipp, Rita M. Cantor, Kelly L. Krass, Eric T.P. Keulen, Bradley E. Aouizerat, Aldons J. Lusis, Jerome I. Rotter. Genome Scan for Blood Pressure in Dutch Dyslipidemic Families Reveals Linkage to a Locus on Chromosome 4p. Hypertension. 2001; 38:773-778.

Hopkins PN, Lifton RP, Hollenberg NK, Jeunemaitre X, Hallouin MC, Skuppin J, Williams CS, Dluhy RG, Lalouel JM, Williams RR, Williams GH. Blunted renal vascular response to angiotensin II is associated with a common variant of the angiotensinogen gene and obesity. J Hypertens 1996; 14: 199−207.

Hua H, Zhou S, Liu Y, Wang Z, Wan C, Li H, Chen C, Li G, Zeng C, Chen L, Chao L, Chao J Relationship between the regulatory region polymorphism of human tissue kallikrein gene and essential hypertension. Journal of human hypertension 2005 Sep 19 (9): 715-21.

Hunt SC, Ellison RC, Atwood LD, Pankow JS, Province MA, Leppert MF . Genome scans for blood pressure and hypertension: the National Heart, Lung, and Blood Institute Family Heart Study. Hypertension 2002 : 40:1-6.

Hyndmann ME, Howard G, Subodh V, Bridge PJ, Edworthy S, Jones C, Lonn E, Charbonneau F, Anderson T.The T-786 C Mutation in Endothelial Nitric Oxide Synthase is associated with Hypertension. Hypertension, 2002; 39: 919-922.

Jeng JR, Harn HJ, Jeng CI, Yueh KC, Shieh SM. Angiotensin I converting enzyme gene polymorphism in Chinese patients with hypertension. Amh J Hypertens. 1997; 10:558-61.

Jeunemaitre X, Soubrier F, Kotelevtsev YV, Lifton RP, Williams CS, Charru A, Hunt SC, Hopkins PN, Williams RR, Lalouel JM, et al. Molecular basis of human hypertension: role of angiotensinogen. Cell. 1992; 71(1):169-80.

Jeunemaitre X, Ituro Inoue, Christopher Williams, Anne Charru, Jean Tichet, Mike Powers, Arya Mitra Sharma, Anne-Paule Gimenez-Roqueplo, Akira Hata, Pierre Corvol and Jean-Marc Lalouel· Haplotypes of Angiotensinogen in Essential Hypertension. The American Journal of Human Genetics.1997; 60: Issue 6, 1448-1460.

Jorgenson E and Witte J S, "A gene-centric approach to genome-wide association studies," Nature Reviews Genetics, 2006 7(11), pp. 885–891.

Julier C et al., Genetic susceptibility for human familial essential hypertension in a region of homology with blood pressure linkage on human chromosome 17, Hum Mol.Genet.1997:6 (12), 2077-2085

Kamide K, Kokubo Y, Yang J, Tanaka C, Hanada H, Takiuchi S, Inamoto N, Banno M, Kawano Y, Okayama A, Tomoike H, Miyata T. Hypertension susceptibility genes on chromosome 2p24-p25 in a general Japanease population. Journal of hypertension.2005; 23(5):955-60.

Kamitani A, Rakugi H, Higaki J, Yi Z, Mikami H, Miki T, Ogihara T. Association analysis of a polymorphism of the angiotensinogen gene with essential hypertension in Japanese. J Hum Hypertens. 1994; 8(7):521-4.

Kato N, Genetic Analysis in Human Hypertension, Hypertens Res 2002, 25: 319-327.

Kearney PM, Whelton M, Reynolds K, et al. Global burden of hypertension: analysis of worldwide data. Lancet. 2005; 365:217-223.

Kiema T.R, Kauma H, Rantala A.O, Lilja M, Reunanen A, Kesaniemi Y.A, Savolainen M.J. Variation at angiotensinconverting enzyme gene and angiotensinogen gene loci in relation to blood pressure. Hypertension. 1996; 28:1070–1075.

Kristjansson K, Manolescu A, Kristinsson A, et al. Linkage of essential hypertension to chromosome 18q. Hypertension 2002; 39:1044–1049.

Krushkal J, Ferrell R, Mockrin SC, Turner ST, Sing CF, Boerwinkle E. Genome-wide linkage analyses of systolic blood pressure using highly discordant siblings. Circulation 1999; 99:1407–1410.

Kumar A, Li Y, Patil S, Jain S. A haplotype of the angiotensinogen gene is associated with hypertension in african americans. Clin Exp Pharmacol Physiol. 2005; 32(5-6):495-502.

Levy D, Ehret G B, Rice K, et al., "Genome-wide association study of blood pressure and hypertension," Nature Genetics, 2009 41(6), pp. 677–687.

Lifton RP, Gharavi AG, Geller DS. Molecular Mechanisms of Human Hypertension. Cell. 2001; 104: 545-556.

Lifton, R. P.; Hunt, S. C.; Williams, R. R.; Pouyssegur, J.; Lalouel, J. M. : Exclusion of the Na(+)-H+ antiporter as a candidate gene in human essential hypertension. *Hypertension* 1991; 17: 8-14.

Litchfield WR; Steven C. Hunt; Xavier Jeunemaitre; Naomi D. L. Fisher; Paul N. Hopkins; Roger R. Williams; Pierre Corvol; ; Gordon H. Williams. Increased urinary free cortisol: a potential intermediate phenotype of essential hypertension. Hypertension. 1998; 31: 569–574.

Liu Y, Jin W, Jiang ZW, Zhang KX, Sheng HH, Jin L, Sheng YY, Huang W, Yu JD. Relationship between six single nucleotide polymorphisms of angiotensinogen gene and essential hypertension. Zhonghua Yi Xue Yi Chuan Xue Za Zhi. 2004; 21(2):116-9.

Lockette W, Ghosh S, Farrow S, MacKenzie S, Baker S, Miles P, Schork A, Cadaret L.. Alpha 2-adrenergic receptor gene polymorphism and hypertension in blacks. Am J Hypertens. 1995; 8(4):390-4.

Longini IM, Higgins MW, Minton PC, Moll PP, Keller JB: Environmental and genetic sources of familial aggregation of blood pressure in Tecumseh, Michigan. *Am J Epidemiol. 1984;* 120:131–144.

Matsubara M, Sato T, Nishimura T, Suzuki M, Kikuya M, Metoki H, et al. CYP11B2 polymorphisms and home blood pressure in a population-based cohort in Japanese: the Ohasama study. Hypertens Res 2004; 27: 1-6.

Mettimano M, Launi A, Migneco A, Specchia ML, Romano-Spica V, Savi L. Angiotensin related genes involved in essential hypertension: allelic distribuition in an Italian. Ital Heart J. 2001; 2 (8): 289-93.

Mimura G Study of twins with hypertension Singapore Medical Journal 1973; 14(3)278-281

Mondry A, Loh M, Liu P, Zhu AL, Nagel M. Polymorphism of the insertion/deletion ACE and M235T AGT genes and hypertension: surprising new findings and meta-analysis of data. BMC Nephrol. 2005; 6 (1): 1-11.

Nakayama M, Yasue H, Yashimura M, Shimasaki Y,Kugiyama K, Ogawa H, et al. T786C mutation in the 5´-flanking region of the endothelial nitric oxide synthase Gene is associated with coronary spasm. Circulation 1999; 99: 2864 70.

Nakno Y, Oshima T, Hiraga H, Matsuure H, Kajiyama G, Kambe M. Genotype of Angiotensin I Converting Enzyme Gene is a Risk Factor for Early Onset of Essential Hypertension in Japanese. J Lab Clin Med. 1998; 131(6):502-6.

Naoharu Iwai, MD; Tomohiro Katsuya, MD; Kazuhiko Ishikawa, MD; Toshifumi Mannami, MD; Jun Ogata, MD; Jitsuo Higaki, MD; Toshio Ogihara, MD; Tadashi Tanabe, PhD; Shunroku Baba, MD Human Prostacyclin Synthase Gene and Hypertension The Suita Study Circulation 1999; 100; 2231-2236.

Neel JV, Weder AB, Julius S. Type II diabetes, essential hypertension and obesity as syndromes of impaired genetic homeostasis. The thrifty genotype hypothesis enters the 21st century. Perspect Biol med. 1998; 42:44-74

Newton-Cheh C, Johnson T, Gateva V, et al., "Genome-wide association study identifies eight loci associated with blood pressure," Nature Genetics, 2009; 41(6), pp. 666–676.

Niamh Moore; Patrick Dicker; John K. O'Brien; Milos Stojanovic; Ronán M. Conroy; Achim Treumann; Eoin T. O'Brien; Desmond Fitzgerald; Denis Shields; Alice V. Stanton.

Renin Gene Polymorphisms and Haplotypes, Blood Pressure, and Responses to Renin-Angiotensin System Inhibition *Hypertension.* 2007; 50:340.

North KE, Howard BV, Welty TK, Best LG, Lee ET, Yeh JL, Fabsitz RR, Roman MJ, MacCluer JW . Genetic and environmental contributions to cardiovascular disease risk in American Indians: the strong heart family study. Am J Epidemiol: 2003 157: 303-14.

O'Donnell CJ, Lindpaintner K, Larson MG, Rao VS, Ordovas JM, Schaefer EJ, et al. Evidence for association and genetic linkage of the angiotensin-converting enzyme locus with hypertension and blood pressure in men but not women in the Framingham Heart Study. Circulation. 1998; 97: 1766-72.

Okura T, Kitami Y, Hiwada K. Restriction fragment length polymorphisms of the human renin gene: association study with a family history of essential hypertension. J Hum Hypertens. 1993; 7461.□:457.

Org E, Eyheramendy S, Juhanson P, et al., "Genome-wide scan identifies CDH13 as a novel susceptibility locus contributing to blood pressure determination in two European populations," Human Molecular Genetics, 2009; 18 (12) , pp.2288–2296.

Oscar A, Oparil C and Oparil S. Essential Hypertension: Part I: Definition and etiology. Circulation 2000; 101:329-335.

Padmanabhan S, Melander O, Hastie C, et al., "Hypertension and genome-wide association studies: combining high fidelity phenotyping and hypercontrols," Journal of Hypertension, 2008 26(7) pp. 1275–1281.

Pan WH, Chen JW, Fann C, Jou YS, Wu SY: Linkage analysis with candidate genes: the Taiwan young-onset hypertension genetic study. Hum Genet 2000; 107: 210–215.

Pandey R, Quan WY, Hong F, Jie SL. Vaccine for hypertension: modulating the renin angiotensin system. International journal of cardiology. 2009; 134(2):160-8.

Pankaj Sharma, Jennei Fatibene, Franco, Haiyan Jia, Sue Monteith, Chrysothemis Brown, David Clayton, Kevin O'Shaughnessy, Morris J. Brown. Hypertension. A Genome-Wide Search For Susceptibility Loci to Human Essential Hypertension 2002; 35:1291-1296.

Pickering G. The inheritance of arterial pressure. In: Stamler J., Stanley R., Pullman T. (Editors). The Epidemiology of Hypertension. 1967; 18.

Platt R. The Influence of Heredity, in: Stamler, J; Stamler, R; Pullman, TN (eds): The Epidemiology of Hypertension. Grune & Stratton, New York, 1967, 9-17.

Rajan S, Ramu P, Umamaheswaran G, Adithan Association of aldosterone synthase (CYP11B2 C-344T) gene polymorphism & susceptibility to essential hypertension in a south Indian Tamil population. Indian J Med Res 132, October 2010, pp 379-385.

Regan JW, Kobilka TS, Yang-Feng TL, Caron MG, Lefkowitz RJ, Kobilka BK. Cloning and expression of a human kidney cDNA for an alpha 2-adrenergic receptor subtype. Proc Natl Acad Sci U S A. 1988; 85(17):6301-5.

Rice, T., Vogler, G. P., Perusse, L., Bouchard, C. and Rao, D. C. Cardiovascular risk factors in a French Canadian population: resolution of genetic and familial environmental effects on blood pressure using twins, adoptees, and extensive information on environmental correlates. Genet. Epidemiol. 1989; 6, 571–588.

Risch N and Merikangas K, "The future of genetic studies of complex human diseases," Science, 1996; 273(5281), pp. 1516–1517.

Ritchie MD, Hahn LW, Roodi N, Bailey LR, Dupont WD, Fritz FP, Moore JH: Multifactor-Dimensionality Reduction Reveals High-Order Interactions Among Estrogen-Metabolism Genes in Sporadic Breast Cancer. *Am J Hum Genet* 2001, 69:138-147.

Ritchie MD, Hahn LW, Moore JH. Power of multifactor dimensionality reduction for detecting gene-gene interactions in the presence of genotyping error, missing data, phenocopy, and genetic heterogeneity. *Genet Epidemiol.* 2003; 24(2):150-7.

Rutherford, S.; Johnson, M. P.; Griffiths, L. R. : Sibpair studies implicate chromosome 18 in essential hypertension. *Am. J. Med. Genet.* 2004. 126A: 241-247.

Sajjad Rafiq, Sonia Anand & Robert Roberts Genome-Wide Association Studies of Hypertension:Have They Been Fruitful? J. of Cardiovasc. Trans. Res. 2010 3:189–196.

Salah A, Khan M, Esmail N, Habibullah S, Al Lahham Y Genetic polymorphism of S447X lipoprotein lipase (LPL) and the susceptibility to hypertension Journal of critical care 2009 Sep 24 (3): 3.

Sass C, Herbeth B, Siest G, Visvikis S: Lipoprotein lipase (C/G)447 polymorphism and blood pressure in the Stanislas cohort. J Hypertens 2000; 18: 1775–1781.

Sayed-Tabatabaei FA, Schut AFC, Hofman A, Bertoli-Avella AM, Vergeer J, Witteman JCM, et al. A study of gene-environment interaction on the gene for angiotensin converting enzyme: a combined functional and population based approach. J Med Genet. 2004; 41: 99-103.

Schunkert H, Hense HW, Do¨ring A, Riegger GAJ, Siffert W: Association between a polymorphism in the G protein b3 subunit gene and lower renin and elevated diastolic blood pressure.Hypertension 1998; 32: 510–513.

Schuster, H.; Wienker, T. F.; Bahring, S.; Bilginturan, N.; Toka, H. R.; Neitzel, H.; Jeschke, E.; Toka, O.; Gilbert, D.; Lowe, A.; Ott, J.; Haller, H.; Luft, F. C. : Severe autosomal dominant hypertension and brachydactyly in a unique Turkish kindred maps to human chromosome 12. *Nature Genet* 1996; 13: 98-100.

Scott Watkinsa W, Steven C. Hunt, Gordon H. Williams C, Whitney Tolpinrud, Xavier Jeunemaitre, Jean-Marc Lalouel, and Lynn B. Jordea Genotype - phenotype analysis of angiotensinogen polymorphisms and essential hypertension: the importance of haplotypesJ Hypertens. 2010 January ; 28(1): 65–75.

Sethi AA, Nordestgaard BG, Tybjaerg-Hansen A: Angiotensinogen gene polymorphism, plasma angiotensinogen, and risk of hypertension and ischemic heart disease: a meta-analysis. Arterioscler Thromb Vasc Biol 2003, 23:1269-1275.

Sharma A.M. and Jeunemaitre, X.; The future of genetic association studies in hypertension: improving the signal-to-noise ratio, J of Hypetension,, 2000; 18, 811-814.

Sipahi T, Budak M, Sen S, Ay A, Sener S. Association between ACE gene Insertion (I) / Deletion (D) polymorphism and primary hypertension in Turkish patients of Trakya region. Biotechnol. & Biotechnol. Eq. 2006; 20(2).

Skol A. D, Scott L. J, Abecasis G. R, and Boehnke M. "Optimal designs for two-stage genome-wide association studies," Genetic Epidemiology, 2007; 31(7), pp. 776–788.

Soldner A, Spahn-Langguth H, Mutschler E: The renin-angiotensinaldosterone system: focus on its distinct role in arterial hypertension and its various inhibitors as a therapeutic strategy to effectively lower blood pressure. Pharmazie 1996, 51:783-799.

Staessen, J. A., Wang J, Bianchi G et al. Essential hypertension. Lancet, 2003; 361 (9369), 1629-1641.

Stanton, J.L., Braitman, L.E., Riley, A.M., Jr., Khoo, C.S., and Smith, J.L.. Demographic, dietary, life style, and anthropometric correlates of blood pressure. Hypertension. 1982; 4, III135-142.

Stoll M., Kwitek-Black A.E., Cowley A.W. Jr., New target regions for human hypertension via comparative genomics. Genone Res. 2000; 10:473-482

Sudhir Jain, Xiangna Tang, Chittampalli S. Narayanan, Yogesh Agarwal, Stephen M. Peterson, Clinton D. Brown, Jurg Ott and Ashok Kumar. Angiotensinogen Gene Polymorphism at −217 Affects Basal Promoter Activity and Is Associated with Hypertension in African-Americans. Journal of Biological Chemistry. 2002; 277:36889-36896.

Sushma Patkar, BH. Charita, C. Ramesh, T.Padma High risk of essential hypelrtension in males with intron 4 polymorphism of eNos gene Indian J of Hum genet, 2009, May-August 15(2), 49-53.

Sushma Patkar, Bh.Charita, Ramesh.C and Padma.T Risk conferred by 786T>C polymorphism of NOS3 gene to essential hypertension in synergy with smoking and elevated body mass index. International Journal of Current Research 2011; 2(2), pp.097-102.

Thiel BA, Chakravarthi A, Cooper RS, Luke A, Lewis S, Lynn A et al A genome wide linkage analysis investigating the determinants of blood pressure in whites and African amricans Am J hypertens 2003 February; 16(2): 154-7

Timberlake DS, Daniel T, O' Connor and Robert J. Parmer, Molecular Genetics of essential hypertension: recent results and emerging strategies, Curr Ooin Nephrol Hypertens 2001, 10:71-79.

Tomoaki Ishigami; Satoshi Umemura; Kouichi Tamura; Kiyoshi Hibi; Nobuo Nyui; Minoru Kihara; Machiko Yabana;Yasujiro Watanabe; Yoichi Sumida; Toshihiro Nagahara; Hisao Ochiai; ; Masao Ishii. Essential Hypertension and 5' Upstream Core Promoter Region of Human Angiotensinogen Gene. Hypertension. 1997; 30:1325-1330.

Tsai C T; Daniele Fallin; Fu-Tien Chiang; et al. Angiotensinogen gene haplotype and hypertension: interaction with ACE gene I allele. Hypertension. 2003; 41:9-15.

Vasudevan Ramachandran, Patimah Ismail, Johnson S, Norashikin S, Saidin M, Rusni Mohd J. Association of insertion/deletion polymorphism of angiotensin-converting enzyme gene with essential hypertension and type 2 diabetes mellitus in Malaysian subjects. Journal of Renin-Angiotensin-Aldosterone System. 2008; 9 (4):208-214.

Von Wowern, F.; Bengtsson, K.; Lindgren, C. M.; Orho-Melander, M.; Fyhrquist, F.; Lindblad, U.; Rastam, L.; Forsblom, C.; Kanninen, T.; Almgren P.; Burri, P.; Katzman, P.; Groop, L.; Hulthen, U. L.; Melander, O. : A genome wide scan for early onset primary hypertension in Scandinavians. *Hum. Molec. Genet.* 2003; 12: 2077-2081.

Wang H.G., J.L. Wang ; P. Chang; F.L. Cao; X.C. Liu; Y.B. ma; G.X. Zhai and H.Q Gao. Endothelial nitric oxide synthase gene polymorphisms and essential hypertension in Han Chinese. Genetics and molecular research, 2010, 9(3): 1896-1907.

Wang JH, Lin CM, Wang LS, Lai NS, Chen DY, Cherng JM. Association between molecular variants of the angiotensinogen gene and hypertension in Amis tribes of eastern Taiwan. J Formos Med Assoc. 2002; 101(3):183-8.

Williams RR, Hunt SC, Hasstedt SJ, Hopkins PN, Wu LL, Berry TD, Stults BM, Barlow GK, Schumacher MC, Lifton RP, et al Are there interactions and relations between genetic and environmental factors predisposing to high blood pressure? *Hypertension*,1991; 18: I29-37.

Williams GH, Dluhy RG, Lifton RP, Moore TJ, Gleason R, Williams R, Hunt SC, Hopkins PN, Hollenberg NK. Non-modulation as an intermediate phenotype in essential hypertension. Hypertension. 1992; 20: 788–796

Williams SM et al. Combinations of variations in multiple genes are associated with hypertension. Hypertension 2000; 36(1): 2-6.

Williams, P. D., Puddey I. B, Martin N.G, Beilin L. J. Platelet cytosolic free calcium concentration, total plasma calcium concentration and blood pressure in human twins: a genetic analysis. Clinical Science (London, England), 1992; 82(5), 493–504.

Wowern VF, Bengtsson K, Lindblad U, Rastam L, Melander O. Functional variant in the (alpha)2B adrenoceptor gene, a positional candidate on chromosome 2, associates with hypertension. Hypertension.. 2004; 43: 592–597.

Wu DA, Bu XD, Warden CH, et al: Quantitative trait locus mapping of human blood pressure to a genetic region at or near the lipoprotein lipase gene locus on chromosome 8p22. J Clin Invest 1996; 97: 2111–2118.

Wu SJ, Fu-Tien Chiang, Wei J. Chen, et al. Three single nucleotide polymorphisms of the angiotensinogen gene and susceptibility to hypertension: single locus genotype vs. haplotype analysis. Physiol Genomics. 2004; 17:79-86.

Wu SJ, Chiang FT, Jiang JR, Hsu KL, Chern TH, Tseng YZ.. The G-217A variant of the angiotensinogen gene affects basal transcription and is associated with hypertension in a Taiwanese population. J Hypertens. 2003; 21(11):2061-7.

Xin Tu, Jinwen Tu, Xiuying Wen, Jinming Wang, Daoliang Zhang A study of lipoprotein lipase gene intron 8 polymorphisms in Chinese Han race essential hypertension patients.International journal of cardiology 2005 Mar 99 (2): 263-7.

Xu, X.; Rogus, J. J.; Terwedow, H. A.; Yang, J.; Wang, Z.; Chen, C.; Niu, T.; Wang, B.; Xu, H.; Weiss, S.; Schork, N. J.; Fang, Z. : An extreme-sib-pair genome scan for genes regulating blood pressure. *Am. J. Hum. Genet.* 1999; 64: 1694-1701.

Yan Gui W, Yan-hua W, Qun X, Wei-jun T, Ming-Ling G, Jian W, et al. Associations between RAS gene polymorphisms, environmental factors and hypertension in Mongolian people. Eur J Epidemiol. 2006; 21: 287-92.

Zhao.Y.Y; Jie Zhou; Chittampalli S. Narayanan; Yanning Cui; Ashok Kumar. Role of C/A Polymorphism at -20 on the Expression of Human Angiotensinogen Gene. *Hypertension*. 1999; 33:108-115.

Zhu, X.; Luke, A.; Cooper, R. S.; Quertermous, T.; Hanis, C.; Mosley, T.; Gu, C. C.; Tang, H.; Rao, D. C.; Risch, N.; Weder, A.: Admixture mapping for hypertension loci with genome-scan markers. *Nature Genet.* 37: 177-181, 2005.

# 7

# Candidate Genes in Hypertension

Hayet Soualmia
*High Institut of Medical Technologies of Tunis,*
*Biochemistry Laboratory LR99ES11, Rabta University Hospital, Tunis,*
*Tunisia*

## 1. Introduction

Essential hypertension (EH) is a polygenic and multifactorial disorder that results from genetic and/or environmental factors (Lifton et al., 2001). This disease has no identifiable origin, but results from a disturbance of systems regulating blood pressure (BP) such as several circulating and local neurohumoral and vasoactive factors. Genetic variations of these factors could play a role in the genesis of EH which represents a major risk factor for ischemic heart disease, stroke, peripheral vascular disease and progressive renal damage (Mesrati, 2007). EH rises with age, and it aggregates with other cardiovascular risk factors, such as dyslipidaemia, glucose intolerance, hyperinsulinaemia, abdominal obesity, and hyperuricaemia. Other environmental factors influence this disease like high dietary intake of sodium, alcohol, and stress. Family history, appears to play a major role because EH is more likely to develop in individuals when there is a strong family history. Several studies have identified a variety of candidate genes in EH as well as their interaction with one another and with the environment. Among these hypertension-predisposition genes investigated, genes involved in the renin-angiotensin-aldosterone system, catecholaminergic/adrenergic function, genes of signal transduction system as G protein β3-subunit, sodium channel system, α adducin and atrial natriuretic peptides. Several other biomarkers have been reported to increase the ability to predict EH such as hormone receptors like glucagon receptor and insulin like growth factor 1 (O'Shaughnessy, 2001, Timberlake et al., 2001) and other systems as endothelin, apolipoprotein and cytokine systems. In this chapter, we expose the genetic markers of EH and their expression related to lifestyle through several strategies such as investigation of specific candidate genes, genome-wide searches, use of intermediate phenotypes, comparative genomics and a combination of these methods (Timberlake et al., 2001)

## 2. Candidate genes in hypertension

A large number of candidate genes previously known and novel candidate genes that mediate susceptibility to hypertension are identified. The notion that hypertension is a polygenic disease, is reinforced by advanced biotechnological tools, and data are provided as to the actual number of genes involved, gene-gene interaction or gene-environment-interaction. The renin-angiotensin-aldosterone system is widely implicated and other gene systems are also emerging.

### 2.1 The renin-angiotensin-aldosterone system

The renin-angiotensin-aldosteron system (RAAS) is implicated in the control of BP and sodium balance. This system plays a key role in the regulation of kidney function. Genetic variations of components of the RAAS such as the renin (REN), angiotensinogen (AGT), angiotensin II-type 1 receptor (AGTR1), angiotensin-converting enzyme (ACE) (Allikmets et al., 1999) and aldosterone (CYP11B2) genes have been shown to be associated with susceptibility to EH.

#### 2.1.1 Renin

Renin is the catalytic enzyme acting on angiotensinogen. It is encoded by the renin (REN) gene located at the 1q32 region. Several studies prove that the REN gene increases BP and susceptibility to hypertension. REN gene insertion/deletion (I/D) polymorphism is found to be associated with EH (Ying et al., 2010) and multiple REN SNPs are significantly associated with risk for hypertension. In the single SNP analysis, the strongest association with hypertension was seen with rs6693954, which is in high linkage disequilibrium with rs2368564 located at intron 9 (Sun et al., 2001). The REN-5312T allele has been reported to be associated with elevated diastolic BP (Vangjeli et al., 2010). Furthermore, the Bgl I variant in intron 1 and the 10501G/A SNP in exon 9 were associated with hypertension in US white and Gulf Arabs group from the United Arab Emirates (Frossard et al., 2001, Ahmad et al., 2005). In addition, an association of C-4021T and C-3212T with hypertension has been identified in African Americans (Zhu et al., 2003) and a SNP in intron 4 (54620025A/C) was shown to be associated with elevated BP and hypertension in Spanish women (Mansego et al., 2008). All these studies provide evidence that renin is an important candidate gene for EH.

#### 2.1.2 Angiotensinogen

Angiotensinogen (AGT) gene located on chromosome 1q42-43, contains five exons spanning 13 kb (Gaillard et al., 1989). AGT is cleaved by renin to the decapeptide angiotensin (Ang) I precursor of Ang II. Significant evidence supporting the genetic susceptibility of the AGT locus for hypertension has been provided by many studies in various ethnic groups. A number of associated single nucleotide polymorphisms (SNPs) has been identified including M235T (rs669), T174M (rs4762), and G-217A (rs5049). Several studies have reported that the 235T and T174 allele increased the risk of EH (Jeunmaitre, 2008, Kunz et al., 1997, Fang et al., 2010, Sethi et al., 2003). Moreover, mutation in the promoter region that involves the presence of an adenine (A) instead of a guanine (G) 6 bp upstream from the transcription initiation site (G-6A) has been reported to have a positive correlation with hypertension (Wang et al., 2002). This mutation has been identified in a Taiwanese aboriginals, where the prevalence of the -6A and 235T variants of the AGT gene are high and are significantly associated with hypertension (Wang et al., 2002). Among all these AGT polymorphisms gene, the M268T variant is the most studied in several populations and representes a candidate gene for EH (Gopi-Chand et al., 2011).

#### 2.1.3 Angiotensin-converting-enzyme

The angiotensin-converting-enzyme (ACE) is located on chromosome 17q23. In addition to increasing the production of Ang II, it is also responsible for the degradation of bradikinin, a vasodilating and natriuretic substance. Several polymorphisms were present in the ACE gene but the prominent of these polymorphisms is the insertion or deletion (I/D) of 287 pb in intron 16 of this gene. Previous studies have reported that this polymorphism affected both serum ACE concentration and BP (Rigat et al., 1990), and DD genotype carriers have twice as high as ACE concentration compared to II genotype carriers, while subjects with ID genotype has intermediate or moderate ACE plasma concentration. In several studies, the D allele showed statistically significant relationship with hypertension in different populations. Thus, the ACE gene is a candidate gene for EH in humans.

### 2.1.4 Angiotensin II type 1 receptor

The human gene for angiotensin II type 1 receptor (AGTR1) located at chromosome 3q21-25, has a length of > 55 kb, is composed of five exons and four introns. A single nucleotide polymorphism (SNP) has been described in which there is either an adenine (A) or a cytosine (C) base (A/C) transversion in position 1166 in the 3′ untranslated region of the gene (Bonnardeaux et al., 1994). The +1166A/C polymorphism is the most studied and evaluated. Nine other SNPs influencing AGTR1 expression were described (Erdmann et al., 1999) and seven other SNPs reported in the 5′ flanking region of the gene, were not in linkage equilibrium with +1166A/C polymorphism (Poirier et al., 1998, Takahashi et al., 2000). Moreover, the SNP at nucleotide position +573 was investigated in hypertension and diabetes (Doria et al., 1997, Chaves et al., 2001) and several other new SNPs have been described, however, not all of them are associated with hypertension. In some studies, a linkage disequilibrium was shown betweeen these new SNPs and the +1166 A/C polymorphism, in particular the -153 A/G polymorphism (Lajemi et al., 2001). In addition, the +1166 A/C variant in the AGTR1 gene was associated with the severe form of EH (Bonnardeaux et al., 1994; Kainulainen et al., 1999) and in Caucasian hypertensive subjects with a strong family history, the C allele was over-represented (Wang et al., 1997) and more frequent in women with pregnancy induced hypertension. Several other studies have reported significant interaction between the AGTR1 +1166A/C polymorphism and hypertension in different populations (Wang &Staessen, 2000, Henskens et al., 2003). So, the 1166 A/C polymorphism in the AGTR1 gene is a biomarker for EH.

### 2.1.5 Angiotensin II type 2 receptor

The angiotensin II type-2 receptor (AGTR2) gene is located on the X-chromosome. It consists of 3 exons and 2 introns, with the entire open reading frame of the AGTR2 located on exon 3 (Martin & Elton 1995). The AGTR2 is thought to oppose the growth promoting effect of the AGTR1 and was the mediator for vasodilatation, natriuresis and apoptosis of smooth muscle cells. A commonly occurring intronic polymorphism has been described at a lariat branch-point in intron 1 (Nishimura et al. 1999). Its position, described relative to the translation initiation site of the human AGTR2 gene, is (−1332A/G) (Nishimura et al. 1999), although it has also been previously described by others (Erdmann et al., 2000) as (+1675). It is located 29 bp before exon 2, close to the region that is important for transcriptional activity (Warnecke et al. 1999). The AGTR2 A1675G polymorphism was shown to be involved in the development of EH in male (Zivkovic et al., 2007, Delles et al. 2000, Jin et al., 2003a, Alfakih et al., 2004), whereas the G4599A polymorphism located in exon 3 of the AGTR2 gene was associated with hypertension in women. Other SNPs in the

AGTR2 gene were identified by Zhang et al. (2003) suggesting a relationship between the 1334T/C polymorphism and the development of hypertension in a Chinese population.

### 2.1.6 Aldosterone synthase

The enzyme aldosterone synthase (CYP11B2) is the key enzyme in the final steps of aldosterone biosynthesis. It is encoded by the CYP11B2 gene located on chromosome 8q22 (Hilgers & Schmidt, 2005, Brand et al., 1998). Several polymorphisms have been identified in the CYP11B2 gene (White & Rainey, 2005). Among them, the promoter region C-344T polymorphism (rs id 1799998) is the best evaluated. This polymorphism either increases aldosterone to renin ratio in essential hypertensives or decreases aldosterone production, leading to sodium wasting and decreased excretion of potassium (Nicod et al., 2003, Matsubara et al., 2004). Furthermore, several studies have shown that the C-344T polymorphism is implicated in the risk of EH (Kumar et al., 2003, Gu et al., 2004) and other cardiovascular parameters. So the CYP11B2 gene is associated with the development of EH.

## 2.2 Sodium system

Several studies have examined the genetic influence on BP responses to dietary sodium and potassium intake in different populations. These studies have identified many candidate genes related to salt sensitivity of BP (Beeks et al., 2004). With the use of association or linkage studies, it appears that mutations increasing renal sodium reabsorption raise BP. The majority of these genes encode for renal ion channels and transporters or for components of hormonal or paracrine systems participating in the regulation of renal sodium reabsorption. All the genes involved in BP control are described in humans and in mice.

### 2.2.1 Epithelial Sodium channel

Epithelial sodium channel (Enac) is an amiloride sensitive epithelial sodium channel, composed of three subunits: α, β, and γ and encoded by different genes. SCNNIA gene coded for subunit α, located on human chromosome 12p13, and involved in aldosteronism and pseudohypoaldosteronism type I. SCNNIB and SCNNIG genes coded respectively for β, and γ subunits are related to monogenic form of salt sensitive hypertension (Kamida et al., 2004). The SCNNIA G2139 allele (Iwai, 2002, Wong, 1999) and Thr663Ala were reported to be associated with hypertension. A variety of mutations Gly589Ser, Thr594Met, Arg597His, Arg624Cys, Glu632Gly, Gly442Val and Val434Met has been shown in the SCNNIB gene and were implicated in the pathogenesis of systolic BP. In black individuals, the T594M mutation of the β subunit of this gene increases the risk of hypertension (Baker et al., 1998, Dong et al., 2002). In addition, a Japanese study (Matsubara et al., 2002) indicated a linkage between systolic BP and microsatellite markers on chromosome 16p12.3, a region close to the gene coding for the β and γ subunits of Enac gene (Wong et al.; 1999). Another study (Hyun-Seok et al., 2010) identified several SNPs in SCNNIB, SCNNIG genes and showed a link between hypertension and these polymorphisms. A recent study (Zhao et al., 2011) reported multiple common SNPs in SCNNIG associated with BP response to sodium intervention.

### 2.2.2 Thiazide sensitive Na+Cl- cotransporter

The sodium chloride cotransporter (NCC) is the thiazide sensitive Na-Cl cotranporter (TSC) located at the apical membrane of the distal convoluted tubule of the nephron (Plotkin et al., 1996), accounts for the absorption of 5% of the salt filtered at the glomerulus (Obermuller et al., 1995). The TSC gene, consisting of 26 exons that encode 1021 amino acid residus, is located on chromosome 16q13. Mutations in the human TSC gene is associated with a loss of TSC function, as seen in Gitelman's syndrome, an autosomal recessive disease that affects BP regulation (Simon et al., 1996). Several TSC gene variants have been reported in different populations. TSC gene polymorphisms (C2736A, C1420T, G816C) were identified in Swedish population and only homozygous A2736 and T1420 alleles were significantly associated with EH in this population (Melander et al., 2000), whereas the G2736A was related to hypertension in Japanese women. Other SNPs of TSC gene rs7204044 and rs13306673 were studied in Mongolian and Han populations. TSC gene rs 7204044 is a genetic factor for EH in these two ethnicities, but rs13306673 is a genetic factor for EH only in Han population (Chang et al., 2011).

### 2.2.3 NEDD4L

NEDD4L is a ubiquitin ligase that controls the expression of the kidney epithelial sodium channels. The NEDD4L gene located on human chromosome 18q21, is an attractive candidate gene in pathogenesis for hypertensive disorders (Pankow et al., 2000). Several SNPs, including a common SNP (rs4149601) known to result in abnormal splicing, are identified in African Americans, American whites, and Greek whites with EH (Russo et al., 2005). In Swedish subjects, the rs4149601 polymorphism and an intronic NEDD4L marker (rs2288774) were associated with systolic and diastolic BP, as a consequence of altered NEDD4L interaction with EnaC (Fava et al., 2006). Moreover, SNP (rs513563) in NEDD4L was associated with hypertension in both African and Caucasian whites (Russo et al., 2005). In Chinese Hans, another rs3865418 variant of NEDD4L gene was implicated in the prevalence of EH in this population (Wen et al., 2008).

### 2.2.4 Na+ K+ /ATPase

The Na+K+/ATPase (NAK) is an integral membrane protein responsible for establishing and maintaining the electrochemical gradients of Na+ and K+ across the plasma membrane. The NKA is characterized by a complex molecular heterogeneity consisting of α, β and γ subunits. Four different α-polypeptides (α1, α2, α3, and α4) and three distinct β-isoforms (β1, β2, and β3) have been identified in mammalian. The α1 subunit is ubiquitous and predominates in the kidney, whereas the α2 subunit is most prevalent in the brain, heart, and muscle cells (Sweadner, 1989). The NAK catalytic subunit is encoded by multiple genes (Lalley et al., 1978) and separate genes encoding the α isoforms were identified in human (Shull & Lingrel, 1987). In mouse, the gene encoding the α1 subunit (ATP1A1) has been assigned to mouse chromosome 3. The α2 subunit gene (ATP1A2) is located on mouse chromosome 7 but the gene encoding the α3 subunit is located on mouse chromosome 1. The Na+K+/ATPase β3 subunit gene, which also exhibits a distinctive and complex tissue-specific pattern of expression (Mercer et al., 1986), maps to the same region of chromosome 1, but is not tightly linked to the α3 subunit gene. Genetic studies have reported that the 3'end of the gene for the α2 subunit (ATP1A2) and the β subunits (ATP1B1) variants were associated with BP and hypertension (Shull et al., 1990, Kasantsev et al., 1992, Masharani & Frossard, 1988, Glenn et al., 2001) but the Bgl II ATP1A1 polymorphism gene in the first intron is associated with diabetic neuropathy (Vague et al., 1997). In addition, SNPs has been described, close to the ATP1A1 gene (D1S453, 160 kb) in Sardinian hypertensive and normotensive cohort (Glorioso et al., 2001). This study has identified an interaction of ATP1A1 and Na+K+2Cl-Cotransporter genes in Human EH.

### 2.3 Adducin

Adducin is a cytoskeleton protein that promotes the binding of spectrin with actin and may modulate a variety of other cell functions such as ion transport (Matsuoka et al., 2000). It is an heterodimeric protein consisting of an α-subunit and β-subunit or and α-subunit and γ-subunit, composed of three different subunits: adducin α, β, and γ which are encoded by three genes (ADD1, ADD2, ADD3) located on different chromosomes (Matsuoka et al., 2000). Adducin is one among the proteins that regulate Na+K+/ATPase activity. Abnormalities in adducin by genetic mutation have been shown to influence the surface expression and maximum velocity of Na+K+/ATPase and subsequently faster renal tubular Na+ reabsorption (Mische et al., 1987). Clinical and experimental studies have reported that the α adducin gene mutations could affect renal Na+ transport and explain a large proportion of BP variation (Bianchi et al., 1994, Barlassina et al., 1997), suggesting the involvement of mutated adducin variants in sodium-dependent hypertension. In animal models, single nucleotide polymorphisms (SNPs) in the ADD1 gene lead to increased tubular Na+ reabsorption and hypertension (Tripodi et al., 1996). In humans, a guanine to thymine SNP at nucleotide 614 in exon 10 of the ADD1 gene (rs4961) leads to a glycine (Gly) to tryptophan (Trp) change at amino acid position 460. This polymorphism has been associated with elevated untreated BP (Lanzani et al., 2005) and hypertension salt sensitivity (Barlassina et al., 2000, Turner et al., 2003).

#### 2.3.1 ADD1

The gene encoding human ADD1 is mapped onto the chromosome location 4p16.3. Two missense mutations G460W and S586C in the human α adducin gene (ADD1) were shown to be associated with EH (Cusi et al., 1997). The common molecular variant of the ADD1 gene causing the substitution of tryptophan instead of glycine (Gly460Trp) at amino acid position 460 was found to be associated with increased risk of hypertension in different population (Cusi et al., 1997, Ju et al., 2003).

#### 2.3.2 ADD2

C1797T ADD2 gene silent polymorphism in exon 15 was reported to be associated with hypertension in post menopausal women (Wang et al., 2002), in oral contraceptive users and in high salt intake populations. In Polish and Russian subjects (Tikhonoff et al., 2003), BP and the prevalence of hypertension were associated with the C1797T polymorphism in the β (ADD2), particularly in post menopausal women (Cwynar et al., 2005).

#### 2.3.3 ADD 3

In ADD3 gene, the A to G substitution polymorphism located in intron 11 (IVS11 þ386A>G -rs3731566) exists but neither previous publications nor genome browser databases provided any suggestion about its functional role. Previous studies on populations and patients have demonstrated that the ADD1 Gly460Trp polymorphism, alone or in combination with variation in the ADD3 (IVS11 þ386A>G) or ACE (I/D) genes, influences the peripheral and central BP (Cwynar et al., 2005). Indeed, mean arterial pressure increased to the largest extent in patients carrying both the mutated ADD1Trp allele and the ADD3 GG genotype. Interaction between the ADD1 and ADD3 genes, which are located on different chromosomes, is in keeping with the heterodimeric structure of the adducin protein and strengthens the role of these genes compared with that of other loci mapping near to the adducin subunits (Kuznetsova et al., 2008).

### 2.4 Natriuretic peptides

The natriuretic peptide system (NP), with its diverse actions on renal and hemodynamic function and vasoactive hormone activity continues to attract attention as a potentially major regulator of body fluid volume and arterial pressure. The atrial natriuretic peptide (ANP), mainly produced by right atria in response to volume expansion, influences BP and body fluid homeostasis (Ogawa et al., 1995). This system consists of a family of three peptidic hormones A-type NP (ANP), B-type NP (BNP), and C-type NP (CNP) that interact with three receptors NP receptor A (NPRA), NP receptor B (NPRB) and NP clearance receptor (NPRC). The NPRC is encoded by the NPR3 gene and is a determinant of NP plasma concentration.

Genetic variants of the ANP system are involved in the etiology of hypertension (Rutlege et al., 1995, Kato et al., 2000), for this reason ANP is proposed as a candidate gene with salt-sensitive HT in some studies (Rutlege et al., 1995, Ciechnowicz et al., 1997). Several polymorphisms have been described in the human ANP gene: -C664G, G1837A, T2238C polymorphisms and a microsatellite marker of both NPRA and BNP genes were characterized (Rubattu et al., 2006). The T2238C ANP and the G1837A ANP intronic gene polymorphisms have been reported to be associated with left ventricular mass in human EH (Schmieder et al., 1996) and increased risk of ischemic stroke (Rubattu & Volpe, 2001). An I/D polymorphism at position 15129 of the 3′UTR of NPRA gene deletion variant is associated with hypertensive family history and higher systolic BP.

In the BNP gene, a variable number of tandem repeat (VNTR) polymorphism in the 5′-flanking region (-1241 nucleotides from the major transcriptional initiation site) was discovered. This VNTR polymorphism is a tandem repeat of the 4-nucleotide sequence TTTC appears to be a useful genetic marker of EH in females (Kosuge et al., 2007).

In CNP gene, four polymorphisms are identified : G733A, G1612C, G2347T and G2628A, two polymorphisms in the promoter region, one polymorphism in the coding region (exon 2) that accompanied an amino acid change from Gly to Val at amino acid position 61, and one polymorphism in the 3′-non coding region. Only the G2628A genotype in 3′-UTR was associated with BP and made greater contribution to hypertension (Ono et al., 2002). Overall these observations, suggested that atrial gene peptides could be considered candidate markers in EH.

### 2.5 Signal transduction pathways genes

The basic signal transduction steps are mediated through specific receptors binding, G protein coupled receptors and some growth factors. Specific receptors like adrenergic receptors, glucagon receptor and growth factors as insulin-like growth factor 1 (IGF-I) genes are assumed to be important mediator in the pathophysiological response to BP increase. Mutation into the genes encoding signal transduction pathways have been associated with hypertension.

### 2.5.1 G Proteins

The main role of G proteins is to translate signals from the cell surface into a cell (Siffert, 2003) to mediate the intracellular effects of many hormones and peptides. A polymorphism C3T at nucleotide 825 in exon 10 of the β3 subunit of GTP binding protein (GNB3/C825T) has been identified (Bohm et al., 1997). This polymorphism is associated with enhanced intracellular signal transduction (Siffert et al., 1998) and has been reported to be associated with a variety of cardiovascular risk factors, including hypertension (Siffert et al., 1998, Schunkert et al., 1998, Benjafield et al., 1998), obesity (Siffert et al., 1999, Casiglia et al., 2008), diabetes (Bluthner et al., 1999) or dyslipidemia (Ishikawa et al., 2000, Hayakawa et al., 2007). A significantly higher frequency of the T allele has been identified in EH (Beige et al., 1999, Siffert, 1996). The mechanism whereby the 825T variant may lead to hypertension remains unknown, but it may involve an increase of Na-H exchanger activity (Siffert, 1996) which enhanced renal sodium reabsorption and induced the BP increase. Several studies have demonstrated that the 825T allele of GNB3 is associated with hypertension (Benjafiel et al., 1998, Beige et al., 1999, Dong et al., 1999, Hengstenberg et al., 2001, Timberlake et al., 2001, Casiglia et al., 2008). Together, these studies highlight the importance of the GBN3/C825T variant gene in EH.

### 2.5.2 Glucagon receptor

The glucagon is involved in the regulation of electrolyte and water homeostasis. The effects of glucagon are mediated through its binding to a specific receptor (GCG-R), a 480-amino acid protein, which belongs to the superfamily of G protein-coupled transmembrane receptors (Laburthe et al., 1996). A Gly40Ser missense mutation in exon 2 of this receptor induced a lower affinity of the receptor for glucagon and a reduced cAMP response in transfected cells (Hansen et al., 1996). In humans, carriers of the mutation have a significantly lower increased plasma glucose concentration in response to glucagon infusion (Tonolo et al., 1997). A decrease in receptor activity in vivo might contribute to common EH by reducing the renal natriuretic effect of glucagon. Several studies have shown that the GCG-R plays a role in the predisposition to EH (Chambers & Morris, 1996, Tonolo et al., 1997). Other studies have reported significant association of the Gly40Ser polymorphism in hypertensive women with family history of hypertension in both parents (Chambers & Morris, 1996, Morris et al., 1997), whereas in French people, the Gly40Ser GCG-R variant was associated with hypertension only in men (Brand et al., 1999). Therefore, the glucagon receptor gene (*GCG-R*) could be a candidate gene for predisposition to human EH.

### 2.5.3 Insulin-like growth factor 1

The insulin-like growth factor 1 (IGF-I) is assumed to be an important mediator in the pathophysiological response to increased BP in the vessel wall, and low circulating IGF-I levels have been associated with cardiovascular disease development (Juul et al., 2002). The absence of the 192 bp allele in the promoter region of the IGF-I gene variant was associated with low circulating IGF-I levels and linked to systolic BP. An increased risk of developing atherosclerosis was shown in hypertensive subjects with this IGF-I polymorphism. The genetic variation of the IGF-I receptor may affect the susceptibility to ischemic stroke (Cheng et al., 2008) and the diversity of left ventricular structure in hypertensives (Horio et al., 2010). The (IGF-I) is a mediator in limiting the damaging effects of high BP on the EH.

### 2.6 Noradrenergic system

The sympathetic nervous system acts through two main groups of adrenergic receptors, α and β with several subtypes α1 and α2 receptors and β receptors have the subtypes β1, β2 and β3, all linked to Gs proteins. The adrenergic system affects blood pressure by cardiac output and peripheral resistance regulation. Several studies have identified the implication of the β adrenergic receptors in the genesis of hypertension and many candidate gene studies have evaluated the association of one or more polymorphisms of adrenergic receptors in cardiovascular diseases, suggesting involvement of adrenergic pathways in EH.

#### 2.6.1 β1-adrenergic receptor

The β1 adrenergic receptor (ADRB1), is a 7-transmembrane Gs protein coupled receptor. The ADRB1 is located on chromosome 10 (Hoehe et al., 1995) and is expressed in cardiac myocytes (Strader et al., 1994). Several polymorphisms of the ADRB1 exist, but two major single nucleotide Ser49Gly and Arg389Gly (Maqbool et al., 1999) are associated with BP. Arg389Gly variant is located in the intracellular cytoplasmic tail near the seventh transmembrane region of the receptor, which is a Gs-protein binding domain. The Arg389 polymorphism mediates a higher isoproterenol-stimulated adenylate cyclase activity than the Gly389 variant in vitro (Moore et al., 1999). The Ser49Gly polymorphism is located in the extracellular amino-terminal region of the receptor (Moore et al., 1999), but the potential functional consequence of this polymorphism is unknown. The genetic variants of the β1 adrenergic receptor could play an important role in the development of hypertension, because the β1 adrenergic receptor is essential in cardiac output regulation and the ADRB1 inhibitor reduces BP. Several studies have investigated the effects of these polymorphisms on resting haemodynamics and the incidence of hypertension, showing significantly higher diastolic BP and heart rates than siblings carrying either one or two copies of the 389G allele (Bengtsson et al., 2001).

#### 2.6.2 β2-adrenergic receptor

The β2-adrenergic receptor (ADRB2) is responsible for vasodilatation in the vasculature via the cAMP pathway in smooth muscle cells or by release of nitric oxide (NO) from vascular endothelium (Eisenach et al., 2002). This receptor is implicated in the pathogenesis of hypertension. The ADRB2 gene located on chromosome 5q, is intronless, and codes for 413 amino acids. The most common SNPs in the ADRB2 gene include amino acid position 16, which contains either glycine or arginine (major/minor allele: Gly16/Arg), and amino acid position 27, which contains either glutamine or glutamic acid (Gln27/Glu). Some studies have shown that these two polymorphisms are associated with resistance to desensitization (Green et al., 1994, Green et al., 1995), but others have reported that the Gly16 variant ADRB2 gene is associated with EH in different populations (Lang et al., 1995, Svetkey et al., 1997, Kotanko et al., 1997, Timmermann et al., 1998, Lou Y et al., 2011). Moreover, another variant, the A46G in the ADRB2 gene is significantly associated with EH risk only in male among the Northern Han Chinese population (Lou et al., 2011). Therefore, the β2 adrenergic receptor gene is considered a candidate gene for the development of EH.

#### 2.6.3 β3-adrenergic receptor

The β3-adrenergic receptor (ADRB3) gene is located on chromosome 8p and codes for 396 amino acids. The ADRB3 gene contains a SNP that encodes either tryptophan or arginine (Trp64/Arg). This polymorphism is considered most relevant to lipolysis and thermogenesis. The ADRB3 genotype appears to have some influence in the development of obesity and appears to impact insulin resistance and the development of diabetes. So, The ADRB3 gene is not implicated in the risk of EH.

### 2.7 Endothelin system

Potent vasoconstrictor peptides, composed of three member family of peptides, namely endothelin-1 (ET-1), endothelin-2 (ET-2), endothelin-3 (ET-3) and their receptors, have a convincing role in EH. High circulating endothelin plasma levels have been reported in EH and genetic variants identified in the different component of endothelin system genes are involved in the etiology of hypertension.

#### 2.7.1 Endothelin 1

Endothelin (ET)-1, produced by vascular endothelial cells, is a potent vasoconstrictor that acts as a modulator of vasomotor tone, cell proliferation, and vascular remodeling (Yanagisawa et al., 1988, Levin, 1995). The biological actions of ET-1 are mediated by two different receptors, ET-A receptor (ET-A) and ET-B receptor (ET-B). The interaction of ET-1 with ET-A in vascular smooth muscle cells is primarily responsible for ET-1–mediated vasoconstriction, whereas endothelial cell expressing ET-B promotes vasodilation (Haynes et al., 1995, Hirata et al., 1993). ET-1 is implicated in the pathogenesis of hypertension, heart failure, atherosclerosis, chronic kidney disease, and diabetes (MacGregor et al., 2000). High circulating endothelin plasma levels have been reported in EH. Human ET-1 gene is located on chromosome 6 and encodes a 21-amino acid peptide. Several SNPs in the endothelin system genes have been shown to have functional relevance and association with cardiovascular phenotypes and/or diseases (Taupenot et al., 2003). A G5665T polymorphism named Lys198Asn polymorphism of the preproendothelin-1 gene has been shown to be associated with higher BP in Caucasians and in Japanese populations with the T allele (Asai et al., 2001, Jin et al., 2003b). Therefore, the ET-1 is a candidate responsible for EH.

#### 2.7.2 Endothelin 2

ET-2 is expressed in the right atria. A single A985G base change in the '3-UTR of the ET-2 gene was identified in hypertensives when BP was assessed as a quantitative trait. The difference in genotype and allele frequencies between the extremes of BP suggests that the ET-2 locus influences the severity rather than the initial development of hypertension (Sharma et al., 1999).

### 2.7.3 Endothelin-converting enzyme

Endothelin-converting enzyme (ECE) is a main component in endothelin (ET) biosynthesis, leading to the generation of ET-1, a potent vasoconstricting peptide, and contributing to BP control. Two different ECE genes, ECE-1 (Xu & Yanagisawa, 1994) and ECE-2 (Emoto & Yanagisawa, 1995), have been identified, but only ECE-1 expression is altered in human cardiovascular diseases. The gene is located at chromosome 1 (Albertin et al., 1996), has a length of 120 pb and is consisting of 20 exons (Schweizer et al., 1997, Valdenaire et al., 1999, Funke-Kaiser et al., 2000). Human ECE-1 is expressed in four different isoforms: ECE-1a, ECE-1b, ECE-1c and ECE-1d (Shimada et al., 1995, Valdenaire et al., 1999) generated from an additional prometers (Valdenaire et al., 1995, Valdenaire et al., 1999). The ECE-1b isoform expressed in endothelial and vascular smooth muscle cells (Valdenaire et al., 1999, Orzechowski et al., 1997), may contribute to vascular ET generation and BP regulation.

Several polymorphisms have been described in the human ECE-1b promoter gene, but only combinations of two common variants within the 5'-flanking region (T-839G, C-338A) were significantly associated with high BP values in non-treated hypertensive females (Funke-Kaiser et al., 2003). The -338A allele showed an increase in promoter activity compared with the wild-type promoter. Some studies conducted in African-American hypertensives have reported higher ECE-1 activity compared with white hypertensive patients (Grubbs et al., 2002), indicating that genetic variability in the ET system, e.g. ECE-1 gene, could be linked with severity of EH (Funke-Kaiser et al., 2003). So, the ECE-1 gene is a candidate gene in EH.

### 2.7.4 Endothelin receptors

ET-1 acts through two receptors ET-RA and ET-RB. Several single SNPs spanning the ET-RA gene were typed. The substitution of a thymine for a cytosine located in the untranslated part of exon 8 of the ET-RA gene was associated with pulse pressure and hypertension (Benjafield et al., 2003). In addition, an association was reported between genotype at the rs5335 (C+70G) SNP and night systolic BP and diastolic BP (Rahman et al., 2008). In this study the rs5335 (C+70G) polymorphism of the ET-RA receptor gene has small effects on the risk of hypertension. In another study (Ormezzano et al., 2005), the T allele of the ET-RA A/C+1222T polymorphism is associated with a reduction of baroreflex sensitivity in both healthy and hypertensive subjects. Likewise, a common polymorphism G1065A revealed that the AA+GA genotypes were significantly more frequent in salt-resistant than in salt-sensitive individuals, suggesting a protective role for the A allele (Caprioli et al., 2008).

### 2.7.5 Endothelial nitric oxide synthase

Nitric oxide synthase (eNOS) synthesizes nitric oxide (NO), a potent vasodilator produced by endothelial cells. The eNOS gene (NOS3) is located at the 7q35-q36 region, has a length of 21 kb and consisted of 26 exons. Variants of this gene have been investigated for association with hypertension and other cardiovascular disorders (Casas et al., 2006). Among them, three polymorphisms have been widely examined for clinical relevance (Casas et al., 2006, Cooke et al., 2007). A G894T substitution in exon 7 resulting in a remplacement of Glu to Asp substitution at codon 298 (rs1799983), an insertion-deletion in intron 4 (4a/b) consisting of two alleles (the a-deletion which has four tandem 27-pb repeats and the b-insertion having five repeats), and a T786C substitution in the promotor region (rs2070744). Several studies have shown significant association of the eNOS3 polymorphisms gene with hypertension (Uwabo et al., 1998, M. Shoji et al., 2000, Jachymova et al., 2001, Hyndman et al., 2002). In the Chinese population, a significant and independent association between the eNOS-G894T polymorphism and EH has been shown (Men et al., 2001). In addition, a meta-analysis of 33 studies have examined the eNOS G894T, 4a4b, T-786C, and G23T polymorphisms and their relationship to susceptibility for hypertension, and reported that: the allele 4b under a recessive model provided evidence of protection (Zintzaras et al., 2006). Thus, the eNOS gene is a risk factor for EH.

### 2.8 Apolipoproteins

Apolipoproteins are large complexes of molecules that transport lipids through the blood. They play a major role in lipid metabolism. Genetic variations identified in apolipoprotein genes have been shown to be involved in the risk of EH.

#### 2.8.1 Apolipoprotein B

Apolipoprotein B (ApoB) is the main apolipoprotein of chylomicrons and low density lipoproteins (LDL), which occurs in the plasma in two main forms, ApoB48 and ApoB100. ApoB100 is synthesized in the liver and is present in very low density lipoproteins and their metabolic products. It is a principal ligand for low density lipoprotein (LDL) receptors (Boerwinkle et al., 1989) which mediate the uptake of LDL from the liver and peripheral cells. Like this, ApoB100 plays an important role in cholesterol homeostasis and a positive relationship has been established between coronary heart disease and LDL cholesterol with ApoB (Brunzell et al., 1984). The ApoB gene located at the 2p24 region (Knott et al., 1985), has a lengh of 42 kb, is composed of 29 exons (Blackhart et al., 1986). The 3' end of the ApoB gene exhibits a variable number of tandemly repeated (VNTR) short, A+T rich DNA sequences (Knott et al., 1986). Several studies have reported that ApoB 3'VNTR alleles is associated with EH (Philippe et al., 1999, Friedl et al., 1990).

#### 2.8.2 Apolipoprotein C3

Genetic variation in the apolipoprotein C (ApoC3) gene, is associated with an increased risk of coronary heart diseases (CDH) (Sacks et al., 2000). ApoC3 is a protein of 79 amino acids, a constituent of triglyceride rich lipoprotein, including very low density lipoprotein (VLDL), chylomicron (CM), and high density lipoprotein (HDL) (Windler et al., 1985). It inhibits the lipoprotein lipase-induced hydrolysis of those particles (Ashavaid et al., 2002). ApoC3 exists in three different isoforms, according to the sialylation degree of the protein. Previous studies have shown that low ApoC3 levels may be associated with reduced CHD risk. Two polymorphisms located at positions −455 (T to C) and −482 (C to T) in the 5′ ApoC3 gene promoter region, have been shown to be associated with elevated levels of serum triglyceride and with a negative insulin response element (Dammerman et al., 1993). Another study has reported that the ApoC3 3206GG genotype was associated with a decrease in diastolic BP while the ApoC3 -482T allele was associated with a decrease in pulse pressure levels.

#### 2.8.3 Apolipoprotein E

Apolipoprotein E (ApoE) gene situated on chromosome 19, appears in humans in three different forms named E2, E3 and E4 differing from each other by amino acid substitution in two various positions (varying Cys112Arg and Arg158Cys) and coded by three alleles ε2, ε3 and ε4 at a single gene locus. ApoE polymorphism is one of the common genetic factors responsible for inter-individual variations in lipid and lipoprotein levels. ApoE4 has a higher and ApoE2 much lower affinity to the LDL receptor. The ε2 allele is associated with the lowest while the ε4 allele with the highest plasma cholesterol levels. Therefore, ApoE4 may be considered atherogenic (Curtiss & Boisvert, 2000), while ApoE2 seems to show a protective effect (Davignon et al., 1988). Some study has reported correlation between ApoE4 polymorphism and the incidence of CAD (Baroni et al., 2003). ApoE also seems to play a role in BP regulation. The ε4 allele influences the BP increasing effect of alcohol consumption. This gene environment interaction may have marked implications for the prevention and treatment of hypertension (Kauma et al., 1998).

### 2.8.4 Lipoprotein lipase

Lipoprotein lipase (LPL) is the main enzyme responsible for the hydrolysis of triglyceride (TG) present in circulating lipoproteins, and regulates high density lipoprotein concentrations. LPL gene located on chromosome 8p22 (Sparkes et al., 1987), has a length of 30 kb (Deeb & Peng, 1989), is composed of 10 exons. Mutations in locus intron 6 of LPL gene (Oka et al., 1989, Zuliani & Hobbs, 1990) lead to hypertriglyceridemia, dyslipidemia leading to various disorders as coronary artery disease, hypertension and obesity. The association betweeen hypertension and the LPL locus (8p22) was reported by several studies (Chen et al., 2005, Yang et al., 2003). Significant evidence for linkage of systolic BP, but not diastolic BP has been associated with LPL locus located on the short arm of chromosome 8 (8p22) (Du-An et al., 1992). Another study has identified a S447X polymorphism in exon 9 of LPL gene that results from replacement of serine amino acid with a stop codon creating a restriction site. This study has reported that the more common SS genotype is associated with a lower LPL activity compared with the infrequent SX/XX genotype and carriers of (SS) genotype were at high risk of developing hypertension (Salah et al., 2009). Another study, has suggested that a high concentration of triglyceride and/or low concentration of HDL-cholesterol are associated with high systolic BP and pulse pressure in hypertensive patients with the X447 allele of the LPL gene (Liu et al., 2004). Therefore, the LPL gene is considered as a candidate gene that could contribute to the development of EH.

## 2.9 Cytokines

Interleukin-6 (IL-6) is a multifunctional cytokine involved in inflammation, potentially influencing BP. The human IL-6 gene is located on chromosome 7p21 (Bowcock et al., 1988). Genetic variations of the IL-6 gene have been reported, and the commonly studied polymorphism is the functional variant -174G>C (Fishman et al., 1998). Association of this polymorphism with coronary artery diseases has been reported in some studies (Rauramaa et al. 2000, Berg et al., 2009, Pola et al 2002). In addition, this polymorphism has been shown to be associated in vivo with high levels of IL-6 (Jenny et al., 2002, Brull et al., 2001). Previous studies (Ridker et al., 2000, Chae et al., 2001) have reported that increased IL-6 levels is correlated with high BP and may be an independent risk factor for hypertension. Moreover, in Japanese women, a weak association was reported between hypertension and other IL-6 gene promotor variants, the C/G substitution at −634, the G/A substitution at 4391 in a 3- non-coding portion of exon 5, and the A/T variation in the −447 position (Nakajima et al., 1999).

### 2.10 Neuropeptide Y

Neuropeptide Y (NPY) is a sympathetic cotransmitter with catecholamines (Takiyyuddin et al., 1994). It exhibits a vasoconstricting action and has multiple receptors, Y1-Y5. NPY interacts with the Y1 receptor (NPY1R) to control adrenergic activity and BP (Michalkiewicz et al., 2005). The gene encoding the NPY1R coupled with G proteins is located on chromosome 4q31.3-q32 (Eva et al., 2006). Genetic variation at the NPY1R locus has implications for heritable autonomic control of the circulation, and systemic hypertension (Wang et al., 2009). Several NPY1R variants have been identified in EH. Both the promoter A-585T and the 3'-UTR A+1050G variants had important effects upon both diastolic BP and systolic BP and interacted to determine diastolic BP. Homozygous for both the promoter variant major allele (A/A at A-585T) and the 3'-UTR variant minor allele (G/G at A +1050G) had dramatic BP elevation (Wang et al., 2009). Moreover, other studies have reported that hypertension is influenced by the NPY T1128C polymorphism in South Indian population (Bhaskar et al., 2010) and in a Swedish hypertensive population (Wallerstedt et al., 2004). Therefore, the NPY gene is a candidate marker in EH.

## 3. Gene-gene interactions in EH

Large numbers of gene variants have been described in EH, and the pathogenic role of gene-gene interaction has received increasing attention. Some study (Bell et al., 2006) has reported that the presence of epistatic interactions and locus heterogeneity in the underlying genetics of hypertension may explain the lack of replicated linkage (Williams, 2004). The developped linkage tests for multiple susceptibility loci applied to human data (Cordell, H.J., 1995, Cox, N.J., 1999) have contributed to advance of the gene-gene interactions studies, but these methods have examined only pre-selected regions. Thus, by two dimensional genome-scan approach, Bell et al., (2006) have identified significant evidence for loci on chromosomes 5, 9, 11, 15, 16 and 19, which influence hypertension when gene-gene interactions are taken into account (5q13.1 and 11q22.1, two-locus lod score 5 5.72; 5q13.1 and 19q12, two-locus lod score 5 5.35; 9q22.3 and 15q12, two-locus lod score 5 4.80; 16p12.3 and 16q23.1, two-locus lod score 5 4.50). Another study (Williams et al., 2000) has examined the effects of allele interactions at 4 candidate loci. Three of the loci are in the renin-angiotensin-system: angiotensinogen, ACE, and AGTR1, and they have been associated with hypertension. The fourth locus studied is a previously undescribed locus, named FJ. In total, seven polymorphic sites at these loci were analyzed for their association with hypertension in normotensive and hypertensive age-matched individuals. There were no significant differences between the 2 phenotypic classes with respect to either allele or genotype frequencies. In this report, when authors have tested for nonallelic associations (linkage disequilibrium), they found that of the 120 multilocus comparisons, 16 deviated significantly from random in the hypertensive class, but there were no significant deviations in the normotensive group. This study suggests that genetic interactions between multiple loci rather than variants of a single gene underlie the genetic basis of hypertension. The relation of many polymorphisms has been examined also in Chinese hypertensive patients (Dongfeng et al., 2006), in several candidate genes with the risk of hypertension: (1) renin-angiotensin-aldosterone system, including ACE, AGTR1, and CYP11B2, (2) sympathetic nervous system, including α-1 adrenergic receptor 1A (ADRA1), ADRB2, and tyrosine hydroxylase (TH); (3) lipoprotein metabolism, including LPL; (4) intracellular messengers, including GNB3 and NOS3 ; and (5) sodium and electrolyte balance, including G protein-coupled receptor kinase 4 (GRK4) and protein kinase lysine- deficient 4 (WNK4). Both single-locus and multilocus analyses revealed that two genes from the sympathetic system (TH and ADRB2) and one gene affecting the sodium balance (GRK4) were independently associated with the significant risk of hypertension in the Chinese Han population. In addition to these 3 individual predictors, an interaction between CYP11B2 and AGTR1, both from RAAS, was also found to be involved in the relationship with hypertension. These findings support the recognized understanding that complex genetic interactions account for hypertension risk. Additional studies have genotyped hypertensives at the AGT M235T, ACE I/D, CYP11B2 C-344T, REN, AGTR1 and/or ADD loci, have reported that combinations of polymorphisms at several of these loci steadily increase the odds ratio of predicting hypertension (Agachan B et al., 2003, Vasku A et al., 1998, Tsai CT et al., 2003). Another study (Tomaszewski et al., 2006) revealed epistatic interaction between ADRB2 and NPY in regulation of LDL levels in hypertensive subjects. The effect of NPY locus appears to be altered by ADRB2. Specifically, Leu7Leu genotype within NPY SNP was associated with increased concentrations of LDL only in the presence of Arg16Gln27. Taken together all these studies provide evidence that several functional polymorphisms within candidate genes act individually or together in the etiology of EH.

## 4. Conclusion

The actual number of candidate genes detected in EH studies reinforced the highly polygenic nature of this disease. Knowing the genes responsible for this condition is an important prerequisite to prevent the expression of these disease markers related to lifestyle, especially for predisposed subjects at risk. From a large series of studies conducted in humans and animals, the renin-angiotensin-aldosterone system constitued risk genes and other systems like sodium system genes, signal transduction system genes, endothelial system genes, and neurohormonal and adrenergic genes were involved in genetic predisposition of EH. In addition, several lessons could be learned from these genetic studies and applied to other additional candidate genes that would be necessary to identify in EH. Actual strategies used for genetic studies showed some limitations. As well the candidate gene strategy (which assumes that a given gene, or a set of genes involved in a specific function, might contribute in BP variation) as linkage and/or association studies suffered from limited sample sizes and a low prior probability of the selected candidate genes being associated with hypertension. Moreover, the sequence variants influencing the phenotype of EH have remained elusive, but with better mapping techniques, better phenotyping methods and systems biology approach, and potential gene-gene interactive model, we should begin to discover those variants that could lead to its enhanced prevention, detection, and treatment of EH.

## 5. References

Agachan, B. ; Isbir, T. ; Yilmaz , H. & Akoglu E. (2003). Angiotensin converting enzyme I/D, angiotensinogen T174M-M235T and angiotensin II type 1 receptor A1166C gene polymorphisms in Turkish hypertensive patients. *Exp Mol Med* 35: 545-9

Ahmad, U.; Saleheen, D.; Bokhari, A. & Frossard, PM. (2005). Strong association of a renin intronic dimorphism with essential hypertension. *Hypertens Res* 28: 339-344

Albertin, G.; Rossi, GP.; Majone, F.; Tiso, N.; Mattara, A.; Danieli, GA.; Pessina, AC. & Palu, G. (1996). Fine mapping of the human endothelin-converting enzyme gene by fluorescent in situ. *Biochem Biophys Res Commun* 221:682-687

Alfakih, K.; Maqbool, A.; Sivananthan, M.; Walters, K.; Bainbridge, G.; Ridgway, J.; Balmforth, AJ. & Hall, AS. (2004). Left ventricular mass index and the common, functional, X-linked angiotensin II type 2 receptor gene polymorphism (-1332G/A) in patients with systemic hypertension. *Hypertension* 43:1189

Allikmets, K.; Patrik, T. & Viigimaa, M. (1999). The renin-angiotensin system in essential hypertension: Associations with cardiovascular risk. *Blood Press* 8:70-78

Asai, Y.; Ohkubo, T.; Katsuya, T.; Higaki, J.; Fu, Y.; Fukuda, M.; Hozawa, A.; Matsubara, M.; Kitaoka, H.; Tsuji, I.; Araki, T.; Satoh, H.; Hisamichi, S.; Imai, Y. & Ogihara, T. (2001). Endothelin 1 gene variant associates with blood pressure in overwitht people. *Hypertension* 33:1169-1174

Ashavaid, TF.; Shalia, KK.; Kondkar, AA.; Todur, SP.; Nair, KG. & Nair, SR. (2002). Gene polymorphism and coronary risk factors in Indian population. *Clin Chem Lab Med* 40:975- 985

Baker, EH.; Dong, YB. & Sagnella, GA. (1998). Association of hypertension with T594M mutation in beta subunit of epithelial sodium channels in black people resident in London. *Lancet* 351:1388-1392

Barlassina, C.; Citterio, L.; Bernardi, L.; Buzzi, L.; D'Amico, M.; Sciarrone, T. & Bianchi, G. (1997) Genetics of renal mechanisms of primary hypertension: the role of adducin. *J Hypertens* 15:1567-1571.

Barlassina, C.; Schork, NJ.; Manuta, P.; Citterio, L.; Sciarronre, M.; Lanella, G.; Bianchi, G. & Cusi, D. (2000). Synergistic effect of alpha-adducin and ACE genes causes blood pressure changes with body sodium and volume expansion. *Kidney Int* 57:1083-1090

Baroni, MG.; Berni, A.; Romeo, S.; Arca, M.; Tesorio, T.; Sorropago, G.; Di Mario, U. & Galton, DJ. (2003). Genetic study of common variants at the Apo E, Apo AI, Apo CIII, Apo B, lipoprotein lipase (LPL) and hepatic lipase (LIPC) genes and coronary artery disease (CAD): variation in LIPC gene associates with clinical outcomes in patients with established CAD. *BMC Med Genet* 4:8

Beeks, E.; Kessels, AG.; Kroon, AA.; van der Klauw, MM. & de Leeuw, PW. (2004). Genetic predisposition to salt-sensitivity: a systematic review. *J Hypertens* 22:1243-1249

Beige, J.; Hohenbleicher, H.; Distler, A. & Sharma, AM. (1999). G-Protein β3 subunit C825T variant and ambulatory blood pressure in essential hypertension. *Hypertension* 33:1049-51

Bell, JT.; Wallace, C.; Dobson, R.; Wiltshire, S.; Mein, C.; Pembroke, J.; Brown, M.; Clayton, D.; Samani, N.; Dominiczak, A.; Webster, J.; Lathrop, GM.; Connell, J.; Munroe, P.; Caulfield, M. & Farral M. (2006). Two-dimensional genome-scan identifies novel epistatic loci for essential hypertension. Hum Mol Genet 15: 1365–1374

Bengtsson, K.; Orho-Melander, M.; Lindblad, U.; Melander, O.; Bøg-Hansen, E.; Ranstam, J.; Råstam, L.; Groop, L. (1999). Polymorphism in the angiotensin converting enzyme but not in the angiotensinogen gene is associated with hypertension and type 2 diabetes: the Skaraborg Hypertension and Diabetes Project. *J Hypertens* 17:1569-1575

Benjafield, AV.; Jeyasingam, CL.; Nyholt, DR.; Griffiths, LR. & Morris, BJ. (1998). G-protein β3 subunit gene (GNB3) variant in causation of essential hypertension. *Hypertension* 32:1094-1097

Benjafield, AV.; Katyk, K. & Morris, BJ. (2003). Association of EDNRA, but not WNK4 or FKBP1B, polymorphisms with essential hypertension. *Clin Genet* 64(5):433-8.

Berg, KK.; Madsen, HO.; Garred, P.; Wiseth, R.; Gunnes, S. & Videm, V. (2009). The additive contribution from inflammatory genetic markers on the severity of cardiovascular disease. *Scand J Immunol* 69:36-42

Bhaskar, LV.; Thangaraj, K.; Non, AL.; Praveen, KK.; Pardhasaradhi, G.; Singh, L. & Rao, VR. (2010). Neuropeptide Y gene functional polymorphism influences susceptibility to hypertension in Indian population. *J Hum Hypertens* 24(9):617-22

Bianchi, G.; Tripodi, G.; Casari, G. ; Salardi, S. ; Barber, BR.; Garcia, R. ; Leoni, P. ; Torielli, L. ; Cusi, D. ; Ferrandi, M. (1994). Two point mutations within the adducin genes are involved in blood pressure variation. *Proc Natl Acad Sci USA* 91:3999-4003

Blackhart, BD.; Ludwig, EM.; Pierotti, VR.; Caiati, L.; Onasch, MA.; Wallis, SC.; Powell, L.; Pease, R.; Knott, TJ. & Chu, ML. (1986). Structure of the human apolipoprotein B gene. *Biol Chem* 33:15364-15367

Bluthner, M.; Schmidt, S.; Siffert, W;. Knigge, H.; Nawroth, P. & Ritz, E. (1999). Increased frequency of G protein β3-subunit 825 T allele in dialyzed patients with type 2 diabetes. *Kidney Int* 55:1247-50

Boerwinkle, E.; Xiong, W.; Fourest, E. & Chan, L. (1989). Rapid typing if tandemly repeated hypervariable loci by the polymerase chain reaction: application to the apolipoprotein B 3' hypervariable region. *Proc Natl Acad Sci USA* 86:212-6

Bohm, SK.; Grady, EF. & Bunnet, NW. (1997). Regulatory mechanisms that modulate signaling by G-protein-coupled receptors. *Biochem J* 322:1-18

Bonnardeaux, A.; Davis, E.; Jeunemaître, X. ; Fery, I. ; Charru, A. ; Clauser, E. ; Tiret, L. ; Cambien, F. ; Corvol, P. & Soubrier, F. (1994). Angiotensin II type I receptor gene polymorphisms in human essential hypertension. *Hypertension* 24:63-9

Bowcock, AM.; Kidd, JR.; Lathrop, GM.; Daneshvar, L.; May, LT.; Ray, A.; Sehgal, PB.; Kidd, KK. & Cavalli-Sforza, LLQ. (1988). The human 'interferon-beta 2/hepatocyte stimulating factor/interleukin-6' gene: DNA polymorphism studies and localization to chromosome 7p21. *Genomics* 3: 8-16

Brand, E.; Bankir, L.; Plouin, PF. & Soubrier, F. (1999). Glucagon Receptor Gene Mutation (Gly40Ser) in human essential hypertension the PEGASE study. *Hypertension* 34:15-17

Brand, E.; Chatelain, N.; Mulatero, P.; Féry, I.; Curnow, K.; Jeunemaitre, X.; Corvol, P.; Plouin, PF.; Cambien, F.; Pascoe, L.; Soubrier, F. (1998). Structural analysis and evaluation of the aldosterone synthase gene in hypertension. *Hypertension* 32: 198-204

Brull, DJ.; Montgomery, HE.; Sanders, J.; Dhamrait, S.; Luong, L.; Rumley, A.; Lowe, GD. & Humphries, SE. (2001). Interleukin-6 gene -174g>c and -572g>c promoter polymorphisms are strong predictors of plasma interleukin-6 levels after coronary artery bypass surgery. *Arterioscler Thromb Vasc Biol* 21:1458-63

Brunzell, JD.; Sniderman, AD.; Albers, JJ. & Kwiterovich, PO. (1984). Apoproteins B and AI and coronary artery disease in humans. *Arteriosclerosis* 4:79-83

Caprioli, J.; Mele, C.; Mossali, C.; Gallizioli, L.; Giacchetti, G.; Noris, M.; Remuzzi, G. & Benigni, A. (2008). Polymorphisms of EDNRB, ATG, and ACE genes in salt-sensitive hypertension. *Can J Physiol Pharmacol* 86:505-10

Casas, JP.; Cavalleri, GL.; Bautista, LE. ; Smeeth, L. ; Humphries, SE. & Hingorani , AD. (2006). Endothelial nitric oxide synthase gene polymorphisms and cardiovascular disease: a HUGE review. *Am J Epidemiol* 164:921-35

Casiglia, E.; Tikhonoff, V.; Caffi, S.; Martini, B.; Guidotti, F.; Bolzon, M.; Bascelli, A.; D'Este, D.; Mazza, A. & Pessina, AC. (2008). Effects of the C825T polymorphism of the GNB3 gene on body adiposity and blood pressure in fertile and menopausal women: a population-based study. *J Hypertens* 26:238-43

Chae, CU.; Lee, RT.; Rifai, N & Ridker, PM. (2001). Blood pressure and inflammation in apparently healthy men. *Hypertension* 38:399-403

Chambers, SM. & Morris, BJ. (1996). Glucagon receptor gene mutation in essential hypertension. *Nature Genet* 12:122. Letter

Chang, PY.; Zhao, LG. & Su, XL. (2011). Association of TSC gene variants and hypertension in Mongolian and Han populations. *Genet Mol Res* 10:902-909

Chaves, FJ.; Pascual, JM.; Rovira, E.; Armengod, ME. & Redon, J. (2001). Angiotensin II AT1 receptor gene polymorphism and microalbuminuria in essential hypertension. *Am J Hypertens* 14:364-70

Chen, P.; Jou, YS.; Fann, CS.; Chen, JW.; Wu, SY. & Pan, WH. (2005). Lipoprotein lipase gene is linked and associated with hypertension in Taiwan young-onset hypertension genetic study. *J Biomed Sci* 12:651-8

Cheng, J.; Liu, J.; Li, X.; Peng, J.; Han, S.; Zhang, R.; Xu, Y. & Nie, S. (2008). Insulin-like growth factor-1 receptor polymorphism and ischemic stroke: a case-control study in Chinese population. *Acta Neurol Scand* 118:333-8

Ciechanowicz, A.; Kurzawski, G.; Widecka, K.; Goździk, J.; Adler, G. & Czekalski, S. (1997). The T--C mutation of the nucleotide 2238 in the gene of atrial natriuretic peptide (ANP) precursor and heterogeneity of sodium-sensitive hypertension. Preliminary report. *Pol Arch Med Wewn* 98:501-9

Cooke, GE.; Doshi, A. & Binkely, PF. (2007). Endothelial nitric oxide synthase gene: prospects for treatment of heart disease. *Pharmacogenomics* 8:1723-1734.

Cordell, HJ.; Todd, JA.; Bennett, ST.; Kawaguchi, Y. & Farrall, M. (1995) Two-locus maximum lod scor analysis of a multifactorial trait: joint consideration of IDDM2 and IDDM4 with IDDM1 in type 1 diabetes. *Am J Hum Genet* 57: 920-934

Cox, NJ.; Frigge, M.; Nicolae, DL.; Concannon, P.; Hanis, CL.; Bell, GI. & Kong, A. (1999) Loci on chromosomes 2 (NIDDM1) and 15 interact to increase susceptibility to diabetes in Mexican Americans. *Nat Genet* :21, 213 -215

Curtiss, LK. & Boisvert, WA. (2000). Apolipoprotein E and atherosclerosis. *Curr Opin Lipidol* 11:243-251

Cusi, D.; Barlassina, C.; Azzani, T.; Casari, G.; Citterio, L.; Devoto, M.; Glorioso, N.; Lanzani, C.; Manunta, P.; Righetti, M.; Rivera, R.; Stella, P.; Troffa, C.; Zagato, L. & Bianchi, G. (1997). Polymorphisms of alpha-adducin and salt sensitivity in patients with essential hypertension. *Lancet* 349:1353-1357

Cwynar, M.; Staessen, JA.; Ticha, M.; Nawrot, T.; Citterio, L.; Kuznetsova, T.; Wojciechowska, W.; Stolarz, K.; Filipovský, J.; Kawecka-Jaszcz, k.; Grodzicki, T.; Struijker-Boudier, HA.; Thijs, L.; Van Bortel, L. & Bianchi, G. (2005). On behalf of the European Project on Genes in Hypertension (EPOGH) Investigators. Epistatic interaction between α and γ-adducin influences peripheral and central pulse pressure in White Europeans. *J Hypertens* 23:961-969

Dammerman, M.; Sandkuijl, LA.; Halaas, JL.; Chung, W. & Breslow, JL. (1993). An apolipoprotein CIII haplotype protective against hypertriglyceridemia is specified by promoter and 3′ untranslated region polymorphisms. *Proc Natl Acad Sci USA* 90:4562-4566

Davignon, J.; Gregg, RE. & Sing, CF. (1988) Apolipoprotein E polymorphism and atherosclerosis. *Arteriosclerosis* 8:1-21

Deeb, SS. & Peng, R. (1989). Structure of the human lipoprotein lipase gene. *Biochemistry* 28: 4131-4135

Delles, C.; Erdmann, J.; Jacobi, J,.; Fleck, E.; Regitz-Zagrosek, V. & Schmieder, RE. (2000). Lack of association between polymorphisms of angiotensin II receptor genes and response to short-term angiotensin II infusion. *J Hypertens* 18:1573-8

Dong, Y.; Zhu, H.; Sagnella, GA.; Carter, ND.; Cook, DG. & Cappuccio, FP. (1999). Association between the C825T polymorphism of the G protein beta3-subunit gene and hypertension in blacks. *Hypertension* 34:1193-6

Dong, YB.; Plange-Rhule, J.; Owusu, I.; Micah, F;. Eastwood, JB.; Carter, ND.; Saggar-Malik, AK.; Cappuccio, FP. & Jeffery, S. (2002). T594M mutation of the beta-subunit of the epithelial sodium channel in Ghanaian populations from Kumasi and London and a possible association with hypertension. *Genet Test* 6:63-5

Dongfeng, G.; Shaoyong, S.; Dongliang, G.; Shufeng, C.; Jianfeng, H.; Biao, L.; Runsheng, C. & Boqin Q. (2006). Association study with 33 single-nucleotide polymorphisms in 11 candidate genes for hypertension in Chinese. *Hypertension* 47:1147-1154

Doria, A.; Onuma, T.; Warram, JH. & Krolewski, AS. (1997). Synergistic effect of angiotensin II type 1 receptor genotype and poor glycaemic control on risk of nephropathy in IDDM. *Diabetologia* 40:1293-9

Du-An, W.; Xiangdong, B.; Craig, H.; Warden, D.; Shen, DC.; Jeng, CY.; Wayne, HH.; Sheu, M.; Fuh, MT.; Tomohiro, K.; Victor, JD.; Gerald, MR.; Aldons, JL.; Jerome, IR. & Chen, YD. (1992). Quantitative Trait Locus Mapping of Human Blood Pressure to a Genetic Region at or near the Lipoprotein Lipase Gene Locus on Chromosome 8p22. *J Clin Invest* 97: 2111-2118

Eisenach, JH.; Clark, ES.; Charkoudian, N.; Dinenno, FA.; Atkinson, JL.; Fealey, RD.; Dietz, NM. & Joyner, MJ. (2002). Effects of chronic sympathectomy on vascular function in the human forearm. *J Appl* Physiol 92:2019-2025

Emoto, N. & Yanagisawa, M. (1995) Endothelin-converting enzyme-2 is a membrane-bound, phosphoramidon-sensitive metalloprotease with acidic pH optimum. *J Biol Chem* 270:15262-15268

Erdmann, J., Guse, M., Kallisch, H., Fleck, E. & Regitz-Zagrosek, V. (2000). Novel intronic polymorphism (+1675G/A) in the human angiotensin II subtype 2 receptor gene. *Hum Mutat* 15: 487

Erdmann, J.; Riedel, K.; Rohde, K.; Folgmann, I.; Wienker, T.; Fleck, E. & Regitz-Zagrosek, V. (1999). Characterization of polymorphisms in the promoter of the human angiotensin II subtype 1 (AT1) receptor gene. *Ann Hum Genet* 63:369-74

Eva, C.; Serra, M.; Mele, P.; Panzica, G. & Oberto, A. (2006). Physiology and gene regulation of the brain NPY Y1 Receptor. *Front Neuroendocrinol* 27:308-339

Fang, YJ.; Deng, HB.; Thomas, GN.; Tzang, CH.; Li, CX.; Xu, ZL.; Yang, M. & Tomlinson, B. (2010). Linkage of angiotensinogen gene polymorphisms with hypertension in asibling study of Hong Kong Chinese. *J Hypertens* 28: 1203-1209

Fava, C.; von Wowern, F.; Berglund, G.; Carlson, J.; Hedblad, B.; Rosberg, L.; Burri, P.; Almgren, P. & Melander, O. (2006). 24-h ambulatory blood pressure is linked to chromosome 18q21-22 and genetic variation of NEDD4L associates with cross-sectional and longitudinal blood pressure in Swedes. *Kidney Int* 70:562-9

Fishman, D.; Faulds, G.; Jeffery, R.; Mohamed-Ali, V.; Yudkin, JS.; Humphries, S & Woo, P. (1998). The effect of novel polymorphisms in the interleukin-6 (IL-6) gene on IL-6 transcription and plasma IL-6 levels, and an association with systemic-onset juvenile chronic arthritis. *J Clin Invest* 102:1369-76

Friedl, W.; Ludwig, EH.; Paulweber, B.; Sandhofer, F. & McCarthy, BJ. (1990). Hypervariability in a minisatellite 3' of the apolipoprotein B gene in patients with coronary heart disease compared with normal controls. *J Lipid* Res 31:659-665

Frossard, PM.; Malloy, MJ.; Lestringant, GG. & Kane, JP. (2001). Haplotypes of the human renin gene associated with essential hypertension and stroke. *J Hum Hypertens* 15: 49-55

Funke-Kaiser, H.; Bolbrinker, J.; Theis, S.; Lemmer, J.; Richter, CM.; Paul, M. & Orzechowski, HD. (2000). Characterization of the c-specific promoter of the gene encoding human endothelin-converting enzyme-1 (ECE-1). *FEBS Lett* 466-310-316

Funke-Kaiser, H.; Reichenberger, F.; Ko¨pke, K.; Herrmann, SM.; Pfeifer, J.; Orzechowski, HD.; Zidek, W.; Paul, M. & Brand, E. (2003). Differential binding of transcription factor E2F-2 to the endothelin-converting enzyme-1b promoter affects blood pressure regulation. *Hum Mol Genet* 12:423-33

Gaillard, I.; Clauser, E. & Corvol, P. (1989). Structure of human angiotensinogen gene. *DNA* 8:87-99

Glenn, B.S;. Stewart, WF.; Schwartz, BS. & Bressler, J. (2001). Relation of alleles of the sodium-potassium adenosine triphosphatase α2 gene with blood pressure and lead exposure. *Am J Epidemiol* 153:537-45

Glorioso, N.; Filigheddu, F.; Troffa, C.; Soro, A.; Parpaglia, PP.; Tsikoudakis, A.; Meyers, RH.; Herrera, VLM. & Ruiz-Opazo, N. (2001). Interaction of α1-NaK-ATPase and NaK2Cl-cotransporter genes in human essential hypertension. *Hypertension* 38:204-209

Gopi-Chand, M.; Srinath, J.; Rao, RS.; Lakkakula, BV.; Kumar, S. & Rao, VR. (2011). Association between the M268T polymorphism in the angiotensinogen gene and essential hypertension in a South Indian Population. *Biochem Genet* 49:474-82

Green, SA.; Turki, J.; Bejarano, P.; Hall, IP. & Liggett, SB. (1995). Influence of beta 2-adrenergic receptor genotypes on signal transduction in human airway smooth muscle cells. *Am J Respir Cell Mol Biol* 13:25-33

Green, SA. Turki, J.; Innis, M. & Liggett, SB. (1994). Amino-terminal polymorphisms of the human beta 2-adrenergic receptor impart distinct agonistpromoted regulatory properties. *Biochemistry* 33:9414-9419

Grubbs, AL.; Anstadt, MP. & Ergul, A. (2002) Saphenous vein endothelin system expression and activity in African American patients. *Arterioscler Thromb Vasc Biol* 22:1122-1127

Gu, D.; Ge, D.; He, J.; Li, B.; Chen, J.; Liu, D.; Chen, J. & Chen, R. (2004). Haplotypic analyses of the aldosterone synthase gene *CYP11B2* associated stage-2 hypertension in northern Han Chinese. *Clin Genet* 66 :409-16

Hansen, LH.; Abrahamsen, N.; Hager, J.; Jelinek, L.; Kindsvogel, W.; Froguel, P. & Nishimura, E. (1996). The Gly40Ser mutation in the human glucagon receptor gene associated with NIDDM results in a receptor with reduced sensitivity to glucagon. *Diabetes* 45:725-730

Hayakawa, T.; Takamura, T.; Abe, T. & Kaneko, S. (2007). Association of the C825T polymorphism of the G-protein β3 subunit gene with hypertension, obesity, hyperlipidemia, insulin resistance, diabetes, diabetic complications, and diabetic therapies among Japanese. *Metabolism* 56:44-8

Haynes, WG.; Strachan, FE. & Webb, DJ. (1995). Endothelin ETA and ETB receptors cause vasoconstriction of human resistance and capacitance vessels in vivo. *Circulation* 92:357-363

Hengstenberg, C.; Schunkert, H.; Mayer, B.; Doring, A.; Lowel, H.; Hense, HW.; Fischer, M.; Riegger, GA. & Holmer, SR. (2001). Association between a polymorphism in the G protein beta3 subunit gene (GNB3) with arterial hypertension but not with myocardial infarction. *Cardiovasc Res* 49:820-7

Henskens, LH.; Spiering, W.; Stoffers, HE.; Soomers, FL.; Vlietinck, RF.; de Leeuw, PW. & Kroon, AA. (2003). Effects of ACE I/D and AT1R-A1166C polymorphisms on blood pressure in a healthy normotensive primary care population: first results of the Hippocates study. *J Hypertens* 21:81-6

Hilgers, KF. & Schmidt, BM. (2005). Gene variants of aldosterone synthase and hypertension. *J Hypertens* 23:1957-9

Hirata, Y.; Emori, T.; Eguchi, S.; Kanno, K.; Imai, T.; Ohta, K. & Marumo, F. (1993). Endothelin receptor subtype B mediates synthesis of nitric oxide by cultured bovine endothelial cells. *J Clin Invest* 91:1367-1373

Hoehe, MR.; Otterud, B.; Hsieh, W-T.; Martinez, MM.; Stauffer, D.; Holik, J.; Berrettini, WH.; Byerley, WF.; Gershon, ES. & Lalouel, JM. (1995). Genetic mapping of adrenergic receptor genes in humans. *J Mol Med* 73:299-306

Horio, T.; Kamide, K.; Takiuchi, S.; Yoshii, M.; Miwa, Y.; Matayoshi, T.; Yoshihara, F.; Nakamura, S.; Tokudome, T.; Miyata, T. & Kawano, Y. (2010). Association of insulin-like growth factor-1 receptor gene polymorphisms with left ventricular mass and geometry in essential hypertension. *J Hum Hypertens* 24:320-6

Hyndman, MF.; Parsons, HG.; Verma, S.; Bridge, PJ.; Edworthy, S.; Jones, C.; Lonn, E.; Charbonneau, F. & Anderson, TJ. (2002). The $T^{-786}$ C mutation in endothelial nitric oxide synthase is associated with hypertension. *Hypertension* 39:919-922

Hyun-Seok, J.; Kyung-Won, H.; Ji-Eun, L.; Sue-Yun, H.; Sang-Ho, L.; Chol, S.; Hun Kuk, P. & Bermseok, O. (2010). Genetic Variations in the Sodium Balance-Regulating Genes ENaC, NEDD4L, NDFIP2 and USP2 Influence Blood Pressure and Hypertension. *Kidney Blood Press Res* 33:15-23

Ishikawa, K.; Imai, Y.; Katsuya, T.; Ohkubo, T.; Tsuji, I.; Nagai, K.; Nakata, Y.; Satoh, H.; Hisamichi, S.; Higaki. J. & Ogihara ,T. (2000). Human G-protein β3 subunit variant is associated with serum potassium and total cholesterol levels but not with blood pressure. *Am J Hypertens* 13:140-5

Iwai, N.; Iwai, N.; Baba, S.; Mannami, T.; Ogihara, T. & Ogata, J. (2002). Association of sodium channel alpha subunit promoter variant with blood pressure. *J Am Soc Nephrol* 13:80-85

Jachymova, M.; Horky, K.; Bultas, J.; Kozich, V.; Jindra, A.; Peleska, J. & Martásek, P. (2001). Association of the Glu298Asp polymorphism in the endothelial nitric oxide synthase gene with essential hypertension resistant to conventional therapy. *Biochem Biophys Res Commun* 284:426-430

Jenny, NS.; Tracy, RP.; Ogg, MS.; Luongle, A.; Kuller, LH.; Arnold, AM.; Sharrett, AR. & Humphries, SE. (2002). In the elderly, interleukin-6 plasma levels and the _174G>C polymorphism are associated with the development of cardiovascular disease. *Arterioscler Thromb Vasc Biol* 22:2066-71

Jeunemaitre, X. (2008). Genetics of the human renin angiotensin system. *J Mol Med* 86:637-641.

Jeunemaitre, X.; Soubrier, F.; Kotelevtsev, YV. ; Lifton, RP.; Williams, CS.; Charru, A.; Hunt, SC.; Hopkins, PN.; Williams, RR. & Lalouel, JM. (1992). Molecular basis of human hypertension: role of angiotensinogen. *Cell* 71:169-180

Jin, JJ.; Nakura, J.; Wu, Z.; Yamamoto, M.; Abe, M.; Chen, Y.; Tabara, Y.; Yamamoto, Y.; Igase, M.; Bo, X.; Kohara, K .& Miki, T. (2003a). Association of angiotensin II type 2 receptor gene variant with hypertension. *Hypertens res* 26:547-52

Jin, JJ.; Nakura, J.; Wu, Z.; Yamamoto, M.; Abe, M. ; Tabara, Y.; Yamamoto, Y.; Igase, M.; Kohara, K. & Miki, T. (2003b). Association of endothelin-1 gene variant with hypertension. *Hypertension* 41:163-7

Ju, Z.; Zhang, H. ; Sun, K. ; Song, Y. ; Lu, H. ; Hui, R. & Huang, X. (2003). Alpha-adducin gene polymorphism is associated with essential hypertension in Chinese: A case-control and family-based study. *J Hypertens* 21:1861-8

Juul, A.; Scheike, T.; Davidsen, M.; Gyllenborg, J. & Jorgensen, T. (2002). Low serum insulin-like growth factor I is associated with increased risk of ischemic heart disease: a population-based case-control study. *Circulation* 106:939-944

Kainulainen, K.; Perola, M.; Terwilliger, J.; Kaprio, J.; Kaskenvuo, M.; Syvänen, AC.; Vartianen, I.; Peltonen, L. & Kontula, K. (1999). Evidence for the involvement of the type 1 angiotensin II receptor locus in essential hypertension. *Hypertension* 33:844-9

Kamida, K.; Tanaka, C.; Takiuchi, S.; Miwa, Y.; Yoshii, M.; Horio, T.; Kawano, Y. & Miyata, T. (2004). Six missense mutations of the epithelial sodium channel: β and γ subunits in Japanese Hypertensives. *Hypertens Res* 27:333-38

Kato, N.; Sugiyama, T.; Morital, H.; Morital, H.; Nabikas, T.; Kurihara, H.; Yamori, Y. & Yazaki, Y. (2000). Genetic analysis of the atrial natriuretic peptide gene in essential hypertension. *Clin Sci* 98:251-8

Kauma, H.; Savolainen, MJ.; Rantala, AO. ; Lilja, M.; Kervinen, K.; Reunanen, A. & Kesäniemi, YA. (1998). Apolipoprotein E phenotype determines the effect of alcohol on blood pressure in middle-aged men. *Am J Hypertens* 11:1334-43

Kazantsev, A.; Yamaoka, LH. & Roses, AD. (1992). A dinucleotide repeat polymorphism in the human NaKATPase, alpha subunit (ATP1A3) gene. *Nucleic Acids Res* 20:1164

Knott, TJ.; Rall, SCJr.; Innerarity, TL.; Jacobson, SF.; Urdea, MS.; Levy-Wilson, B.; Powell, LM.; Pease, RJ.; Eddy, R.; Nakai, H.; Byers, M.; Priestley, LM.; Robertson, E.; Rall, LB.; Betsholtz, C.; Shows, TB.; Mahley, RW. & Scott, J. (1985). Human apolipoprotein B: structure of carboxyl-terminal domains, sites of gene expression, and chromosomal localization. *Science* 230:37-43

Knott, TJ.; Wallis, SC.; Powell, LM.; Pease, RJ.; Lusis, AJ.; Blackhart, B.; McCarthy, BJ.; Wilson, B. & Scott, J. (1986). A hypervariable region 3' to the human apolipoprotein B gene. *Nucleic acids research* 14:7501-7503

Kosuge, K.; Soma, M.; Nakayama, T.; Aoi, N.; Sato, M.; Isumi, Y. & Matsumoto, K. (2007). A novel variable number of tandem repeat of the natriuretic peptide precursor B gene's 5'-flanking region is associated with essential hypertension among Japanese females. *Int J Med Sci* 4:146-152

Kotanko, P.; Binder, A.; Tasker, J.; DeFreitas, P.; Kamdar, S.; Clark, AJL.; Skrabal, F. & Caulfield, M. (1997). Essential hypertension in African Caribbeans associates with a variant of the b-2 adrenoceptor. *Hypertension* 30:773-776

Kumar, NN.; Benjafield, AV.; Lin, RC.; Wang, WY.; Stowasser, M. & Morris, BJ. (2003). Haplotype analysis of aldosterone synthase gene (CYP11B2) polymorphisms shows association with essential hypertension. *J Hypertens* 21:1331-7

Kunz, R.; Kreutz, R.; Beige, J.; Distler, A. & Sharma, AM. (1997). Association between the angiotensinogen 235T variant and essential hypertension in whites: a systematic review and methodological appraisal. *Hypertension* 30:1331-1337

Kuznetsova, T.; Citterio, L.; Herbots, L.; Carpini, SD.; Thijs, L.; Casamassima, N.; Richart, T.; Fagard, RH.; Bianchi, G. & Staessen, JA. (2008). Effects of genetic variation in adducin on left ventricular diastolic function as assessed by tissue doppler imaging in a Flemish population. *J Hypertens* 26:1229-1236

Laburthe, M.; Couvineau, A.; Gaudin, P.; Maoret, JJ. ; Rouyer-Fessard, C. & Nicole, P. (1996). Receptors for VIP, PACAP, secretin, GRF, glucagon, GLP-1, and other members of their new family of G protein-linked receptors: structure-function relationship with special reference to the human VIP-1 receptor. *Ann NY Acad Sci* 805:94-109

Lajemi, M.; Labat, C.; Gautier, S.; Lacolley, P.; Safar, M.; Asmar, R.; Cambien, F.; & Benetos, A. (2001). Angiotensin II type 1 receptor-153A/G and 1166A/C gene polymorphisms and increase in aortic stiffness with age in hypertensive subjects. *J Hypertens* 19:407-13

Lalley, PA.; Francke, U. & Minna, JD. (1978). Homologous genes for enolase, phosphogluconate dehydrogenase, phosphoglucomutase, and adenylate kinase are syntenic on mouse chromosome 4 and human chromosome 1p. *Proc Natl Acad Sci USA* 75:2382-2386

Lang, CC.; Stein, CM.; Brown, RM.; Deegan, R.; Nelson, R.; He, HB.; Wood, M. & Wood, AJ. (1995). Attenuation of isoproterenol-mediated vasodilatation in blacks. *N Engl J Med* 333:155-160

Lanzani, C.; Citterio, L.; Jankaricova, M.; Sciarrone, MT.; Barlassina, C.; Fattori, S.; Messaggio, E.; Serio, CD., Zagato,L.; Cusi, D.; Hamlyn, JM.; Stella, A., Bianchi, G. & Manunta, P. (2005). Role of the adducin family genes in human essential hypertension. *J Hypertens* 23:543-549

Levin, ER. (1995). Endothelins. *N Engl J Med* 333:356-363

Lifton, RP.; Gharavi, AG. & Geller, DS. (2001). Molecular mechanisms of human hypertension. *Cell* 104:545-556

Liu, A.; Lee, L.; Zhan, S.; Cao, W.; Lv, J.; Guo, X. & Hu, Y. (2004). The S447X polymorphism of the lipoprotein lipase gene is associated with lipoprotein lipid and blood pressure levels in Chinese patients with essential hypertension. *J Hypertens* 22:1503-9

Lou, Y.; Liu, J.; Li, Y.; Liu, Y.; Wang, Z.; Liu, K.; Wu, H.; Niu, Q.; Gu, Y.; Guo, Y.; Li, Z. & Wen, S. (2011). Association Study of the b2-Adrenergic Receptor Gene Polymorphisms and Hypertension in the Northern Han Chinese. In: *PloS one*,

01.08.2011, Available from http: // www.plosone.org 6 April 2011 | Volume 6 | Issue 4 | e18590

MacGregor, AJ.; Snieder, H.; Schork, NJ. & Spector, TD. (2000). Twins: novel uses to study complex traits and genetic diseases. *Trends Genet* 16:131-134

Mansego, ML.; Redon, J.; Marin, R.; Gonzalez-Albert, V.; Martin-Escudero, JC.; Fabia, MJ.; Martinez, F. & Chaves, FJ. (2008). Renin polymorphisms and haplotypes are associated with blood pressure levels and hypertension risk in postmenopausal women. *J Hypertens* 26:230-23

Maqbool, A.; Hall, AS.; Ball, SG. & Balmforth, AJ. (1999). Common polymorphisms of β1-adrenoceptor: identification and rapid screening assay. *Lancet* 353:897

Martin, MM. & Elton, TS. (1995). The sequence and genomic organization of the human type 2 angiotensin II receptor. *Biochem Bioph Res Commun* 209:554-62

Masharani, U. & Frossard, PM. (1988). MspI and HindIII restriction fragment length polymorphisms at the human Na,K-ATPase betasubunit (ATP1B) gene locus. *Hum Genet* 80:308

Matsubara, M.; Metoki, H.; Suzuki, M.; Fujiwara, T.; Kikuya, M.; Michimata, M.; Ohkubo, T.; Hozawa, A.; Tsuji, I.; Hisamichi, S.; Araki, T. & Imai, Y. (2002). Genotypes of the betaENaC gene have little influence on blood pressure level in the Japanese population. *Am J Hypertens* 15:189-92

Matsubara, M.; Sato, T.; Nishimura, T.; Suzuki, M.; Kikuya, M.; Metoki, H.; Michimata, M.; Tsuji, I.; Ogihara, T. & Imai, Y. (2004). CYP11B2 polymorphisms and home blood pressure in a population-based cohort in Japanese: the Ohasama study. *Hypertens Res* 27:1-6

Matsukawa, N.; Grzesik, WJ.; Takahashi, N.; Pandey, KN.; Pang, S.; Yamauchi, M. & Smithies, O. (1999). The natriuretic peptide clearance receptor locally modulates the physiological effects of the natriuretic peptide system. *Proc Natl Acad Sci* 96:7403-7408

Matsuoka, Y.; Li, X. & Bennett, V. (2000) Adducin: structure, function and regulation. Cell Mol Life Sci 57:884-895

Melander, O.; Ortho-Melander, M.; Bengtsson, K.; Lindblad, U.; Râstam, L.; Groop, L. & Hulthén, UL. (2000). Genetic variants of thiazide-sensitive NaCl-cotransporter in Gitlman's syndrome and primary hypertension. *Hypertension* 36:389-394

Men, C.; Tang, K.; Lin, G.; Li, J. & Zhan, Y. (2001). ENOS-G894T polymorphism is a risk factor for essential hypertension in China. *Indian J Biochem* 48:154-7

Mercer, RW.; Schneider, JW.; Savitz, A.; Emanuel, J.; Benz, EJ Jr. & Levenson, R. (1986). Rat-brain Na,K-ATPase beta-chain gene: primary structure, tissue-specific expression, and amplification in ouabain-resistant HeLa C+ cells. *Mol Cell Biol* 6:3884-3890

Mesrati, FH. (2007). Essential hypertension. *Lancet* 370:591-603

Michalkiewicz, M.; Zhao, GQ.; Jia, Z;. Michalkiewicz, T. & Racadio, MJ. (2005). Central neuropeptide Y signaling ameliorates N(omega)-nitro-L-arginine methyl ester hypertension in the rat through a Y1 receptor mechanism. *Hypertension* 45:780–785

Mische, SM.; Mooseker, MS. & Morrow, JS. (1987). Erythrocyte adducin : A calmodulin-regulated actin-bundling protein that stimulates spectrin-actin binding. *J Cell Biol* 105:2837-2845

Moore, JD.; Mason, DA.; Green, SA.; Hsu, J. & Liggett, SB. (1999). Racial differences in the frequencies of cardiac β 1-adrenergic receptor polymorphisms: analysis of c145A3G and c1165G3C. *Hum Mutat* 14:271

Morris, BJ.; Jeyasingam, CL.; Zhang, W.; Curtain, RP. & Griffiths, LR. (1997). Influence of family history on frequency of glucagon receptor Gly40Ser mutation in hypertensive subjects. *Hypertension* 30:1640-1641

Nakajima, T.; Ota, N.; Yoshida, H.; Watanabe, S.; Suzuki, T. & Emi, M. (1999). Allelic variants in the interleukin-6 gene and essential hypertension in Japanese women. *Genes Immun* 1:115-119

Nicod, J.; Bruhin, D.; Auer, L.; Vogt, B.; Frey, FJ. & Ferrari, P. (2003). A biallelic gene polymorphism of CYP11B2 predicts increased aldosterone to renin ratio in selected hypertensive patients. *J Clin Endocrinol Metab* 88:2495-500

Nishimura, H.; Yerkes, E.; Hohenfellner, K.; Miyazaki, Y.; Ma, J.; Hunley, TE.; Yoshida, H.; Ichiki, T.; Threadgill, D.; Phillips, JA.; Hogan, BM.; Fogo, A.; Brock, JW.; Inagami, T.& Ichikawa, I. (1999). Role of the angiotensin type 2 receptor gene in congenital anomalies of the kidney and urinary tract, CAKUT, of mice and men. *Mol Cell* 3:1-10

O'Shaughnessy, KM. (2001). The genetics of essential hypertension. *Br J Clin Pharmacol* 51:5-11

Obermüller, N.; Bernstein, P.; Velazquez, H.; Reilly, R.; Reilly, R.; Moser, D.; Ellison, DH. & Bachmann, S. (1995). Expression of the thiazide-sensitive Na-Cl cotransporter in rat and human Kidney. *Am J Physiol* 269:F900-F910

Ogawa, Y.; Itoh, H. & Nakao, K. (1995). Molecular bioloby and biochemistry of natriuretic peptide family. *Clin Exp Pharmacol Physiol* 22:49-53

Oka, K;. Tkalcevic, GT.; Stocks, J.; Galton, DJ. & Brown, WV. (1989). Nucleotide sequence of PvuII polymorphic site at the lipoprotein lipase gene locus. *Nucleic Acids Res* 17:6752

Ono, K.; Mannami, T.; Baba, S.; Tomoike, H.; Suga, S. & Iwai, N. (2002). A Single-Nucleotide Polymorphism in C-Type Natriuretic Peptide Gene May Be Associated with Hypertension. *Hypertens Res* 25:727-730

Ormezzano, O.; Poirier, O.; Mallion, JM.; Nicaud, V.; Amar, J.; Chamontin, B.; Mounier-Véhier, C.; François, P. ; Cambien, F. & Baguet, JP. (2005). A polymorphism in the endothelin-A receptor gene is linked to baroreflex sensitivity. *J Hypertens* 23:2019-26

Orzechowski, HD.; Richter, CM.; Funke-Kaiser, H.; Kroger, B.; Schmidt, M.; Menzel, S.; Bohnemeier, H. & Paul, M. (1997). Evidence of alternative promoters directing isoform-specific expression of human endothelin-converting enzyme-1 mRNA in cultured endothelial cells. *J Mol Med* 75:512-521

Pankow, JS.; Rose, KM.; Oberman, A.; Hunt, SC.; Atwood, LD.; Djousse, L.; Province, MA. & Rao, DC.; (2000). Possible locus on chromosome 18q influencing postural systolic blood pressure changes. *Hypertension* 36:471-476

Philippe, MF.; Enyioma, N.; Obineche, G. & Lestringant, G. (1999). Association of an apolipoprotein B gene marker with essential hypertension. *Hypertension* 33:1052-1056

Plotkin, MD.; Kaplan, MR.; Verlander, JW.; Lee, WS.; Xu, ZC.; Lytton, J. & Hebert, SC. (1996). Localization of the thiazide sensitive Na-Cl cotransporter, rTSC1 in the rat kidney. *Kidney Int.* 50:174-183

Poirier, O.; Georges, JL.; Ricard, S.; Arveiler, D.; Ruidavets, JB.; Luc, G.; Evans, A.; Cambien, F. & Tiret, L. (1998). New polymorphisms of the angiotensin II type 1 receptor gene and their associations with myocardial infarction and blood pressure: the ECTIM study. Etude Cas-Témoin de l'Infarctus du Myocarde (1988). *J Hypertens* 16:1443-7

Pola, R.; Flex, A.; Gaetani, E.; Pola, P. & Bernabei, R. (2002). The −174 G/C polymorphism of the interleukin-6 gene promoter and essential hypertension in an elderly Italian population. *J Hum Hypertens* 16:637-640

Rahman, T.; Baker, M.; Hall, DH.; Avery, PJ. & Keavney, B. (2008). Common genetic variation in the type A endothelin-1 receptor is associated with ambulatory blood pressure: a family study. *J Hum Hypertens* 22:282-8

Rauramaa, R.; Väisänen, SB.; Luong, LA.; Schmidt-Trücksäss, A.; Penttilä, IM.; Bouchard, C.; Töyry, J. & Humphries, SE. (2000). Stromelysin-1 and interleukin-6 gene promoter polymorphisms are determinants of asymptomatic carotid artery atherosclerosis. *Arterioscler Thromb Vasc Biol* 20:2657-2662

Ridker, PM.; Rifai, N.; Stampfer, MJ. & Hennekens, CH; (2000). Plasma concentration of interleukin-6 and the risk of future myocardial infarction among apparently healthy men. *Circulation* 101:1767-72

Rigat, B.; Hubert, C.; Alhenc-Gelas, F. ; Cambien, F. ; Corvol, P. & Soubrier, F. (1990). An insertion/deletion polymorphism in the angiotensin I converting enzyme gene accounting for half the variance of serum enzyme levels. *J Clin Invest* 86:1343-6

Rubattu, S.; Bigatti, G.; Evangelista, A.; Lanzani, C.; Stanzione, R.; Zagato, L.; Manunta, P.; Marchitti, S.; Venturelli, V.; Bianchi, G.; Volpe, M. & Stella, P. (2006). Association of atrial natriuretic peptide and type a natriuretic peptide receptor gene polymorphisms with left ventricular mass in human essential hypertension. *J Am Coll Cardiol* 48: 499-505

Rubattu, S. & Volpe, M. (2001). The atrial natriuretic peptide: a changing view. *J Hypertens* 19:1923-31

Russo, CJ.; Melista, E.; Cui, J.; De Stefano, AL.; Bakris, GL.; Manolis, AJ.; Gavras, H. & Baldwin, CT. (2005). Association of NEDD4L Ubiquitin Ligase with Essential Hypertension. *Hypertension* 46:488-491

Rutledge, DR.; Sun, Y. & Ross, EA. (1995). Polymorphisms within the atrial natriuretic peptide gene in essential hypertension. *J Hypertens* 13:953-5

Sacks, FM.; Alaupovic, P.; Moye, LA. ; Cole, TG. ; Sussex, B.; Stampfer, MJ.; Pfeffer, MA. & Braunwald, E. (2000). VLDL, apolipoproteins B, CIII, and E, and risk of recurrent coronary events in the Cholesterol and Recurrent Events (CARE) trial. *Circulation* 102:1886-1892

Salah, A.; Khan, M.; Esmail, N.; Habibullah, S. & Al Lahham, Y. (2009). Genetic polymorphism of S447X lipoprotein lipase (LPL) and the susceptibility to hypertension. *J Crit Care* 24:e11-4

Schmieder, RE.; Martus, P. & Klingbeit, A. (1996). Reversal of left ventricular hypertrophy in essential hypertension. A meta-analysis of randomized double blind studies. *JAMA* 275:1507-13

Schunkert, H.; Hense, HW.; Doring, A.; Riegger, GA; & Siffert, W. (1998). Association between a polymorphism in the G protein β3 subunit gene and lower renin and elevated diastolic blood pressure levels. *Hypertension* 32:510-3

Schweizer, A.; Valdenaire, O.; Nelbock, P.; Deuschle, U.; Dumas, Milne Edwards, JB.; Stumpf, JG. & Loffler, BM. (1997) Human ECE-1: three isoforms with distinct subcellular localizations. *Biochem* J 328:871-877

Sethi, AA.; Nordestgaard, BG.; Tybjaerg-Hansen, A. & Tybjaerg-Hansen, A. (2003). Angiotensinogen gene polymorphism, plasma angiotensinogen, and risk of hypertension and ischemic heart disease: a meta-analysis. *Arterioscler Thromb Vasc Biol* 23:1269-1275

Sharma, P.; Hingorani, A;. Jia, H.; Hopper, R. & Brown, MJ. (1999). Quantitative association between a newly identified molecular variant in the endothelin-2 gene and human essential hypertension. *J Hypertens* 17:1281-7

Shimada, K.; Matsushita, Y.; Wakabayashi, K.; Takahashi, M.; Matsubara, A.; Iijima, Y. & Tanzawa, K. (1995) Cloning and functional expression of human endothelin-converting enzyme cDNA. *Biochem Biophys Res Commun* 207:807-12

Shoji, M.; Tsutaya, S.; Saito, R,.; Takamatu, H. & Yasujima, M. (2000). Positive association of endothelial nitric oxide synthase gene polymorphism with hypertension in northern Japan. *Life Sci* 66:2557-2562

Shull, M.M. & Lingrel, JB. (1987). Multiple genes encode the human Na+,K+-ATPase catalytic subunit (multiple isoforms/genomic library). *Proc Nat Acad Sci USA* 84:4039-4043

Shull, MM.; Pugh, DG. & Lingrel, J. (1990). The human Na,K-ATPase alpha 1 gene characterization of the 5'-flanking region and identification of a restriction fragment length polymorphism. *Genomics* 6:451-60

Siffert, W. (2003). G protein beta 3 subunit 825T allele and hypertension. *Curr Hypertens res* 5:47-53

Siffert, W.; Forster, P.; Jockel, KH.; Mvere, DA.; Brinkmann, B.; Naber, C,.; Crookes, R,.; Du, P.; Heyns, A.; Epplen, JT.; Fridey, J.; Freedman, BI.; Müller, N.; Stolke, D.; Sharma, AM.; Al Moutaery, K.; Grosse-Wilde, H.; Buerbaum, B.; Ehrlich, T.; Ahmad, HR.; Horsthemke, B.; Du Toit, ED.; Tiilikainen, A.; Ge, J. & Wang, Y. (1999). Worldwide ethnic distribution of the G protein β3 subunit 825T allele and its association with obesity in Caucasian, Chinese, and black African individuals. *J Am Soc Nephrol* 10:1921-31

Siffert, W.; Rosskopf, D.; Siffert, G.; Busch, S.; Moritz, A.; Erbel, R.; Sharma, AM.; Ritz, E,.; Wichmann, HE.; Jakobs, KH. & Horsthemke, B. (1998). Association of a human G protein β3 subunit variant with hypertension. *Nat Genet* 18:45-8

Siffert, WG. (1996) proteins, hypertension, and coronary heart disease: novel findings and hypotheses. *Kidney Blood Press Res* 19:71-80

Simon, DB.; Nelson-Williams, C.; Bia, MJ.; Ellison, D.; Karet, FE.; Molina, AM.; Vaara, I.; Iwata, F.; Cushner, HM.; Koolen , M.; Gainza, FJ.; Gitleman, HJ. & Lifton, RP. (1996). Gitelman's variant of Bartter's syndrome, inherited hypokalaemic alkalosis, is caused by mutations in the thiazide-sensitive Na-Cl cotransporter. *Nat Genet* 12:24-30

Sparkes, RS.; Zollman, S.; Klisak, I.; Kirchgessner, TG.; Komaromy, MC.; Mohandas, T.; Schotz, MC. & Lusis, AJ. (1987). Human genes involved in lipolysis of plasma lipoproteins: mapping of loci for lipoprotein lipase to 8p22 and hepatic lipase to 15q21. *Genomics* 1:138-144

Strader, CD.; Fong, TM.; Tota, MR.; Underwood, D. & Dixon, RA. (1994). Structure and function of G protein-coupled receptors. *Annu Rev Biochem* 463:101-132

Sun, B.; Williams, JS.; Pojoga, L.; Chamarthi, B.; Lasky-Su, J.; Raby, BA.; Hopkins, PN.; Jeunemaitre, x.; Brown, NJ,.; Ferri, C. & Williams, GH. (2011). Renin gene polymorphism: its relationship to hypertension, renin levels and vascular responses. *J Renin Angiotensin Aldosterone Syst* April 13. [Epub ahead of print]

Svetkey, LP.; Chen, YT.; McKeown, SP.; Preis, L. & Wilson, AF. (1997). Preliminary evidence of linkage of salt sensitivity in black Americans at the beta-2 adrenergic receptor locus. *Hypertension* 29:918-922

Sweadner, KJ. (1989). Isozymes of the Na/KATPase. *Biochim Biophys Acta* 988:185-220

Takahashi, N.; Murakami, H.; Kodama, K.; Kasagi, F.; Yamada, M.; Nishishita, T. & Inagami, T. (2000). Association of a polymorphism at the 5'-region of the angiotensin II type 1 receptor with hypertension *Ann Hum Genet* 64:197-205

Takiyyuddin, MA.; Brown, MR.; Dinh, TQ.; Cervenka, JH.; Braun, SD.; Parmer, RJ.; Kennedy, B. & O'Connor, DT. (1994). Sympatho-adrenal secretion in humans: factors governing catecholamine and storage vesicle peptide co-release. *J Auton Pharmacol* 14:187-200

Taupenot, L.; Harper, KL. & O'Connor, DT. (2003). The chromogranin-secretogranin family. *N Engl J Med* 348:1134-1149

Tikhonoff, V.; Kuznetsova, T.; Stolarz, K.; Bianchi, G.; Casiglia, E.; Kawecka-Jaszcz, K.; Nikitin, Y.; Tizzoni, L.; Wang, JG. & Staessen, JA. (2003). β-Adducin polymorphisms, blood pressure and sodium excretion in three European populations. *Am J Hypertens* 16:840-846

Timberlake, DS.; O'Connor, DT. & Parmer, RJ. (2001). Molecular genetics of essential hypertension: Recent results and emerging strateries. *Curr Opin Nephrol Hypertens* 10:71-79

Timmermann, B.; Rune, M.; Luft, FC.; Gerdts, B.; Busjahn, A.; Omvik, P.; Guo-Hua, L.; Schuster, H.; Wienker, TF.; Hoehe , M. & Lund-Johansen, P. (1998). β-2 adrenoceptor genetic variation is associated with genetic predisposition to essential hypertension: the Bergen Blood Pressure Study. *Kidney Int* 53:1455-1460

Tomaszewski, M.; Charchar, FJ.; Lacka, B.; Pesonen, U., William Y.S. Wang, WYS.; Zukowska-Szczechowska, E.; Grzeszczak, W. & Dominiczak AF. (2004). Epistatic interaction between _2-adrenergic receptor and neuropeptide Y genes influences LDL-cholesterol in hypertension. *Hypertension* 44:689-694

Tonolo, G.; Melis, MG.; Ciccarese, M.; Secchi, G.; Atzeni, MM.; Maioli, M.; Pala, G.; Massidda, A.; Manai, M.; Pilosu, RM.; Li, LS. & Luthman, H. (1997). Physiological and genetic characterization of the Gly40Ser mutation in the glucagon receptor gene in the Sardinian population: the Sardinian. Diabetes genetic study group. *Diabetologia* 40:89-94

Tripodi, G.; Valtorta, F.; Torielli, L.; Chieregatti, E.; Salardi, S. ; Trusolino, L. ; Menegon, A. ; Ferrari, P. ; Marchisio, PC. & Bianchi, G. (1996). Hypertension associated point mutations in the adducin alpha and beta subunits affect actin cytoskeleton and ion transport. *J Clin Invest* 97:2815-2822

Tsai, CT.; Fallin, D.; Chiang, FT. ; Hwang, JJ. ; Lai, LP.; Hsu, KL. ; Tseng, CD. ; Liau, CS. & Tseng YZ. (2003). Angiotensinogen gene haplotype and hypertension: interaction with ACE gene I allele. *Hypertension* 4:9-15

Turner, ST.; Chapman, AB.; Schwartz, GL. & Boerwinkle, E. (2003). Effects of endothelial nitric oxide synthase, alpha-adducin, and other candidate gene polymorphisms on blood pressure response to hydrochlorothiazide. *Am J Hypertens* 16:834-839

Uwabo, J.; Soma, M.; Nakayama, T. & Kanmatsuse, K. (1998). Association of a variable number of tandem repeats in the endothelial constitutive nitric oxide synthase gene with essential hypertension in Japanese, *Am J Hypertens* 11:125-128

Vague, P.; Dufayet, D.; Coste, T.; Moriscot, C.; Jannot, MF. & Raccah, D. (1997). Association of diabetic neuropathy with Na/K ATPase gene polymorphism. *Bull Acad Natl Med* 181:1811-21

Valdenaire, O.; Lepailleur-Enouf, D.; Egidy, G.; Thouard, A.; Barret, A. ; Vranckx, R. ; Tougard, C. & Michel, JB. (1999). A fourth isoform of endothelin-converting enzyme (ECE-1) is generated from an additional promoter. *Eur J Biochem* 264:341-349

Valdenaire, O.; Rohrbacher, E. & Mattei, MG. (1995). Organization of the gene encoding the human endothelin-converting enzyme (ECE-1). *J Biol Chem* 270:29794-29798

Vangjeli, C.; Clarke, N.; Quinn, U.; Dicker, P.; Tighe, O.; Ho, C.; O'Brien, E. & Stanton, AV. (2010). Confirmation That the Renin Gene Distal Enhancer Polymorphism REN-5312C/T Is Associated With Increased Blood Pressure. *Circ Cardiovasc Genet* 3: 53-59

Vasků, A.; Soucek, M.; Znoji, l V.; Rihácek, I.; Tschöplová, S.; Strelcová, L.; Cídl, K.; Blazková, M.; Hájek, D.; Hollá, L. & Vácha, J. (1998). Angiotensin I-converting enzyme and angiotensinogen gene interaction and prediction of essential hypertension. *kidney Int* 53:1479-82

Wallerstedt, SM.; Skrtic, S.; Eriksson, AL.; Ohlsson, C. & Hedner, T. (2004). Association analysis of the polymorphism T1128C in the signal peptide of neuropeptide Y in a Swedish hypertensive population. *J Hypertens* 22(7):1277-81

Wang, JG. & Staessen, JA. (2000). Genetic polymorphisms in the renin-angiotensin system: relevance for susceptibility to cardiovascular disease. *Eur J Pharmacol* 410:289-302

Wang, JG.; Staessen, JA. Barlassina, C.; Fagard, R.; Kuznetsova, T.; Struijker-Boudier, HA.; Zagato, L.; Citterio, L.; Messaggio, E. & Bianchi, G. (2002). Association between hypertension and variation in the α- and β-adducin genes in a white population. *Kidney Int* 62:2152-2159

Wang, L.; Rao, F.; Zhang, K.; Mahata M.; Rodriguez-Flores, JL.; Fung, MM.; Waalen, J.; Cockburn, MG.; Hamilton, BA.; Mahata, SK. & O'Connor, DT. (2009). Neuropeptide Y1 receptor NPY1R: Discovery of naturally occurring human genetic variants governing gene expression in cella as well as pleiotropic effects on autonomic activity and blood pressure in vivo. *J Am Coll Cardiol* 54:944-954

Wang, WY.; Zee, RYL. & Morris, BJ. (1997). Association of angiotensin II type I receptor gene polymorphism with essential hypertension. *Clin Genet* 51:31-4

Warnecke, C.; Willich, T.; Holzmeister, J.; Bottari, SP.; Fleck, E. & Regitz-Zagrosek, V. (1999). Efficient transcription of the human angiotensin II type 2 receptor gene requires intronic sequence elements. *Biochem J* 340:17-24

Wen, H.; Lin, R.; Jiao, Y.; Wang, F.; Wang, S.; Lu, D.; Qian, J.; Jin, L. & Wang, X. (2008). Two polymorphisms in NEDD4L gene and essential hypertension in Chinese Hans - a population-based case-control study. *Clin Exp Hypertens* 30:87-94

White, PC. & Rainey, WE. (2003). Polymorphisms in CYP11B genes and 11-hydroxylase activity. *J Clin Endocrinol Metab* 90:1252-5

Williams, SM.; Addy, JH.; Phillips, JAIII.; Dai,DM.; Kpodonu J, Afful, J.; Jackson, H.; Joseph, K.; Eason, F.; Murray, MM.; Epperson, P.; Aduonum, A.; Wong, LJ.; Jose, PA.; &

Felder RA.(2000). Combinations of variations in multiple genes are associated with hypertension. *Hypertension* 36:2-6

Williams, SM.; Ritchie, MD.; Phillips, JAIII.; Dawson, E.; Prince, M.; Dzhura, E.; Willis, A.; Semenya, A.; Summar, M.; White, BC.; Addy JH.; Kpodonu J.; Wong LJ.; Felder RA.; Jose PA. & Moore JH. (2004). Multilocus analysis of hypertension: a hierarchical approach. *Hum Hered* 57:28-38

Windler, E. & Havel, RJ. (1985). Inhibitory effects of C apolipoproteins from rats and humans on the uptake of triglyceride-rich lipoproteins and their remnants by the perfused rat liver. *J Lipid Res* 26:556-65

Wong, ZY.; Stebbing, M.; Ellis, JA.; Lamantia, A. & Harrap, SB. (1999). Genetic linkage of beta and gamma subunits of epithelial sodium channel to systolic blood pressure. *Lancet* 353:1222-1225

Xu, D. & Yanagisawa, M. (1994) ECE-1: a membrane-bound metalloprotease that catalyzes the proteolytic activation of big endothelin-1. *Cell* 78:473-485

Yanagisawa, M.; Kurihara, H.; Kimura, S.; Tomobe, Y.; Kobayashi, M.; Mitsui, Y.; Yazaki, Y.; Goto, K. & Masaki, T. (1988). A novel potent vasoconstrictor peptide produced by vascular endothelial cells. *Nature* 332:411-415

Yang, W.; Huang, J.; Ge, D.; Yao, C.; Duan, X.; Gan, W.; Huang, G.; Zhao, J.; Hui, R.; Shen, Y.; Qiang, B. & Gu, D. (2003). Variation near the region of the lipoprotein lipase gene and hypertension or blood pressure levels in Chinese. *Hypertens Res* 26:459-64

Ying, CQ.; Wang, YH.; Wu, ZL.; Fang, MW.; Wang, J.; Li, YS.; Zhang, YH. & Qiu, CC. (2010). Association of the renin gene polymorphism, three angiotensinogen polymorphism and the haplotypes with essentiel hypertension in the Mongolian population. *Clin Exp Hypertens* 32:293-300

Zhang, Y.; Zhang, KX.; Wang, GL.; Huang, W. & Zhu, DL. (2003). Angiotensin II type 2 receptor gene polymorphisms and essential hypertension. *Acta Pharmacol Sin* 24:1089-93

Zhao, Q.; Gu D.; Hixson, JE.; Liu, DP.; Rao, DC.; Jaquish, CE. ; Kelly, TN.; Lu, F.; Ma, J.; Mu, J.; Shimmin, LC.; Chedn, J.; Mei, H.; Hamm, LL. & He, J. (2011). Common variants in epithelial sodium channel genes contribute to salt-sensitivity of blood pressure: the GenSalt study. *Circ Cardiovasc Genet* (Epub ahead of print)

Zhu, X.; Chang, YP.; Yan, D.; Weder, A.; Cooper, R.; Luke, A.; Kan, D. & Chakravarti, A. (2003). Associations between hypertension and genes in the renin-angiotensin system. *Hypertension* 41:1027-1034

Zintzaras, E.; Kitsios, G. & Stefanidis, I. (2006). Endothelial NO synthase gene polymorphisms and hypertension: a meta-analysis. *Hypertension* 48:700-710

Zivković, M.; Djurić, T.; Stancić, O.; Alavantić, D. & Stanković, A. (2007). X-linked angiotensin II type 2 receptor gene polymorphism -1332A/G in male patients with essential hypertension. *Clin Chim Acta* 386:110-3

Zuliani, G. & Hobbs, HH. (1990). Tetranucleotide repeat polymorphism in the LPL gene. *Nucleic Acids Res* 18:4958

# 8

# Mitochondrial Mutations in Essential Hypertension

Haiyan Zhu and Shiwen Wang
*General Hospital of Chinese PLA*
*China*

## 1. Introduction

Hypertension is a common condition, a risk factor for heart disease, renal failure and stroke, affecting approximately 1 billion individuals worldwide and 200 million in China[1, 2]. Thus, understanding the underlying etiology of hypertension has been a major research focus, especially the genetics of essential hypertension (EH), large proportion of hypertension. Indeed, since the completion of the draft sequence of human genome, geneticists have announced that within 10 years they expect to determine the significance of the genome as related to essential hypertension[3]. Some progress has been made. For example, for systolic blood pressure alone, 27 nuclear loci have been identified in populations of European and African ancestry[3]. However, to date no consistent results have been obtained across ethnicity and races supporting the need for genetic studies in diverse populations [4-8].

While the nuclear genome has been studied extensively with respect to hypertension, much less work has been done with the mitochondrial genome (mtDNA). Yet there is evidence to suggest that mitochondria and mtDNA may be important in hypertension. For example, mitochondria produce reactive oxidative species (ROS) and these ROS can cause hypertension [9-11]. With respect to the evidence of mtDNA, a hallmark of involvement of mtDNA is maternal inheritance. Multiple studies have identified strong maternal inheritance of blood pressure, with one study suggesting that over one-third of hypertension could be attributed to mtDNA variation [12-14]. Interestingly, a variant in mitochondrial $tRNA^{Ile}$ has been identified in a single family which segregated with hypertension and appeared causal [15]. Taken together, this work suggests the importance of looking at mtDNA variation to further our understanding of the underlying etiology of EH.

## 2. Mitochondria

### 2.1 Biogenesis and bioenergetics

Matrilineal inheritance in EH pedigrees support the hypothesis that mitochondrial genes are also implicated in the pathogenesis of EH. Mitochondria evolved from protobacteria that inhabited primordial eukaryotic cells about 1.5 billion years ago and were first observed more than100 years ago by Altmann. It's a small symbiotic (0.5-1μm) organelle combined with aerobic bacteria and primordial eukaryotic cells. 37 genes make up a mitochondrion within which thousands of mtDNA forming double-stranded 16569 base-pair.(Fig. 1) Of these genes, 24 encode RNAs necessary for protein synthesis (22 tRNAs and 2 rRNAs), The remaining 13 genes encode proteins that are critical subunits of the respiratory chain.

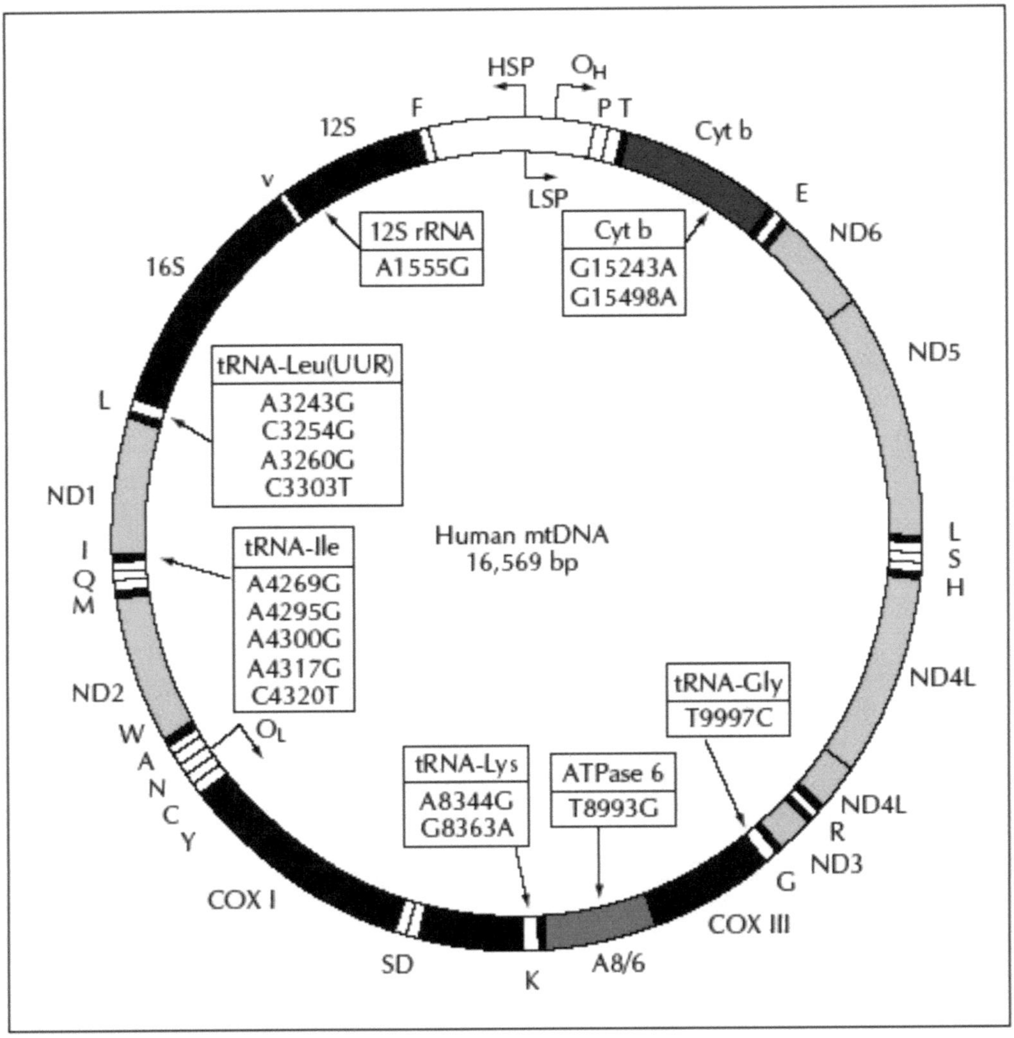


Fig. 1. Human mitochondrial DNA (mtDNA) map showing location of selected pathogenic mutations associated with left ventricular hypertrophy or hypertrophic cardiomyopathy. Human mtDNA is a 16569 base pair circular molecule that codes for 7(ND1,2,3,4,4L,5 and 6) of 43 subunits of complex I; 1 (cytochrome b) of 11 subunits of complex III; 3 (COI, II and III) of 13 subunits of complex IV; and 2( ATPase 6 and 8) of 16 subunits of complex V. It also codes for small and large rRNAs and 22tRNAs, with adjacent letters indicating cognate amino acids. (Adapted from Hirano M et al. Mitochondria and the heart. Current Opinion in Cardiology 2001, 16:201–210.)

The mitochondrion contains an inner and an outer membrane which defines the matrix and the intermembrane space. The outer membrane is permeable to small molecules (up to 10 kDa ) whereas the inner membrane is freely permeable to oxygen and carbon dioxide. This relative impermeability of the inner membrane is essential for maintaining a proton gradient necessary for the synthesis of adenosine triphosphate (ATP). There are several unique features of mtDNA and mitochondrial genetics which are distinct from the features of nuclear genes and the principles of nuclear inheritance. First, mammalian mtDNA does not contain introns which make mtDNA mutations affect phenotype of diseases much more easily comparing to nuclear genes. Second, several mitochondrial genetic codons differ from the universal nuclear genetic code. UCG codes for tryptophan and not termination, AUA codes for methionine not isoleucine, and AGA and AGG are termination rather than arginine codons. AUA are possibly AUU are initiation codons as well as AUG. Third, only the mother contributes to the mtDNA pool of the offspring, It dues mostly to the fact to a large extent that sperm contains only 100 mtDNA while egg contains approximately 10,000 mtDNA[16]. Fourth, the fixation of mtDNA mutations is more than 10 times higher in comparison with the nuclear DNA mutation rate [17]. A possible explanation for this difference is the lack of protective histones and the absence of effective DNA repair systems within mitochondria. In addition, by being exposed to tremendous fluxes of oxygen, mtDNA may also be a target for the reactive oxygen species produced as by-products of oxidative phosphorylation. Fifth, an individual may carry several allelic forms of mtDNA, present in different proportions in different tissues [18,19]. The coexistence of more than one type of mtDNA within a cell, wide-type accompany with mutant type, is called heteroplasmy. Sixth, there is as yet no conclusive evidence demonstrating that orthodox recombination occurs between individual mtDNA molecules. New mtDNA alleles can thus only arise through spontaneous mutations. In spite of striking difference of morphological and inherited characteristics from nuclear genes, mitochondria have three major functions which associated with pathogenesis of diseases synergically. (energetic, reactive oxygen species, apoptosis). First, mitochondria offer about 90%-95% energy to cells through oxidative phosphorylation(OXPHOS). Five multipolypeptide enzyme complexes make up OXPHOS(Fig.2) as follows.: Complex I(NADH:ubiqunone oxidoreductase), II(succinate: uiquinone oxidoreductase), III(ubiquinol: ferrocytochrome C oxidoreductase), IV (cytochrome C oxidase) constitute electron transport train(ETC).Through ETC, energy is released to pump protons from inside the mitochondrial matrix across the mitochondrial inner membrane into the intermembrane space . And the electrochemical gradient($\triangle\psi$) results from ETC offers energy for complex V ($H^+$- translocating ATP synthase) to produce adenosine triphosphate.

Second, toxic by-products, reactive oxygen species(ROS) including $O_2^-$, $H_2O_2$ and $\cdot OH$, derived from mitochondrial OXPHOS do harm to cells to variable extents according to different period of time exposure to ROS. Short-term exposure to ROS can reduce the activity of ETC and slow down the metabolism while long-term exposure will induce irreversible oxidative damage thus cause markedly reduction of mitochondrial function.

Third, mitochondria are implicated in the initiation of apoptosis in specific circumstances through opening mitochondrial permeability transition pore (mtPTP) within the membrane. Program cell death activates for the leaking of apoptosis-promoting factors located in matrix such as cytochrome c. apoptosis-initiation factor(AIF) and kinds of caspases by mtPTP.

### 2.2 Mitochondria and heart diseases

For the three basic functions of mitochondria indicated above, the hypothesis of mitochondria participates in pathogenesis of heart diseases have been supported by both experimental and clinical evidences.

In 1988, the first disease-causing mutation of mtDNA were found that patients with mitochondrial myopathy identified a variety of functional defects of the mitochondrial respiratory chain, predominantly affecting complex I (NADH-CoQ reductase) or complex III (ubiquinol–cytochrome c reductase) in adult cases[20, 21].This discovery led to a rapid surge in the research into mitochondrial disorders, and there are now more than 200 different mtDNA mutations linked to human disease (http://www.mitomap.org) Given the fact that heart is a second largest oxygen-consumed organ within body with 12 % oxygen necessary to work averagely just less than brain, it follows that heart should be a harrowing victim for oxygen deficiency in vivo. Actually, Every heart beat consumes 2% of total cellular ATP. And 90% of its ATP is produced by mitochondrial oxidative phosphorylation. Thus, mitochondria are assumed to be implicated in the pathogenesis of multiple cardiovascular diseases, with regard to the basic functions of the organelle[22].

Mitochondria are found to influence all of the four major features of cadiomyocytes: excitability, contractility, conductibility and autorhythmicity to certain degree. The rate and force of contraction of heart muscle change according to ATP utilization. Patients with mtDNA deletions named sporadic rearrangements often develop atrioventricular blocks, which progress from mild to severe (type I to type III )[23, 24], respectively. Kearns-Sayre Syndrome (KSS) and Chronic Progressive External Ophthalmoplegia(CPEO) are the major multisystemic disorders which affect cardiac conductive system particularly. Diversity of cardiac conduction defects including prolonged intraventricular conductiontime, bundle-branch block, and atrioventricular block often lead to sudden cardiac death. 4.9kb "common" deletion loci from ATP6 through COIII, ND3, ND4L, ND4, to ND5 contribute to KSS[25]. While A3243G mutation associates with maternally inherited PEO with RRF[26] and diabetes and deafness[27].Aon MA, et al introduced a novel conception "mitochondrial criticality" to describe the state in which the mitochondrial network of cardiomyocytes becomes very sensitive to small perturbations in reactive oxygen species (ROS), resulting in the scaling of local mitochondrial uncoupling and $\Delta\Psi_m$ loss to the whole cell, and the myocardial syncytium. The energetic changes are translated into effects on the electrical excitability of the cell, inducing temporal heterogeneity of excitability in the heart, underlies the genesis of potentially lethal cardiac arrhythmias [28].

Except for arrhythmia and excitability, mitochondrial dysfunction has also been suggested to reduce contraction of heart thus result in heart failure and age-associated decline in heart function [29-32].

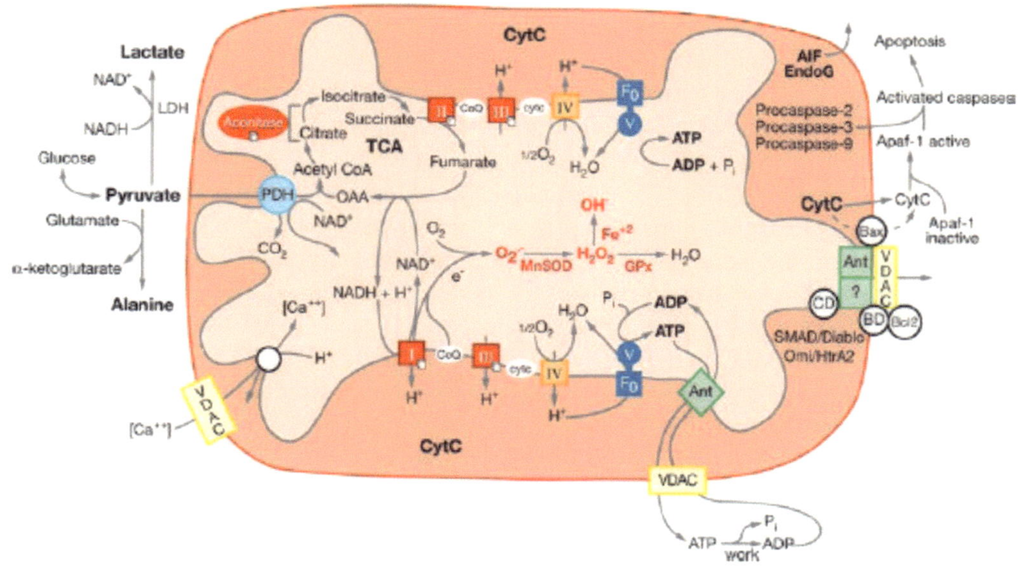


Fig. 2. Diagram showing the relationships of mitochondrial oxidative phosphorylation (OXPHOS) to (a) energy (ATP) production, (b) reactive oxygen species (ROS) production, and (c) initiation of apoptosis through the mitochondrial permeability transition pore (mtPTP). The OXPHOS complexes, designated I to V, are complex I (NADH: ubiquinone oxidoreductase) encompassing a FMN (flavin mononucleotide) and six Fe-S centers (designated with a cube); complex II (succinate: ubiquinone oxidoreductase) involving a FAD (flavin adenine dinucleotide), three Fe-S centers, and a cytochrome b; complex III (ubiquinol: cytochrome c oxidoreductase) encompassing cytochromes b, c1 and the Rieske Fe-S center; complex IV (cytochrome c oxidase) encompassing cytochromes a + a3 and CuA and CuB; and complex V (H+-translocating ATP synthase). Pyruvate from glucose enters the mitochondria via pyruvate dehydrogenase (PDH), generating acetylCoA, which enters the TCA cycle by combining with oxaloacetate (OAA). Cis-aconitase converts citrate to isocitrate and contains a 4Fe-4S center. Lactate dehydrogenase (LDH) converts excess pyruvate plus NADH to lactate. Small molecules defuse through the outer membrane via the voltage-dependent anion channel (VDAC) or porin. The VDAC together with ANT, Bax, and the cyclophilin D (CD) protein are thought to come together at the mitochondrial inner and outer membrane contact points to create the mtPTP. The mtPTP interacts with the pro-apoptotic Bax, anti-apoptotic Bcl2 and the benzodiazepine receptor (BD). The opening of the mtPTP is associated with the release of several pro-apoptotic proteins. Cytochrome c (cytc) interacts with and activates cytosolic Apaf-1, which then binds to and activates procaspase-9. The activated caspase-9 then initiates the proteolytic degradation of cellular proteins. Apoptosis initiating factor (AIF) and endonuclease G (EndoG) have nuclear targeting peptides that are transported to the nucleus and degrade the chromosomal DNA. (Adapted from Wallance DC. Mitochondrial diseases in man and mouse. Science. 1999;283:1482-8.)

# 3. Genetic basis of EH

## 3.1 Nuclear genes

Previous studies of hypertension in humans and experimental animal models have identified a number of candidate genes that have been implicated as possibly contributing to essential hypertension. The renin-angiotensin-aldosterone system may play a prominent role in the genesis of hypertension, and polymorphisms of the genes coding for angiotensinogen, angiotensin-converting enzyme, angiotensin II type 1 and 2 receptors, and aldosterone synthase have been widely studied. Other mechanisms may involve the KLK 1 gene of tissue kallikrein, gene variants of endothelial nitric oxide synthase and polymorphisms of the endothelin-1 gene. A number of studies have highlighted the potential contribution of polymorphisms of genes coding for inflammatory cytokines, adrenergic receptors and intracellular G proteins, which can activate Na+/K+ exchangers. Multiple researches found that the genetic findings may vary greatly according to the populations studied and the causal relationship between candidate genes and EH were difficult to establish firmly[33-35]. Further studies found that mitochondrial variants in EH were heatedly discussed in late 5 years.

# 4. Mitochondrial genes

## 4.1 Clinical researches of mtDNA mutation in EH

Schwartz F, et al[36] investigated the contribution of the mitochondrial genome to hypertension and quantitative blood pressure (BP) phenotypes in the Framingham Heart Study cohort. Longitudinal BP values of 6421 participants (mean age, 53 years; 46% men) from 1593 extended families were analyzed. The role of mitochondrial influence in the hypertensives was 35.2% (95% confidence interval, 27-43%, P < 10) The mitochondrial heritabilities for multivariable-adjusted long-term average systolic BP and diastolic BP were, respectively, 5% (P < 0.02) and 4% (P = 0.11). Schwartz F, et al[37] compared maternal and paternal contributions to the familial aggregation of hypertension in 344 hypertensive probands.Among them, 69 were African American, 153 US Caucasian, 122 Greek Caucasian. It was found that the proportion of hypertensive mothers (81.7, 65.0 and 84.8% for African Americans, US Caucasians and Greek Caucasians, respectively) of these probands was significantly greater than the proportion of hypertensive fathers (50.0, 44.9 and 48.3%, respectively) in all three ethnic groups. The lifetime risk of hypertension was significantly greater for mothers compared with fathers of these hypertensive probands (p<0.001). Examination of the proband's siblings indicated that maternal history of hypertension was associated with greater lifetime risk for hypertension than paternal history (p<0.01).Thus, it drew the conclusion maternal influence on blood pressure suggested involvement of mitochondrial DNA in the pathogenesis of EH. Muscari A, et al [38] hypothesized that hypertension is a condition resulted from elevated levels of reactive oxygen (ROS) and nitrogen (RNS) species. Mitochondria are important sites of ROS production, and a mitochondrial dysfunction, preceding endothelial dysfunction, might favor the development of hypertension. ROS production may also be induced by RNS, which inhibit the respiratory chain and may be generated through the action of a mitochondrial NO synthase. Mitochondrial uncoupling proteins are involved in both experimental and human hypertension. Finally, an excessive production of ROS may damage mitochondrial DNA, with resultant impairment in the synthesis of some components of the respiratory chain and further ROS production, a vicious cycle that may be implicated in hypertensive states.

## 5. Our studies of mtDNA mutation in EH

To determine the relationship between mitochondrial genomic variation and essential hypertension, we performed a systematic and extensive screening of mitochondrial genes at the Institute of Geriatric Cardiology, Chinese PLA General Hospital in a large Chinese cohort. We focused on this Chinese population because of the high morbidity of essential hypertension in Chinese adults (nearly 11.8%)[2] and the limited amount of research on this racial group. We used a population instead of family-based strategy for two reasons: 1) Large numbers of hypertensives without family history are not detected in China, and they might be overlooked for lacking of medical knowledge and regular checks. 2) The morbidity of essential hypertension is not totally family-based; 50-60% of hypertensives are sporadically distributed.[2]

We sequenced mitochondrial genomes in 306 age and gender balanced Chinese hypertensives and controls. In the 153 hypertensives, putative functional changes included 4 changes in rRNA genes, 11 changes in tRNA genes and 25 amino acid substitutions. The remaining variants were synonymous changes or non-coding regions. In the 153 controls, 1 base change in the tRNA genes and 8 amino acid substitutions were found. A8701G in ATP6 gene (belongs to haplogroup M) (P=0.0001) and C8414T in ATP8 gene (belongs to haplogroup D) (P=0.0001) were detected significantly different in the cases and controls. Interestingly, the cases were more likely to have two or more amino acid changes and RNAs variants as compared to the controls (24.75% versus 7.94%, P=0.0001). In addition, several variants were highly conserved and/or specifically located at the 3′ end adjacent to the anticodon, which may contribute to the stabilization of structure thus lead to the decrease of tRNA metabolism. In the cohort of hypertensives, there were several variants that occurred too infrequently to have sufficient statistical power but that have biologic plausibility. T4363C localized at the 3′ end adjacent to the anticodon, which contributed to the stabilization of structure thus lead to the decrease of tRNA metabolism. A4263G at the initial part of tRNAIle may influence the transcription of tRNA herein affect the steady-level of protein synthesis. And some other novel RNAs variants (C3168CC, G3173A, A3203G, T3290C, A4263G, T4363C, C4410A, T8311C) in 16s RNA, $tRNA^{Leu(UUR)}$, $tRNA^{Ile}$, $tRNA^{Met}$, $tRNA^{Gln}$ and $tRNA^{Lys}$ only found in hypertensives but not controls. In coding regions, even though a novel point variant G8720C in ATP6 gene, with high conservation among species was not significant in epidemiological perspective. Synergetic interaction between mitochondrial mtSNPs and/or haplogroups is needed to be investigated in the future[39]. Sequence analysis then performed in tRNA genes, hot spots for cardiovascular diseases, in 270 Chinese Han essential hypertensives and 270 controls. Lymphoblastoid cell lines were immortalized by transformation with the Epstein-Barr virus. Rates of oxygen consumption in intact cells were determined with a YSI 5300 oxygraph (Yellow Springs Instruments) on samples, harboring variants in tRNA genes. In the study, environmental factors including age, gender, BMI, fasting blood sugar and blood lipids, contributing a lot to high blood pressure [40,41] didn't exhibit difference between cases and controls. It was presumed that hereditary factors may associate with the pathogenesis of hypertension in the Chinese Han population. There were 26 variants in tRNA genes were found in hypertensives and these variants were not in controls. Functional analysis found that these variants may lead to deficiencies in tRNA 3′ end metabolism (3' end cleavage, CCA addition and aminoacylation) and/or impairment of critical subunits of the respiratory chain, which help understanding of molecular mechanisms of mitochondrial tRNA genes in essential hypertension as follows: C3254T and A8348G mildly reduced the efficiency of aminoacyl-tRNA synthetase (aaRS) [42]; A4295G reduced efficiency of tRNA 3′-processing endoribonuclease (tRNAseZ) and aaRS [43]; A4317G reorganized T-stem which markedly reduced the efficiency of tRNA 3′-processing endoribonuclease tRNAseZ, aaRS, and tRNA nucleotidyl transferase (CCAse) [44]. The other possible effects of tRNA mutations on tRNA modifications may be the reduction of efficiency of the binding properties of aminoacyl-tRNAs to mitochondrial elongation factor Tu (Ef-Tu) [45]. All of the above variants influenced the process of aminoacylation which affected tRNA metabolism and impaired the synthesis of protein ultimately. Most importantly, eight of these variants were highly conserved from bacteria to human beings (A4263G, A4295G, A4316TA, A4343G, A4388G, C4392T, C4410A and A4435G) thus minor changes in charge or structure may result in impairment of translation and affect the synthesis of protein. In addition, A4295G, A4435G and T4363C all localized at the 3' end adjacent to the anticodon, which contributed to the stabilization of structure thus lead to the decrease of tRNA metabolism. Otherwise, a novel variant A4263G at the initial part of $tRNA^{Ile}$ may influence the transcription of tRNA herein affect the steady-level of protein synthesis. It also possible that such mutations could affect the tRNAs correct decoding of the mRNA in the ribosome (by increase in frameshifting for example) and, particularly in the case of T4363C, could also interfere with aminoacylation, since glutaminyl-tRNA synthetases are known to interrogate the anticodon loop of $tRNA^{Gln}$ during catalysis [46]. And some other novel tRNA variants (T4277C, T4353C, C4410A, T8311C) in $tRNA^{Leu(UUR)}$, $tRNA^{Ile}$, $tRNA^{Met}$, $tRNA^{Gln}$ and $tRNA^{Lys}$ need to be further investigated in the future. Interestingly, functional analysis found significant reduction of oxygen consumption rate in two mutant cell lines carrying variants T4454C and A4263G. Oxygen consumption is a classical means of assessing energy expenditure, one component of energy balance [47, 48]. Cells and organisms are able to trigger an adaptive response to hypoxic conditions that is aimed to help them to cope with these threatening conditions [49]. Failing to keep the balance of oxygen consumption and production may cause cardiovascular diseases and is of particular significance in the pathogenesis of essential hypertension. A variant in mitochondrial $tRNA^{Ile}$ has been identified in a single family which segregated with hypertension and appeared causal [14]. Interestingly, we deduced that except the A4263G and T4454C variants, there were other amino acid changes may contributing to hypertension by entire mitochondrial genome sequencing of the cells. This finding would suggest that there may be a threshold effect with some of these mtDNA variants. Such that often variability at a single locus will not be sufficient to increase hypertension risk. This is consistent with previous work that essential hypertension is controlled by multiple genetic loci, each with a relatively weak effect in the population at large [50]. Most importantly, the oxygen consumption rate in cells harboring variants T4454C (P=0.0010) and A4263G (P=0.0001) decreased as compared to the average level of control cell lines. The findings suggested that variants located in mitochondrial tRNA genes may have biologic plausibility to implicate in the pathogenesis of Chinese essential hypertension.

## 6. Prospects

The mitochondrial influence in EH remains a lot of questions to be answered. The mitochondrial variants always seem to be infrequent and perhaps even private, relationship between nuclear genes and mitochondrial genes is obscure, enviromental influence somehow affects results of studies of mitochondria. All in all, there's still a long way to go to disclose the secret of mitochondria and EH.

## 7. References

[1] Chobanian AV, Bakris GL, Black HR, et al. The Seventh Report of the Joint National Committee on Prevention, Detection, Evaluation, and Treatment of High Blood Pressure: the JNC 7 report. Jama 2003; 289:2560-72.

[2] Liu LS. 2005 Guidelines for prevention and treatment of hypertension in China. People's medical publishing house, Beijing, 2007; pp 1-8.

[3] Harrap SB. Where are all the blood-pressure genes? Lancet 2003; 361:2149-51.

[4] Bonnardeaux A, Davies E, Jeunemaitre X, et al. Angiotensin II type 1 receptor gene polymorphisms in human essential hypertension. Hypertension 1994; 24:63-9.

[5] Caulfield M, Munroe P, Pembroke J, et al. Genome-wide mapping of human loci for essential hypertension. Lancet 2003; 361:2118-23.

[6] Kamide K, Kokubo Y, Fukuhara S, et al. Protein tyrosine kinase 2beta as a candidate gene for hypertension. Pharmacogenet Genomics 2007; 17:931-9.

[7] Banno M, Hanada H, Kamide K, et al. Association of genetic polymorphisms of endothelin-converting enzyme-1 gene with hypertension in a Japanese population and rare missense mutation in preproendothelin-1 in Japanese hypertensives. Hypertens Res 2007; 30:513-20.

[8] Kulah E, Dursun A, Aktunc E, et al. Effects of angiotensin-converting enzyme gene polymorphism and serum vitamin D levels on ambulatory blood pressure measurement and left ventricular mass in Turkish hypertensive population. Blood Press Monit 2007; 12:207-13.

[9] Wallace DC. Mitochondrial diseases in man and mouse. Science 1999; 283:1482-8.

[10] Hirano M, Davidson M, DiMauro S. Mitochondria and the heart. Curr Opin Cardiol 2001; 16:201-10.

[11] Lassègue B, Griendling KK. Reactive oxygen species in hypertension; An update. Am J Hypertens 2004;17:852-60.

[12] Hutchinson, J., Crawford, M.H. Genetic determinants of blood pressure level among the Black Caribs of St Vincent. Human Biology 1981; 53:453-66.

[13] DeStefano AL, Gavras H, Heard-Costa N, et al. Maternal component in the familial aggregation of hypertension.Clin Genet 2001;60:13-21.

[14] Yang Q, Kim SK, Sun F, et al. Maternal influence on blood pressure suggests involvement of mitochondrial DNA in the pathogenesis of hypertension: the Framingham Heart Study. J Hypertens 2007; 25:2067-73.

[15] Wilson FH, Hariri A, Farhi A, et al. A cluster of metabolic defects caused by mutation in a mitochondrial tRNA. Science 2004; 306:1190-4.

[16] Zeviani M, Bonilla E, Devivo DC, Dimauro S. Mitochondrial diseases. Neurol Clin. 1989, 7:123-56.

[17] DiMauro S, Moraes CT. Mitochondrial encephalomyopathies. Arch Neurol. 1993, 50:1197-208

[18] Singh MM, Sinha A. Mitochondrial diseases: relevance to a physician. Postgrad Med. 1998, 12:148-61

[19] Vladutiu GD. Advances in the genetic mechanism of mitochondrial diseases. Curr Opin Neurol. 1997, 10:512-8.

[20] Holt IJ, Harding AE, Morgan-Hughes JA. Deletions of muscle mitochondrial DNA in patients with mitochondrial myopathies. Nature. 1988, 331: 717-9.

[21] Wallace DC, Singh G, Lott MT et al. Mitochondrial DNA mutation associated with Leber's hereditary optic neuropathy. Science. 1988, 242: 1427-30.

[22] Harris DA, Das AM.Control of mitochondrial ATP synthesis in the heart. Biochem J. 1991, 280:561-73.

[23] Hirano M, DiMauro S: Clinical features of mitochondrial myopathies and encephalomyopathies. In Handbook of Muscle Disease. Edited by Lane RJM. New York: Marcel Dekker Inc. USA, 1996,479–504.

[24] Moraes CT, Shanske S, Tritschler HJ, et al.: MtDNA depletion with variable tissue expression: A novel genetic abnormality in mitochondrial diseases. Am J Hum Genet. 1991, 48:492–501.

[25] Alemi M, Prigione A, Wong A, Schoenfeld R, et al. Mitochondrial DNA deletions inhibit proteasomal activity and stimulate an autophagic transcript. Free Radic Biol Med. 2007, 1,42(1):32-43.

[26] Moraes CT, Ciacci F, Silvestri G, et al. Atypical clinical presentations associated with the MELAS mutation at position 3243 of human mitochondrial DNA. Neuromusc Disord. 1993, 3:43–50.

[27] van den Ouweland JM, Lemkes HH, Ruitenbeek W, et al. Mutation in mitochondrial tRNA(Leu)(UUR) gene in a large pedigree with maternally transmitted type II diabetes mellitus and deafness. Nat Genet. 1992 ,1(5):368-71.

[28] Aon MA, Cortassa S, Akar FG, O'Rourke B. Mitochondrial criticality: a new concept at the turning point of life or death. Biochim Biophys Acta. 2006 ,1762(2):232-40.

[29] Hattori K, Tanaka M, Sugiyama S et al. Age-dependent increase in deleted mitochondrial DNA in the human heart: possible contributory factor to presbycardia. Am Heart J. 1991, 121: 1735-42.

[30] Melov S, Shoffner JM, Kaufman A, et al. Marked increase in the number and variety of mitochondrial DNA rearrangements in aging human skeletal muscle. Nucl Acids Res. 1995, 23: 4122-6.

[31] Clayton D, Williams R, Liang I. Meeting highlights: mitochondrial DNA mutations and cardiomyopathy, heart failure, and ischemic heart disease.Circulation. 1995,92:2022–3.

[32] Ide T, Tsutsui H, Hayashidani S, Kang D, et al. Mitochondrial DNA damage and dysfunction associated with oxidative stress in failing hearts after myocardial infarction. Circ Res. 2001, 88(5):529-35.

[33] Niu T, Xu X, Cordell HJ,et al. Linkage analysis of candidate genes and gene-gene interactions in chinese hypertensive sib pairs.Hypertension. 1999 ,33(6):1332-7.

[34] Corvol P, Persu A, Gimenez-Roqueplo AP, et al. Seven lessons from two candidate genes in human essential hypertension: angiotensinogen and epithelial sodium channel. Hypertension. 1999 ,33(6):1324-31.

[35] Matsubara M. Genetic determination of human essential hypertension. Tohoku J Exp Med. 2000 ,192(1):19-33.

[36] Yang Q, Kim SK, Sun F, et al. Maternal influence on blood pressure suggests involvement of mitochondrial DNA in the pathogenesis of hypertension: the Framingham Heart Study. J Hypertens. 2007,25(10):2067-73.

[37] DeStefano AL, Gavras H, Heard-Costa N, et al. Maternal component in the familial aggregation of hypertension.Am J Hypertens. 2011 Jul 28. doi: 10.1038/ajh.2011.131. [Epub ahead of print]

[38] Puddu P, Puddu GM, Cravero E,et al. The putative role of mitochondrial dysfunction in hypertension. Clin Exp Hypertens. 2007 ,29(7):427-34.

[39] Zhu HY, Wang SW, Martin LJ, er al. The role of mitochondrial genome in essential hypertension in a Chinese Han population. Eur J Hum Genet. 2009,17(11):1501-6.

[40] Levinger L, Morl M, Florentz C. Mitochondrial tRNA 3' end metabolism and human disease. Nucleic Acids Res 2004; 32:5430-41.

[41] Staessen JA, Wang J, Bianchi G, et al. Essential hypertension .Lancet 2003; 361: 1629-41.

[42] Hong Y, de Faire U, Heller DA, et al. Genetic and environmental influences on blood pressure in elderly twins. Hypertension 1994; 24:663-70.

[43] Modi P, Imura H, Angelini GD, et al. Pathology-related troponin I release and clinical outcome after pediatric open heart surgery. J Card Surg 2003; 18:295-300.

[44] Tomari Y, Hino N, Nagaike T, et al. Decreased CCA-addition in human mitochondrial tRNAs bearing a pathogenic A4317G or A10044G mutation. J Biol Chem 2003; 278:16828-33.

[45] Hong KW, Ibba M, Weygand-Durasevic I, et al. Transfer RNA-dependent cognate amino acid recognition by an aminoacyl-tRNA synthetase. EMBO J 1996; 15:1983-91.

[46] Nagao A, Suzuki T, Suzuki T. Aminoacyl-tRNA surveillance by EF-Tu in mammalian mitochondria. Nucleic Acids Symp Ser (Oxf) 2007; 51:41-2.

[47] Ritz P, Berrut G. Mitochondrial function, energy expenditure, aging and insulin resistance. Diabetes Metab 2005; 2:5S67-73.

[48] Zhu HY, Wang SW, Liu L, et al. A mitochondrial mutation A4401G is involved in the pathogenesis of left ventricular hypertrophy in Chinese hypertensives.Eur J Hum Genet 2009; 17:172-8.

[49] Clayton D, Williams R, Liang I. Meeting highlights: mitochondrial DNA mutations and cardiomyopathy, heart failure, and ischemic heart disease. Circulation 1995; 92: 2022–3.

[50] Zhu HY, Wang SW, Liu L,et al. Genetic variants in mitochondrial tRNA genes are associated with essential hypertension in a Chinese Han population. Clinica Chimica Acta. 2009.410(1-2):64-9.

9

# Mitochondrial Mutations in Left Ventricular Hypertrophy

Haiyan Zhu and Shiwen Wang
*General Hospital of Chinese PLA*
*China*

## 1. Introduction

Left ventricular hypertrophy (LVH) is one of the vicious organ damages of essential hypertension. It contributes a lot to high mortality of essential hypertension due to sudden cardiac death, ventricular arrhythmia and heart failure. Multi-factors involve in the pathogenesis of hypertension-induced LVH including inherited variants as well as environmental factors. For the genetic influence, nucleus' involvement has been discussed for years. However, much fewer interest has been put in the other inherited system—mitochondrion. To make clear the relationship of mitochondria and LVH, we try to illustrate the clinical and pathological characteristics of LVH, the structure and function of mitochondria and mitochondrial role in LVH as follows:

## 2. Left ventricular hypertrophy

### 2.1 Definition, diagnostic standard, diversity in phenotypes

Left ventricular hypertrophy (LVH) is a common complication of hypertension (the prevalence varies from 14 to 44% screening by echocardiography)[1] with multiple morphological and pathological characteristics which divide to subgroups as eccentric and concentric, asymmetric and symmetric hypertrophy according to heterogeneity in the pattern and extent of left ventricular wall thickening (see Fig. 1.)

Echocardiography is often used as a sensitive screening and surveillance tool for LVH, especially to concentric and symmetric hypertrophy. Based upon a classic equation deduced by Devereux, R.B. (1987)[2]:

$$\text{LV mass}=1.04[(\text{IVST}+\text{LVID}+\text{PWT})^3-\text{LVID}^3]0.001-13.6$$

$$\text{BSA}=0.006\text{H}+0.0128\text{W}-0.1529$$

$$\text{LVMI}=\text{LVM}/\text{BSA}$$

Left ventricular mass index (LVMI) over 134g/m$^2$ in men and above 110g/m$^2$ in women are identified left ventricular hypertrophy.

LVMI≤145 g/m$^2$ is considered as mild, 145<LVMI≤165 g/m$^2$ as moderate, LVMI >165g/m$^2$ as severe[3]. Interventricular Septal Thickness(IVST)/Posterior wall

Thickness(PWT)≥1.3 is considered asymmetric hypertrophy; IVST/PWT≤1.3 identified symmetric; End Diastolic Diameter(EDD)＞50mm considered eccentric hypertrophy, EDD＜50mm identified concentric hypertrophy. In spite of diversity of phenotype LVH encompassed, the morbidity as well as mortality of cardiovascular events increase when induction of LVH.

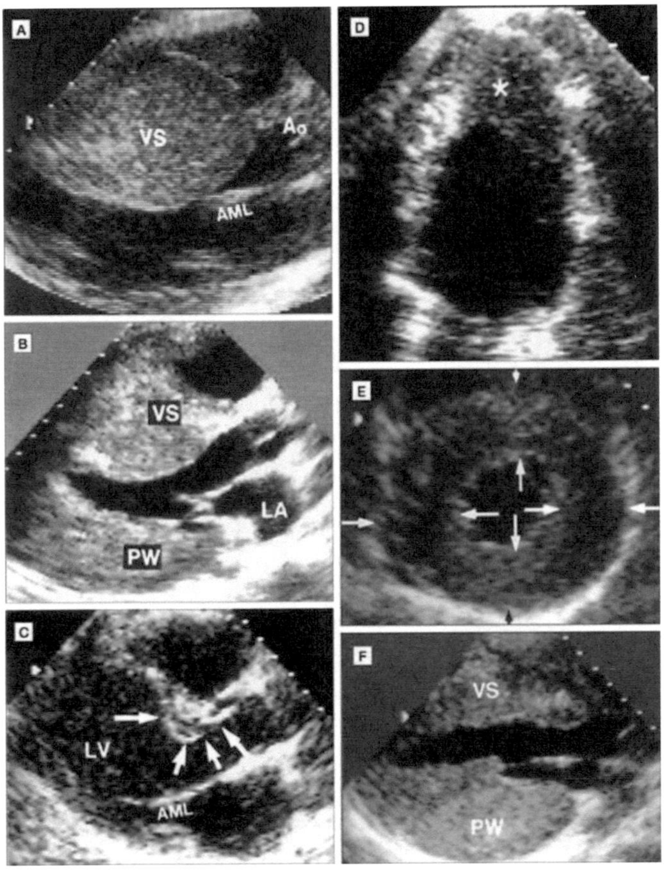


Fig. 1. Heterogeneity in the Pattern and Extent of Left Ventricular (LV) Wall Thickening in HCM Echocardiographic parasternal long-axis stop-frame images obtained in diastole showing A, massive asymmetric hypertrophy of ventricular septum (VS) with wall thickness >50 mm; B, pattern of septal hypertrophy in which the distal portion is considerably thicker than the proximal region at mitral valve level; C, hypertrophy sharply confined to basal (proximal) septum just below aortic valve (arrows); D, hypertrophy confined to LV apex (asterisk), consistent with the designation of apical hypertrophic cardiomyopathy (HCM); E, relatively mild hypertrophy in a concentric (symmetric) pattern with each segment of ventricular septum and LV free wall showing similar or identical thicknesses (paired arrows); F, inverted pattern of hypertrophy in which anterior VS is less substantially thickened than the posterior free wall (PW), which is markedly hypertrophied (i.e., 40 mm). Calibration marks are 1 cm apart. AO indicates aorta; AML, anterior mitral leaflet; and LA, left atrium. Reproduced from Maron BJ. Hypertrophic cardiomyopathy: a systematic review. JAMA. 2002, 287(10): 1308-20.

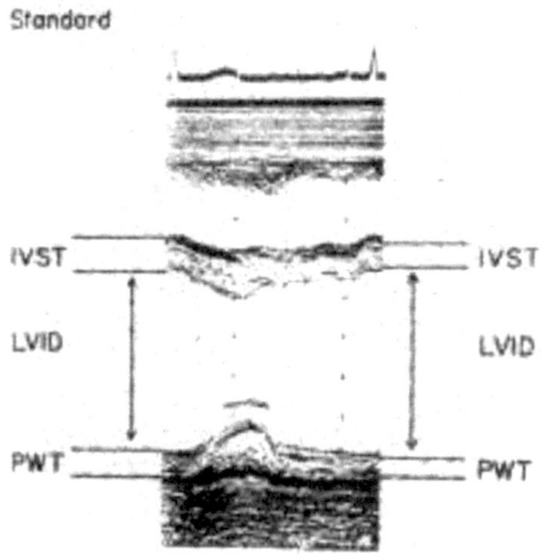


Fig. 2. M-mode echocardiogram of the left ventricle illustrating the standard measurement conventions. IVST= interventricular septal thickness; LVID= left ventricular internal dimension; PWT=posterior wall thickness ( Edited from Devereux, R.B. (1987) Detection of left ventricular hypertrophy by M-mode echocardiography. Anatomic validation, standardization, and comparison to other methods. Hypertension., 9 (Suppl II) , II-19-II-26.)

Essential hypertensive patients with left ventricular hypertrophy increase their mortality rates due to all cardiovascular events from 2 to 10 times more than hypertensives without signs of cardiac hypertrophy [4]. Serving as an independent predictor of cardiovascular events in patients with hypertension, LVH is also a prognostic indicator of hypertension. Patients with normal left ventricular geometry have the best prognosis, those with concentric remodeling or eccentric hypertrophy have intermediate, and those with concentric left ventricular hypertrophy are identified the worst prognosis [5].

Given the fact that left ventricular hypertrophy is an end-organ stage of hypertension, scientists have been striving for the pathogenesis and reversal strategies of left ventricular hypertrophy for years.

## 3. Genetic background

### 3.1 Nuclear genes

Plethoras of evidences support the hypothesis that multiple nuclear genes contribute to left ventricular hypertrophy[6]. It is identified that LVH is influenced by polygenic mutations susceptibility to hemodynamic disorders such as salt-sensitivity, obesity and insulin-resistance etc. Brendan AI. reported a genetic locus on chromosome 2 of the spontaneously hypertensive rat affects relative LV mass independently of blood pressure [7].Yasuyuki Tsujita indicated both genes on chromosome 7 and 17 that influences LVM in a manner dependent on blood pressure [8]. Interestingly, left ventricular hypertrophy shared the same pathological changes with hypertrophic cardiomyopathy such as myocyte disarray, interstitial fibrosis and artery wall thickness. Moreover, hypertrophic cardiomyopathy can result from mutations in 11 genes that encode sarcomere proteins, loci where genes encoding contractile, cytoskeletal, and calcium regulatory proteins. Thus, we can rule out the possibility of indicated genes contribute to hypertrophy cardiomyopathy involving in hypertension-induced left ventricular hypertrophy [9].

## 4. Mitochondrial and left ventricular hypertrophy

### 4.1 mtDNA mutations

In the early stage of hypertension-reduced LVH, ventricular hypertrophy is an important compensatory response to increased load, accompanied by increased amounts of mitochondria [10], which makes it likely that upregulation of cardiac energy production is a mechanism allowing increased cardiac work. However, the mitochondrial function is impaired and the efficiency of mtDNA ultimately decreases dramatically with time passing by. Then, the equilibrium between oxygen offering and consuming will be broken as mitochondrial energy under specific thresholds. The hypothesis of biogenesis of LVH has been supported by plethora of mtDNA mutations. Majamaa-Voltti K et al [11] reported that 3243A>G mtDNA mutation is associated with LVH. Lin Z, et al [12] found G8584A mtDNA mutation may influence LVH in hypertensives. In particular, several point mutations such as G4284A [13], A4295G [14], A4269G[15], A4317G[15] and A4300G[16] located in $tRNA^{Ile}$ contribute to hypertrophic cardiomyopathy to certain degree. A systematic and extended mutational screening for the mitochondrial genome has been initiated in a large cohort of Chinese population by the Geriatric Cardiology Clinic at the Chinese PLA General Hospital, Beijing, China. Specific mutations within the mitochondria were further evaluated. Changes of tRNAs were measured by northern blotting using nonradioactive digoxigenin (DIG)-labeled oligodeoxynucleotides specific for each RNA. Rates of oxygen consumption in intact cells were determined with av YSI 5300 oxygraph. Sequence analysis of mitochondrial DNA in one Chinese pedigree identified a novel A-G transition at position 4401 (A4401G) at the junction of $tRNA^{Met}$ and $tRNA^{Gln}$. The non-coding region mutation appeared to affect the processing of precursors in these mitochondrial tRNAs. The reduction in the rate of respiration and marked decreases in the steady-state levels of $tRNA^{Met}$ and $tRNA^{Gln}$ were detected in the cells carrying this mutation. The novel mutation was absent in 270 Chinese control subjects. In conclusion, the non-coding region (A4401G) mutation was involved in the pathogenesis of left ventricular hypertrophy in Chinese hypertensives[17].

MtDNA mutations can divide into rearrangement mutations and base substitutions. And base substitution mutations are subcategorized into missence mutations (protein coding genes alterations) and protein synthesis mutations (RNAs genes changes).

### 4.2 Rearrangement mutations

Rearrangements of mtDNA due to deletions or duplications generally occur in sporadic patients. Duplications are probably not directly pathogenic, but it produces deleted mtDNA molecules, which implicated into different diseases [18,19]. The most prominent multi-systemic disorders involved in cardiomyopathy are Kearn-Sayre Syndrome (KSS) and Chronic Progressive External Ophthalmoplegia(CPEO) The characteristic symptoms of KSS are cardiac conduction block, cardiomyopathy and caridoembolic stroke with ocular damage including ophthalmoplegia, ptosis, pigmentary degeneration of retina. Compared with cardiac conduction blocks, cardiomyopathy is a much less frequent and late-onset symptom in KSS caused by the relatively low abundance of rearranged mtDNA molecules in the myocardium. Fromenty and colleagues [20] demonstrated that duplications represented an unusually high proportion (41-91%) of all rearranged molecules in hearts from two KSS patients. Because of the preferential accumulation of duplicated rather than deleted mtDNA molecules, the cardiomyopathy may be relatively spared in KSS.CPEO is another rearrangement mtDNA mutation represents a series of abnormalities covering ocular myopathy, mitochondrial myopathy, renal failure and diabetes mellitus [21]. McComish M found the changes of hypertrophy via endomyocardial biopsy on light microscopy[22].

### 4.3 Missence mutaions

Leigh's syndrome is a most severe missence mutation with neural, spinal and cardiac defects. Hypertrophic cardiomyopathy, as a kind of cardiac defect of Leigh's syndrome，results from series of genes involving OXPHOS including MTAP6, NARP8993G and A3243G mutation[23]. Missence mutations in the gene that encodes γ-2 regulatory subunit of the adenosine monophosphate-activated protein kinase(PRKAG2) have been reported to cause familial Wolff-Parkinson-White syndrome associated with conduction abnormalities and LVH [24,25].

### 4.4 Protein synthesis mutations

Myoclonic epilepsy with ragged-red fibers (MERRF) is most frequently caused by an A8344G mutation in the $tRNA^{Lys}$ gene. In a review of 62 reported MERRF patients, about one third had clinical cardiomyopathy; 22% had Wolff-Parkinson-White syndrome[26]. Cardiac evaluation of two MERRF patients revealed asymmetric septal hypertrophy with diffuse hypokinesis of the left ventricle. [27] The G8363A mutation has been identified in two families with MERRF[28,29]. However, in two other families harboring this mutation, hypertrophic cardiomyopathy overshadowed the co-existing encephalopathy and hearing loss[30]. Another protein synthesis mutation is mitochondrial myopathy, lactic acidosis, stroke-like episode(MELAS) which accelerates the process of LVH secondary to vasculopathy[31]. After thorough review of database in Medline, we found that there are 16 mitochondrial genes associated with hypertrophic cardiomyopathies derived from isolated or multisystemic disorder indicated in Table 1 . Thirteen point mutations are in tRNA genes, which do have very specific structural properties that allow an optimal positioning of signals for interaction with various partners such as the cognate aminoacyl-tRNA synthetases (the enzymes that charge the correct amino acid to the 3′ end of the specific tRNAs), translational initiation or elongation factors, and the ribosomal machinery. Three of these are $tRNA^{Leu(UUR)}$ , $tRNA^{Ile}$ and $tRNA^{Lys}$, seem to be hot spots for cardiomyopathies. It is striking that most mutations in $tRNA^{Ile}$ are associated with diseases that present primarily or exclusively with cardiomyopathy.A prime example of a $tRNA^{Leu(UUR)}$ mutation associated with a multisystem disorder is A3243G, the most common cause of mitochondrial encephalomyopathy, lactic acidosis and stroke-like episodes (MELAS) syndrome[32,33]. In a review of 110 reported MELAS patients, cardiac manifestations included congestive heart failure in 18%, Wolff-Parkinson-White syndrome in 14%, and cardiac conduction block in 6%[34].The cardiomyopathy is most commonly hypertrophic[35,36]. Atypical presentations of the A3243G mutation have included maternally inherited PEO with RRF and diabetes and deafness[37]. In addition, isolated cardiomyopathy can be the presenting manifestation of this mutation.[38-40]. Three other point mutations in the tRNA$^{Leu(UUR)}$ have been associated with cardiomyopathies alone (A3260G, C3303T), associated with myopathy (A3260G, C3303T), or as part of the MELAS syndrome (C3254G, A3260G) [38,41-46], The C4320T mutation was also associated with a multiorgan disorder in a child who died at age 7 months of cardiac failure with hypertrophic cardiomyopathy and a severe encephalopathy manifesting as seizures, nystagmus, and spastic tetraparesis[47]. Intriguingly, the three other point mutations in the tRNA$^{Ile}$ gene, A4295G, A4300G, and A4317G, have been identified only in patients with isolated hypertrophic cardiomyopathies [15,48-49] .

| Mutation | Gene | Clinical features | Reference |
|---|---|---|---|
| A3243G | tRNA$^{Leu(UUR)}$ | MELAS;PEO;DM/De; | [32,33, 38,39] |
| C3254G | tRNA$^{Leu(UUR)}$ | Cardiomyopathy(H) | [41] |
| A3260G | tRNA$^{Leu(UUR)}$ | MELAS | [42,43] |
| C3303T | tRNA$^{Leu(UUR)}$ | Myopathy/cardiomyopathy(H); | [44] |
| A4269G | tRNA$^{Ile}$ | MELAS | [50] |
| G4284A | tRNA$^{Ile}$ | Encephalocardiomyopathy(H) | [13] |
| A4295G | tRNA$^{Ile}$ | Cardiomyopathy(H) | [14] |
| A4300G | tRNA$^{Ile}$ | Encephalomyopathy; cardiomyopathy | [16] |
| A4317G | tRNA$^{Ile}$ | Cardiomyopathy(H) | [15] |
| C4320T | tRNA$^{Ile}$ | Cardiomyopathy(H) | [47] |
| A8344G | tRNA$^{Lys}$ | Cardiomyopathy(H+Di) | [51] |
| G8363A | tRNA$^{Lys}$ | Cardiomyopathy(H) | [29-31] |
| G8584A | ATPase 6 | Cardiomyopathy(H)/encephalopathy | [12] |
| T8993G | ATPase 6 | MERRF/De/Cardiomyopathy(H) | [52] |
| T9997C | tRNA$^{Gly}$ | Encephalopathy/cardiomyopathy(H), | [53] |
| G15243A | Cyt b | MERRF | [54] |
| | | NARP/MILS; cardiomyopathy | |
| | | Cardiomyopathy(H)/GI dysmotility | |
| | | Cardiomyopathy(H) | |

AID, aminoglycoside-induced deafness; De, deafness; Di, dilated (cardiomyopathy); DM, diabetes mellitus; GI, gastrointestinal; H, hypertrophic cardiomyopathy; MELAS, mitochondrial encephaomyopathy, lactic acidosis, and strokelike episodes; MERRF, myoclonus epilepsy with raggedred fibers; MILS, maternally inherited Leigh syndrome; NARP, neuropathy, ataxia, retinitis pigmentosa; PEO, progressive external ophthalmoplegia; (Adatpted from Hirano M et al. Mitochondria and the heart. Current Opinion in Cardiology 2001, 16:201–210.)

Table 1. Mitochondrial DNA point mutations associated with hypertrophic cardiomyopathy alone or as a major component of a multisystem disorder

## 5. Defects in mtDNA function

In prior reviews, we noted that several of the cardiomyopathy-associated point mutations in tRNA genes accumulated deficiencies in end maturation, including 3′ end cleavage by tRNAase Z and CCA addition by tRNA ucleotidyl-transferase, and in aminoacylation which affected Trna metabolism thus impaired the synthesis of protein in the end[55-58].

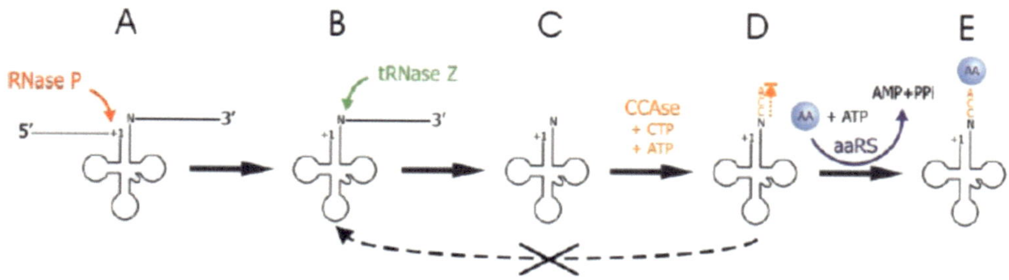


Fig. 3. The tRNA end processing pathway followed by aminoacylation. (A) tRNA is transcribed as a precursor, with a 50 end leader and a 30 end trailer. (B) RNase P has endonucleolytically cleaved the tRNA at +1. (C) tRNAse Z endonucleolytically cleaves the precursor on the 30 side of the discriminator base (N; +73). (D) CCAadding enzyme (CCAse) adds CCA to the 30 end of the tRNA (N) produced by tRNase Z cleavage. (E) tRNA is charged with the cognate amino acid by a specific aminoacyl-tRNA synthetase (aaRS). Dashed line from CCA in (D) to tRNAse Z between (B) and (C) with an X through it indicates that 3'-CCA of mature tRNase Z anti-determinant. (Adapted from Levinger L, et al. Mitochondrial tRNA 3' end metabolism and human disease.Nucleic Acids Res. 2004:11;32(18):5430-41.)

The other genes situated in anticodon stem resulted in missense changes of mitochondria herein influence function of protein variably and implicated in pathogenesis of cardiomyopathy. Of these mtDNA mutations, OXPHOS, ROS and apoptosis, three basic function of mtDNA are estimated as culprits of LVH.

## 6. Oxidative phosphorylation (OXPHOS)

In the early stage of LVH, genes involved in energy transportation including electron transportation chain, tricarboxylic acid (TCA) cycle , glycolysis , fatty acid(FA) metabolism downregulate, while genes devoted to mitochondrial protein transportation and synthesis upregulate. As a result, the expression of cytoskeletal genes increases as well as fetal genes which in line with enhancement of left ventricular mass and size[59]. The compensatory LVH is associated with normalization of myocardial oxygen consumption at the expense of a decrease in the ratio between cardiac work and oxygen consumption (efficiency) [60]. With the time passing by, cardiac working efficiency decreases to a lowest level and heart failure occurs.

## 7. Reactive oxidative species

Since ETC is inhibited, the electrons accumulate in the early stage of the ETC-generating $CoQ_{10}H$: This ubisemiquinone can then donate electrons directly to molecular oxygen (O2) to give superoxide anion(O2·-). Superoxide anion is detoxified by the mitochondrial manganese superoxide dismutase(MnSOD, EC 1.15.1.1) to give $H_2O_2$, and $H_2O_2$ is converted to $H_2O$ by glutathione peroxidase-1(EC1.11.1.9). $H_2O_2$, in the presence of reduced transition metals, can also be converted to the highly reactive hydroxyl radical (·OH). Reactive Oxidative Species potentially has both adaptive and maladaptive signaling consequences. Role of oxidative stress and nitric oxide synthase Growth initiators including angiotensin II, α-agonists, TNF-α, and mechanical strain also promote the formation of reactive oxygen species (ROS) [61]. ROS hypertrophic response at low rates of ROS production to fibrosis [62] and myocyte death at high rates[63]. ROS formation is also stimulated by endothelial nitric oxide synthase (eNOS). In a transgenic eNOS knockout model with low ROS production, severely pressure-loaded hearts developed only modest concentric hypertrophy with little fibrosis and without left-ventricular cavity dilation.[61] Consonant with overall knowledge[63], high rates of ROS production can thus contribute to the transition from left-ventricular hypertrophy to heart failure. Although these findings may be controversial [64], there has been recent confirmation of the concept [65]. Notably, plasma and pericardial markers of oxidative stress are increased in patients with chronic systolic failure of the left ventricle, with these increases related to the clinical severity of heart failure. Controversies in ventricular remodeling.[66]

The chronic release of ROS has been recently linked to the development of left ventricular hypertrophy progression. The chronic release of ROS appears to derive from the nonphagocytic NAD(P)H oxidase and mitochondria. The experimental data are accumulating suggesting that abnormal activation of the nonphagocytic NAD(P)H oxidase in response to neurohormones (angiotensin II, norepinephrine, tumor necrosis factor-a) contribute to cardiac myocyte hypertrophy. In conclusion, the fibrosis, collagen deposition, and metalloproteinase activation involved in the remodeling of failing myocardium are dependent on ROS released. In animal model of chronic pressure overload, apoptosis has revealed as a pivotal trait of myocardial damage together with overproduction of extracellular matrix.

## 8. Programme cell death

Besides contractile disturbances of cardiomyocytes and interstitial and perivascular fibrosis, cardiomyocyte loss is now being considered as one of the determinants of the maladaptive processes implicated in the transition from compensated to decompensate left ventricular hypertrophy. A number of experimental evidence suggests that exaggerated apoptosis may account for the loss of cardiomyocytes in the hypertensive left ventricle. Furthermore, some factors intrinsic and extrinsic to the cardiomyocyte emerge as potential candidates to trigger apoptosis. Increased exposure of ROS accompany with decline in OXPHOS result in the opening of mtPTP, herein, apoptosis-initiated factors leak from inner membrane of mitochondrial to outer membrane. And apoptosis-related factors including procaspase and TNF-α are activated which cause a series pathway of apoptosis[67].

## 9. Variability of phenotypes in left ventricular hypertrophy

Phenotype of LVH is variable even for a same mtDNA mutation due to multiple causes. First, diversity in frequency and efficiency of mitochondria transit from eggs to zygotes. The more mutated mitochondria inherited from mother eggs, the higher probability phenotype will present. Second, difference in mutation load within separated organs cause the diversity in phenotype. Cells will not lose their function until high load of pathogenic mtDNA mutations are present, ranging from 60% to 90%, symptoms arise once mutations over certain threshold and lead to impaired mitochondrial protein synthesis, as well as a severe respiratory chain deficiency. Third, variability of influences derived from nuclear genome. Mitochondrial diseases may result from nuclear DNA mutation (Mendelian mutation) or mitochondrial mutation(maternal inheritance).Mitochondrial synthesis and function require estimated 1000 polypeptides, 37 of which are encoded by mitochondrial (mt) DNA, the rest by nuclear (n) DNA.The nuclear DNA background might also influence phenotypic expression of mtDNA polymorphisms. In fact, Arbustini and colleagues have demonstrated the coexistence of mutations in mtDNA and β-myosin heavy chain (βMHC) in patients with hypertrophic cardiomyopathy, in which mtDNA mutations may contribute to the phenotypic variability of mendelian hypertrophic cardiomyopathies[68].

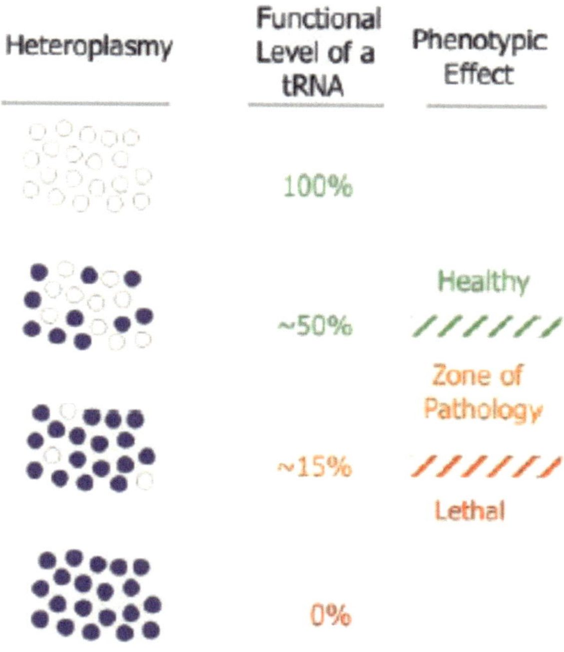


Fig. 4. Heteroplasmy: Mixed (heteroplasmic) populations of wild-type and mutant mitochondrial genomes are present. Filled circles indicate mutant mitochondrial genomes and open circles indicate wild-type. Thresholds: The thresholds for pathology are typically between 15 and 50% of mitochondrial tRNA function, affected by the extent of heteroplasmy. A lower functional level would be lethal and a higher level would be without a phenotype. (Adapted from Levinger L, et al. Mitochondrial tRNA 3' end metabolism and human disease.Nucleic Acids Res. 2004:11;32(18):5430-41.)

## 10. Advances in therapy

Reducing heart load, cutting off vicious cycle of hemodynamic disorders as well as thinning hypertrophic myocardium have been accepted as classic methods to treat LVH. As for the pathogenic involvement of mitochondria, gene therapy is a promising way to improve the outcome of treatment. Nevertheless, there's no effective and consent methods to treat mitochondrial disorders so far. One process under way is to reduce the proportion of mutated mtDNA to subthreshold levels. This could be achieved by adding more wild-type mtDNA, or by removing mutated mtDNA. At the experimental level, some contrary results derived from synthetic wild-type mtDNA transition and gene shifting in skeletal muscles, which help to draw a conclusion that an efficient approach to lead wild-type mtDNA to cells should be further investigated. To remove mutated mtDNA, one approach is to bind specific molecules to mutated mtDNA molecules and prevent them from replicating, while let wild-type mtDNA replication to continue unimpeded. Another approach is to use drugs that select against mutated mtDNA in dividing cells, allowing wild-type mtDNA levels to increase. Otherwise, all the approaches with the goal letting the mutated cells down need to be tested from experimental stages to clinical usage [69]. Recently, antioxidants have been proposed to be important in the pathogenesis of mitochondrial disorders on the basis of ROS involvement [70]. Vitamin B, Vitamin C ,Vitamin E as well as Coenzyme Q has served as scavenger molecules and somewhat has been demonstrated to benefit patients with MELAS and Kearns-Sayre syndrome[71]. Although coenzyme Q10 has shown some early promise in Parkinson's disease and Friedreich's ataxia, such results can only be regarded as provisional at this stage. There have been no large-scale studies to determine the effectiveness of coenzyme Q10 in primary mtDNA diseases [72]. Other molecules involved in ETC may help offering materials for OXPHOS. Moreover, antiapoptosis drugs are beneficial to improving mtDNA diseases in line with the candidate of program cell death.

## 11. Prospects

Left ventricular hypertrophy is a hot spot for improving the life quality of patients with hypertension. The pathogenesis and progression of LVH are tightly linked to mitochondria as we stated above. However, the mechanism of mitochondria implicated into LVH still remain obscure that much more jobs are needed to disclose the secrets of relationship between mitochondria and left ventricular hypertrophy.1) which mtDNA mutation can be served as a marker to predict and indicate the prognosis of LVH? 2) How nDNA influence mtDNA, and to what extent can we use the methods protecting nDNA from damage to attain the role of protecting mtDNA. 3) What steps may we take to reduce frequency and quantity of mutated mtDNA thus cut off the deterioration pathways of LVH.

## 12. References

[1] Julien J, Tranche C, Souchet T. left ventricular hypertrophy in hypertensive patients. Epidemiology and prognosis .Arch Mal Coeur Vaiss. 2004, 97(3):221-7.

[2] Devereux, R.B Detection of left ventricular hypertrophy by M-mode echocardiography. Anatomic validation, standardization, and comparison to other methods. Hypertension.1987,9 (Suppl II):II-19-II-26.

[3] Hu,C.G., Cai,S. The diagnosis and pathological mechanism of left ventricular hypertrophy in hypertensives. Chin. J. Crit. Care. Med.1997,17:55-6.

[4] Coca A, De la Sierra A. Salt sensitivity and left ventricular hypertrophy. Adv Exp Med Biol. 1997, 432:91-101.

[5] Vourvouri EC, Poldermans D, Schinkel AF, et al. Left ventricular hypertrophy screening using a hand-held ultrasound device. Eur Heart J. 2002, 23(19):1516-21.

[6] Post WS, Larson MG, Myers RH, et al. Heritability of left ventricular mass: the Framingham Heart Study.Hypertension. 1997, 30(5):1025-8.

[7] Innes BA, McLaughlin MG, Kapuscinski MK, et al. Independent genetic susceptibility to cardiac hypertrophy in inherited hypertension. Hypertension.1998, 31(3):741-6.

[8] Tsujita Y, Iwai N, Tamaki S, Nakamura Y, et al. Genetic mapping of quantitative trait loci influencing left ventricular mass in rats. Am J Physiol Heart Circ Physiol. 2000 ,279(5):H2062-7.

[9] Ahmad F, Seidman JG, Seidman CE.The genetic basis for cardiac remodeling. Annu Rev Genomics Hum Genet. 2005, 6: 185-216.

[10] Laine H, Katoh C, Luotolahti M, Yki-Järvinen H, et al. Myocardial oxygen consumption is unchanged but efficiency is reduced in patients with essential hypertension and left ventricular hypertrophy. Circulation. 1999,100(24):2425-30.

[11] Majamaa-Voltti, K., Peuhkurinen, K., Kortelainen, M.L., et al. Cardiac abnormalities in patients with mitochondrial DNA mutation 3243A>G. BMC. Cardiovasc Disord. 2002,2:12.

[12] Zhou L, Wan DF, Zhang GY, Li HN, Zhang PP, Zhao XT, Gu JR, Liew CC. Cloning, expression and mutation of mitochondrial ATPase gene of hypertensive patients and rats.ACTA.1999,21:729-732.

[13] Corona P, Lamantea E, Greco M, Carrara F, Agostino A, Guidetti D, Dotti MT, Mariotti C, Zeviani M. Novel heteroplasmic mtDNA mutation in a family with heterogeneous clinical presentations. Ann. Neuro.2002, 51:118-122.

[14] Merante T, Myint T, Benson L, Robinson BH. An additional mitochondrial tRNA-ile point mutation(A-to-G at nucleotide 4295) causing hypertrophic cardiomyopathy. Hum. Mutat.1996, 8: 216-222.

[15] Degoul F, Brule H, Cepanec C, Helm M, Marsac C, Leroux JP, Giege R, Florentz C. Isoleucylation properties of native human mitochondrial tRNA-ile transcripts: implications for cardiomyopathy-related point mutations(4269,4317) in the tRNA-ile gene. Hum Molec. Genet.1998, 7:347-354.

[16] Taylor RW, Giordano C, Davidson MM, et al. A homoplasmic mitochondrial transfer ribonucleic acid mutation as a cause of maternally inherited hypertrophic cardiomyopathy. J Am Coll Cardiol. 2003,41:1786-1796.

[17] Zhu HY, Wang SW, Liu L, Li YH, Chen R, Wang L, Hollimam CJ. A mitochondrial mutation A4401G is involved in the pathogenesis of left ventricular hypertrophy in Chinese hypertensives. Eur J Hum Gene.2009,17:172-8.

[18] Manfredi G, Vu TH, Bonilla E, et al. Association of myopathy with largescale mitochondrial DNA duplications and deletions: which is pathogenic? Ann Neurol. 1997, 42:180–8.

[19] Tang Y, Manfredi G, Hirano M, Schon EA: Maintenance of human rearranged mitochondrial DNAs in long-term cultured transmitochondrial cell lines. Mol Biol Cell. 2000, 11:2349–58.

[20] Fromenty B, Carrozzo R, Shanske S, et al. High proportions of mtDNA duplications in patients with Kearns-Sayre syndrome occur in the heart. Am J Med Genet 1997,71:443–52.

[21] Morgan-Hughes JA, Mair WG. Atypical muscle mitochondria in oculoskeletal myopathy.Brain. 1973, 96(2):215-24.

[22] McComish M, Compston A, Jewitt D. Cardiac abnormalities in chronic progressive external ophthalmoplegia. Br Heart J. 1976,38(5): 526–9.

[23] Wallace DC. Mitochondrial defects in cardiomyopathy and neuromuscular disease. Am Heart J. 2000,139 : 70-85.

[24] Gollob MH, Green MS, Tang AS, et al. Identification of a gene responsible for familial Wolff-Parkinson-White syndrome. N Engl J Med. 2001,344(24):1823-31

[25] Arad M, Benson DW, Perez-Atayde AR, et al. Constitutively active AMP kinase mutations cause glycogen storage disease mimicking hypertrophic cardiomyopathy. J Clin Invest.2002,109(3):357-62.

[26] Hirano M, DiMauro S: Clinical features of mitochondrial myopathies and encephalomyopathies. In Handbook of Muscle Disease. Edited by Lane RJM. New York: Marcel Dekker Inc. USA, 1996:479–504.

[27] Anan R, Nakagawa M, Miyata M, et al. Cardiac involvement in mitochondrial diseases. A study of 17 patients with mitochondrial DNA defects. Circulation.1995, 91:955–61.

[28] Ozawa M, Nishino I, Horai S, et al.: Myoclonus epilepsy associated with ragged-red fibers: a G-to-A mutation at nucleotide pair 8363 in mitochondrial tRNA(Lys) in two families. Muscle Nerve. 1997,20:271–8.

[29] Shtilbans A, Shanske S, Goodman S, et al. G8363A mutation in the mitochondrial DNA transfer ribonucleic acidLys gene: another cause of Leigh syndrome. J Child Neurol. 2000,15:759–61.

[30] Santorelli FM, Mak SC, El-Schahawi M, et al. Maternally inherited cardiomyopathy and hearing loss associated with a novel mutation in the mitochondrial tRNA(Lys) gene (G8363A). Am J Hum Genet. 1996,58:933–9.

[31] Sato W, Tanaka M, Sugiyama S, et al. Cardiomyopathy and angiopathy in patients with mitochondrial myopathy, encephalopathy, lactic acidosis, and strokelike episodes. Am Heart J. 1994,128:733–41.

[32] Pavlakis SG, Phillips PC, DiMauro S, et al. Mitochondrial myopathy, encephalopathy, lactic acidosis, and strokelike episodes: a distinctive clinical syndrome. Ann Neurol. 1984,16:481–8.

[33] Goto Y, Nonaka I, Horai S. A mutation in the $tRNA^{(Leu)(UUR)}$ gene associated with the MELAS subgroup of mitochondrial encephalomyopathies. Nature.1990,348:651-3.

[34] Hirano M, Pavlakis S. Mitochondrial myopathy, encephalopathy,lactic acidosis,and strokelike episodes (MELAS): current concepts. J Child Neurol.1994,9:4–13.

[35] Suzuki Y, Harada K, Miura Y, et al. Mitochondrial myopathy, encephalopathy, lactic acidosis, and stroke-like episodes (MELAS) decrease in diastolic left ventricular function assessed by echocardiography. Pediatr Cardiol.1993,14:162–6.

[36] Okajima Y, Tanabe Y, Takayanagi M, et al. A follow up study of myocardial involvement in patients with mitochondrial encephalomyopathy, lactic acidosis, and stroke-like episodes (MELAS). Heart. 1998,80:292–5.

[37] Moraes CT, Ciacci F, Silvestri G, et al. Atypical clinical presentations associated with the MELAS mutation at position 3243 of human mitochondrial DNA. Neuromusc Disord.1993,3:43–50.

[38] Silvestri G, Bertini E, Servidei S, et al. Maternally inherited cardiomyopathy: a new phenotype associated with the A to G AT nt.3243 of mitochondrial DNA (MELAS mutation). Muscle Nerve. 1997,20:221–5.

[39] Vilarinho L, Santorelli FM, Rosas MJ, et al. The mitochondrial A3243G mutation presenting as severe cardiomyopathy. J Med Genet.1997, 34:607–9.

[40] Hiruta Y, Chin K, Shitomi K, et al. Mitochondrial encephalomyopathy with A to G transition of mitochondrial transfer RNA(Leu(UUR)) 3243 presenting hypertrophic cardiomyopathy. Intern Med. 1995,34:670–3.

[41] Kawarai T, Kawakami H, Kozuka K, et al. A new mitochondrial DNA mutation associated with mitochondrial myopathy: tRNALeu(UUR) 3254 C-to-G.. Neurology.1997,49:598–600.

[42] Zeviani M, Gellera C, Antozzi C, et al. Maternally inherited myopathy and cardiomyopathy:association with mutation in mitochondrial DNA tRNA(Leu)(UUR).Lancet. 1991,338:143-7.

[43] Nishino I, Komatsu M, Kodama S, et al. The 3260 mutation in mitochondrial DNA can cause mitochondrial myopathy, encephalopathy, lactic acidosis, and strokelike episodes (MELAS). Muscle Nerve. 1996,19:1603–4.

[44] Silvestri G, Santorelli FM, Shanske S, et al. A new mtDNA mutation in the tRNA(LeuUUR) gene associated with maternally inherited cardiomyopathy. Hum Mut. 1994,3:37–43.

[45] Mitsuoka T, Kawarai T, Watanabe C, et al. Comparison of clinical pictures of mitochondrial encephalomyopathy with tRNA(Leu(UUR)) mutation in 3243 with that in 3254 No To Shinkei. ?1998,50:1089–92.

[46] Bruno C, Kirby DM, Koga Y, et al. The mitochondrial DNA C3303T mutation can cause cardiomyopathy and/or skeletal myopathy. J Pediatr.1999,135:197–202.

[47] Santorelli FM, El-Shahawi M, Shanske S, et al. A novel mtDNA mutation associated with human cardiomyopathy. Circulation.1995,92(suppl 1):232–3.

[48] Casali C, Santorelli FM, D'Amati G, et al. A novel mtDNA point mutation in maternally inherited cardiomyopathy. Biochem Biophys Res Comm. 1995,213:588–93.

[49] Tanaka M, Ino H, Ohno K, Hattori K, et al. Mitochondrial mutation in fatal infantile cardiomyopathy. Lancet.1990, 2:1452.

[50] Taniike M, Fukushima H, Yanagihara I, et al. Mitochondrial $tRNA^{Ile}$ mutation in fatal cardiomyopathy. Biochem Biophys Res Comm.1992,186:47–53.

[51] Silvestri G, Ciafaloni E, Santorelli F, et al. Clinical features associated with the A>G transition at nucleotide 8344 of mtDNA ("MERRF mutation"). Neurology.1993, 43:1200–6.

[52] Pastores G, Santorelli FM, Shanske S, et al. Leigh syndrome and hypertrophic cardiomyopathy in an infant with a mitochondrial DNA point mutation (T8993G). Am J Med Genet. 1994, 50:265–71.

[53] Merante F, Tein I, Benson L, et al. Maternally inherited hypertrophic cardiomyopathy due to a novel T-to-C transition at nucleotide 9997 in the mitochondrial tRNAglycine gene. Am J Hum Genet. 1994,55:437–46.

[54] Valnot I, Kassis J, Chretien D, et al. A mitochondrial cytochrome b mutation but no mutations of nuclearly encoded subunits in ubiquinol cytochrome c reductase (complex III) deficiency. Hum Genet.1999,104:460–6.

[55] Levinger L, Morl M, Florentz C. Mitochondrial tRNA 3' end metabolism and human disease.Nucleic Acids Res. 2004,32(18):5430-41.

[56] Kelley S, Steinberg S, Schimmel P. Functional defects of pathogenic human mitochondrial tRNAs related to structural fragility. Nature Struct Biol. 2000, 7: 862–5.

[57] Kelley SO, Steinberg SV, Schimmel P. Fragile T-stem in disease-associated human mitochondrial tRNA sensitizes structure to local and distant mutations. J. Biol. Chem.2001,276:10607-11.
[58] Sohm B, Frugier M, Brule H, Olszak K, et al. Towards understanding human mitochondrial leucine aminoacylation identity. J. Mol. Biol.2003, 328:995-1010.
[59] Wilson FH, Hariri A, Farhi A, et al. A cluster of metabolic defects caused by mutation in a mitochondrial tRNA. Science. 2004,306(5699):1190-4.
[60] van den Bosch BJ, Lindsey PJ, van den Burg CM, et al. Early and transient gene expression changes in pressure overload-induced cardiac hypertrophy in mice.Genomics. 2006,88(4):480-8.
[61] Takimoto E, Champion HC, Li M, et al. Oxidant stress from nitric oxide synthase-3 uncoupling stimulates cardiac pathologic remodeling from chronic pressure load. J Clin Invest. 2005, 115: 1221-31.
[62] Siwik DA, Pagano PJ, Colucci WS. Oxidative stress regulates collagen synthesis and matrix metalloproteinase activity in cardiac fibroblasts. Am J Physiol Cell Physiol. 2001, 280: C53-60.
[63] Sawyer DB, Siwik D, Xiao L, Pimentel DR, et al. Role of oxidative stress in myocardial hypertrophy and failure.J Mol Cell Cardiol. 2002, 34: 379-88.
[64] Ichinose F, Bloch KD, Wu JC, et al. Pressure overload-induced LV hypertrophy and dysfunction in mice are exacerbated by congenital NOS3 deficiency. Am J Physiol Heart Circ Physiol 2004,286: H1070-5.
[65] Ruetten H, Dimmeler S, Gehring D, Ihling C, Zeiher AM. Concentric left ventricular remodeling in endothelial nitric oxide synthase knockout mice by chronic pressure overload. Cardiovasc Res 2005, 66: 444-53.
[66] Opie LH, Commerford PJ, Gersh BJ, et al. Controversies in ventricular remodelling. Lancet. 2006,367(9507):356-67.
[67] Gronholm T, Finckenberg T, Palojoki E, et al. Cardioprotective effects of vasopeptidase inhibition in vs. angiotensin type 1-receptor blockade in spontaneously hypertensive rat on a high salt diet. Hypertens Res. 2004,27:609-18.
[68] Fortuño MA, Ravassa S. Apoptosis in hypertensive heart disease. Curr Opin Cardiol. 1998,13(5):317-25.
[69] Hirano M, Davidson M, DiMauro S.Curr Opin Cardiol. Mitochondria and the heart.2001,16(3):201-10.
[70] France-Lanord V, Brugg B, Michel PP, et al. Mitochondrial free radical signal in ceramide-dependent apoptosis: a putative mechanism for neuronal death in Parkinson's disease.J Neurochem. 1997,69(4):1612-21.
[71] Graff C, Clayton DA, Larsson NG. Mitochondrial medicine--recent advances.J Intern Med. 1999 ,246(1):11-23.
[72] Schapira AH. Mitochondrial disease.Lancet. 2006,368(9529):70-82.

10

# Pharmacogenetics of Essential Hypertension

Madhu Khullar and Saurabh Sharma
*Department of Experimental Medicine & Biotechnology,*
*Post Graduate Institute of Medical Education and Research, Chandigarh,*
*India*

## 1. Introduction

Hypertension is one of the most common chronic illnesses effecting more than 1 billion people worldwide and is a major risk factor for coronary artery disease and myocardial infarction, heart failure, stroke and renal failure. By the year 2025, the global prevalence of hypertension is projected to increase to 29.2% in adult population (Kearney et al., 2005). It is well established that reduction in blood pressure is associated with decreased cardiovascular morbidity and mortality (Lewington, Clarke, Qizilbash, Peto, & Collins, 2002). Despite the availability of several antihypertensive drugs which include thiazide diuretics, beta blockers, Angiotensin-Converting Enzyme (ACE) inhibitors, angiotensin receptor blockers (ARB) and calcium channel blockers, global estimates suggest that less than 35% of hypertensives are able to achieve their target systolic and diastolic blood pressure with these drugs (Thoenes et al., 2009). The current strategy of trial and error approach to the management of hypertension is suboptimal and alternative approaches for identifying the optimal antihypertensive regimen in a specific patient are needed. One potential approach for individualizing antihypertensive therapy is through the use of genetic information, or pharmacogenomics, to identify the most appropriate therapy for individual patients. Given the health burden associated with hypertension and the poor rates of BP control, hypertension pharmacogenomics holds great potential. Pharmacogenetics is the science that determines the efficiency and side effects of a medicine based on the genetic make-up of an individual (personalized medicine). Potential benefits of personalized medicines include prescription of drugs based on a patient's genetic profile versus trial and error, hence decreasing the likelihood of adverse reactions and maximizing effectiveness (Centre for Genetics Education, 2007). In the current review, we review genetic association of blood pressure lowering response to different drug classes of antihypertensive therapy in different ethnic populations.

## 2. Meta-analysis for pharmacogenetics of hypertension

In order to compile the current knowledge of pharmacogenetics of anti-hypertensive drugs, we searched PubMed using the MESH terms "Pharmacogenetics+hypertension, Genes + Hypertension, Blood pressure response + hypertension" in Pubmed limiting results to publications on studies in human adults. Similar searches were performed with names of specific antihypertensive drugs including Diuretics, Beta-blockers, ARB and ACE inhibitors. We further identified specific polymorphisms of genes of interest noted in earlier reviews and performed additional PubMed searches based on these candidate genes. Studies on both healthy subjects and patients were included, and there was no time limit on duration of drug administration. Studies with both single and multiple drugs were included. Even if our information of interest was a small part of the study, it was included. Studies that only addressed the association of genetic variants/polymorphisms with hypertension and hypertension-induced end-organ damage but not with blood pressure alterations in response to anti-hypertensive drugs were not included. Reports related to experimental animals, or studies that used manipulated blood pressure (e.g. the attenuation of agonist-induced blood pressure increase) or were in languages other than English, or in which no specific drugs or drug classes were used (i.e. reports on therapy-resistant hypertension in general) were not included. Our aim was to collate the existing body of knowledge on common genetic polymorphisms and their relationship to blood pressure lowering response. We tried to remove bias in the selection of research articles by selecting maximum number of studies and from different ethnic groups. A summary of these findings is shown in the Table (1).

## 2.1 Diuretics

Diuretics are the first-line treatment of hypertension and Thiazides are most commonly prescribed diuretics. Thiazides inhibit Na+/Cl− cotransporter (NCC) in the renal distal convoluted tubule, resulting in decreased sodium re-absorption and increased sodium excretion, which leads to decreased extracellular fluid (ECF) and plasma volume. This volume loss results in diminished venous return, increased renin release, reduced cardiac output and decreased blood pressure (CONWAY & LAUWERS, 1960). Varied Blood pressure (BP) response to diuretics is observed in hypertensive patients. It has been proposed that genetic polymorphisms in several candidate genes such as the Angiotensin-Converting Enzyme (ACE), alpha-adducin (ADD1), G protein b3-subunit (GNB3) gene, angiotensinogen (AGT), angiotensin II receptor1 (AGTR1), etc. may influence blood pressure (BP) response to diuretic therapy (Arnett, Claas, & Glasser, 2006; Gerhard et al., 2008; C.-C. Huang et al., 2011; Luo, Y. Wang, et al., 2009; Sciarrone et al., 2003; Turner, Schwartz, Chapman, & Boerwinkle, 2001; D. Werner et al., 2008). ACE insertion/deletion (ACE I/D) polymorphism has been extensively studied for association with blood pressure lowering response to diuretics (Bozec et al., 2003; Nordestgaard et al., 2010; Scharplatz, Puhan, Steurer, & Bachmann, 2004; Su et al., 2007; Ueda, Meredith, Morton, Connell, & Elliott, 1998; Yu, Zhang, & G. Liu, 2003; Zhou, Wu, J.-Q. Liu, Liang, & G.-F. Liu, 2007); however conflicting results have been reported in different studies. Both, association / lack of association of ACE genotypes with blood pressure-lowering response to diuretics have been reported in different studies (Table). For example, a lack of association between ACE genotypes and adjusted mean difference in diastolic and systolic blood pressure in hypertensive patients on diuretics has been reported in Finnish (Suonsyrjä et al, 2009) and Swedish subjects (Schelleman et al 2006); whereas D allele was found to be associated with greater systolic blood pressure reduction in hypertensive Chinese patients on hydrochlorothiazide (HCTZ)(Jiang et al., 2007; Zhou et al., 2007). Sciarrone et al, 2003, on the other hand, showed that I allele of ACE (I/D) polymorphism was significantly associated with the largest mean blood pressure (MBP) decrease with HCTZ treatment. It has also been observed that response to thiazides may be gender specific (Frazier, S T Turner, G L Schwartz, A B Chapman, & E Boerwinkle, 0000; Zhou, Wu, J.-Q. Liu, Liang, & G.-F. Liu,

2007); for example, Schwartz et al (2002), reported that ACE II homozygosity in women and DD homozygosity in men was associated with the greatest BP lowering responses to HCTZ.

Two other genes, ADD1 and GNB3 genes have also been shown to influence the response to diuretics. α-Adducin is a ubiquitously expressed heterodimeric cytoskeleton protein that modulates a variety of cellular functions, including sodium transport. A genetic variant in ADD1, namely, Gly460Trp polymorphism has been shown to be associated with renal sodium reabsorption, salt-sensitive hypertension and response to diuretic therapy (Glorioso et al., 1999). However, the evidence remains inconsistent between studies and across populations. There are studies showing that use of diuretics in carriers of the 460Trp allele, significantly reduced the risk of cardiovascular outcomes and stroke when compared with other antihypertensive treatments (Cusi et al., 1997); however, negative studies, showing no significant association of ADD1 gene variants with diuretic mediated reduction in adverse cardiovascular events and stroke have also been published (Stephen T Turner, Arlene B Chapman, Gary L Schwartz, & Eric Boerwinkle, 2003). Genetics of Hypertension-Associated Treatment Study (GenHAT) also did not find Gly460Trp polymorphism to be an important modifier of cardiovascular risk. However, female carriers of variant allele treated with diuretics showed an increased risk of CHD, suggesting an interaction between gene variant and gender (Turner et al., 2008). ADD1 Gly460Trp polymorphism has also not been found to influence response to HCTZ in Finnish subjects (Suonsyrjä et al. 2009). A similar study on 5,979 hypertensive patients in USA showed a greater but non-significant association between Gly460Trp polymorphism and BP lowering effect of diuretics (Gerhard et al., 2008).

GNB3 gene, which encodes Beta subunit of Guanine nucleotide-binding protein G(I)/G(S)/G(T) which is associated with signal transduction across cell membranes, has been found to influence BP lowering response in hypertensive patients on diuretics; homozygous carriers of, GNB3 825TT (rs5443) genotype were found to show greater decline in blood pressure than homozygous CC patients in both white Caucasians (190) and African Americans (197) (Turner, Schwartz, Chapman, & Boerwinkle, 2001). In ALLHAT (Antihypertensive and Lipid-Lowering Treatment to Prevent Heart Attack Trial), a multicenter clinical trial conducted in the United States and Canada, minor C allele carriers of natriuretic peptide A gene (NPPA), a gene implicated in the control of extracellular fluid volume and electrolyte homeostasis, were found to respond significantly better to the diuretic chlorthalidone than carriers of other genotypes (Lynch et al., 2008). A recent study has reported that polymorphism in Renin gene may also modulate blood pressure lowering response of thiazide diuretics. In this study, it was seen that Renin CC genotype (rs11240688), Log PRA and baseline Systolic Bloof Pressure (SBP), all contributed to the BP lowering response to Thiazide diuretics in non-diabetic hypertensive Taiwanese patients (Huang et al., 2011).

Several other candidate genes have been also examined for their association with BP lowering response to diuretics. For example, Werner et al., in 2008 have shown that CYP2C9*3 and SLCO1B1 c.521TC genotypes and female gender were significant and independent predictors of the pharmacokinetics of torasemide, a diuretic frequently used in treatment of hypertension in a small set of patients. Organic anion transporter (OAT) 1 and OAT3, encoded by a tightly linked gene pair, plays a key role in renal secretion of diuretics (Nozaki et al., 2007). An intergenic polymorphism between OAT1 and OAT3, rs10792367, has been investigated for BP response to the diuretic HCTZ. In a study on 1,106 Chinese patients, no significant association was found even though it appeared to explain the inter individual variation in response to HCTZ (Han et al., 2011). The NEDD4L gene encodes E3 ubiquitin-protein ligase NEDD4-like enzyme, which reduces renal tubular expression of epithelial Na+ channel (ENaC) and is influenced by a functional rs4149601 G→A NEDD4L polymorphism. As diuretics inhibit renal sodium reabsorption, this polymorphism was studied for an effect on the diuretic efficacy. In Nordic Diltiazem Study (NORDIL) Sweden, the functional NEDD4L rs4149601 polymorphism was found to significantly influence the efficacy of diuretic-based antihypertensive treatment in hypertensive patients (Svensson-Färbom et al., 2011). Similar results have been reported in Chinese patients, where it was found that NEDD4L A-allele carriers showed greater blood pressure reduction than GG carriers with HCTZ (Luo et al., 2009). In yet another study, -344 C/T polymorphism in the CYP11b2 gene, which encodes aldosterone synthase was evaluated for BP response to diuretics in 340 individuals in Brazil; however no significant association between BP response and the polymorphism was observed (Lacchini et al., 2009). A genome wide association study (GWAS) to identify novel SNPs associated with the anti-hypertensive response to the diuretic, hydrochlorothiazide, has shown polymorphisms in two genes, LYZ (rs317689) and YEATS4 (rs315135) to be associated with Diastolic blood pressure lowering response in independent data set of African Americans and Caucasian white subjects (Turner et al., 2008).

Thus, till date, available literature remains inconclusive regarding predictive effect of genotypes on diuretic mediated antihypertensive response, however, with better study designs in future and replication of existing associations, it may be feasible to tailor diuretic therapy based on a patients' specific genetic make up.

### 2.2 β-blockers

β-Blockers are competitive antagonists of the β-adrenergic receptors, thereby modulating activities in this pathway (Reiter, 2004). Although β blockers are among the most widely prescribed of all drug classes for hypertension and various other cardiovascular diseases, β blocker therapy often produces variable responses among patients (Lindholm, Carlberg, & Samuelsson, 2005; Materson et al., 1993). Polymorphisms in various genes involved in sympathetic and renin-angiotensin-aldosterone systems (RAAS) have been investigated for association with variability in blood pressure lowering response to β-Blockers. Existing data suggests that polymorphisms in β1-adrenoceptor gene (ADRB1), namely, Ser49Gly and Arg389Gly may influence blood pressure responses to β-blocker therapy (J. Liu et al., 2006; Aquilante et al., 2008). Homozygosity for ADRB1 Arg389 allele has been shown to be associated with greater decrease in SBP and DBP changes in Caucasians and Chinese hypertensive subjects and ADRB1 Ser49Arg389/Ser49Arg389 haplotype was found to be a predictor of a good SBP response to metoprolol, suggesting its predictability across races (Aquilante et al., 2008; J. Liu et al., 2006). In healthy volunteers with exercise induced heart rate increase, Arg389Arg genotype carriers were also found to show significantly greater reduction in systolic blood pressure than Gly389Gly carriers after 1 day of metoprolol treatment; however, plasma metoprolol concentrations were not significantly different between Arg389Arg and Gly389Gly genotypes 3 hours after metoprolol treatment, suggesting that differences in response were not due to variability in metoprolol pharmacokinetics (J Liu et al., 2003). However, no significant genotype based effects of

ADRB1 Ser49 and Arg389 polymorphism have been observed with dobutamine (Aquilante et al., 2008) or fluoxetine and paoxetine in Caucasian Americans (Turner et al., 2008). ADRB1 Ser49Gly and Arg389Gly and ADRB2 Cys19Arg, Gly16Arg and Gln27Glu polymorphisms were also not found to significantly affect BP response to Atenolol (Filigheddu et al., 2010). In contrast, Pacanowski et al. (2008) found Ser49Gly and Arg389Gly to be significantly associated with response to atenolol in a study of 5,979 patients from 184 sites in the United States and Puerto Rico.

Three SNPs in the GNB3 gene, A3882C, G5249A and C825T have been found to have a significant effect on blood pressure response to atenolol in the female participants in Caucasian Americans (Filigheddu et al., 2010). Carvedilol is a non-selective α and β blocker that reduces the BP by blocking the binding of Norepinephrine to β1- and β2-adrenergic receptors (Stafylas & Sarafidis, 2008). Although polymorphism in CYP2D6 impact pharmacokinetics and pharmacodynamics of carvedilol, it has been shown to have no effect on the blood pressure response to the drug (Sehrt et al. 2011). However, ADRB2 Gln27 carriers were recently reported to show greater reduction in resting BP with carvedilol compared with Glu27carriers in Russian subjects (Tepliakov et al., 2010).

The Glu41Leu polymorphism in GRK5 enhances desensitization of the β1-adrenergic receptor and has been postulated to confer endogenous 'genetic β-blockade' and contribute to an attenuated response to β-blockers in black subjects. Thus GRK5 Gln41Leu variant could contribute to ethnicity base inter-individual variability in response to β-blockade between black and Caucasian individuals (Liggett et al., 2008). Kurnik et al. (2009), however, have observed that GRK5 Gln41Leu polymorphism did not contribute to the ethnic differences in sensitivity to atenolol among Black and Caucasian individuals.

NEDD4L polymorphism has been found to influence renal tubular expression of epithelial Na+ channel (EnaC) (Luo et al., 2009). Gene variants of Gsα (FokI polymorphism), and NEDD4L (rs4149601, G→A) polymorphisms have been investigated for a role in the blood pressure response to β blockers. Gsα genotype was not found to be a significant independent predictor of BP response (Jia et al., 1999); whereas NEDD4L rs4149601 polymorphism was shown to influence the efficacy of β-blockers in the NORDIL study (Svensson-Färbom et al., 2011).

Most of the existing data on pharmacogenetics of β- blockers remains inconclusive and further studies are needed to correlate the genotype -drug response to β- blockers in large populations from different ethnic communities so as to be an effective predictive tool.

### 2.3 ACE inhibitors

ACE inhibitors are one of the most commonly prescribed antihypertensives and block the production of angiotensin II by inhibiting ACE (encoded by the *ACE* gene), an enzyme that converts Angiotensin I to Angiotensin II (Cody, 1997). Polymorphisms in RAAS genes have been shown to influence antihypertensive response of ACE inhibitors, but the results have been contradictory and inconclusive (Lillvis & Lanfear, 2010). The commonly studied variations have been I/D polymorphism in the ACE gene, AGT Met235Thr polymorphism in the AGT gene and AGTR1- A1166C polymorphism (rs5186) (Rosskopf & Michel, 2008; Scharplatz, Puhan, Steurer, & Bachmann, 2004). Both, D and I alleles of ACE I/D Polymorphism were shown to be associated with BP lowering response to ACE Inhibitors in hypertensives in earlier studies (Ueda et al, 1998, Kurland et al, 2001); however, recent studies in larger cohorts have failed to replicate the BP response modulation by ACE inhibitors (Yu, Zhang, & Liu, 2003, D. K Arnett et al., 2005, F. Filigheddu et al., 2008). Recently, another ACE SNP, rs4343, which is located near the ACE I/D and is in linkage disequilibrium with it, has been reported to be strongly associated with BP response to ACE inhibitors in a Genome Wide Association Study (C-M Chung et al., 2010). However this association could not be reproduced in the large randomized placebo controlled EUROPA trial (Brugts et al., 2010).

Besides ACE gene variants, 235T allele of AGT (M235T) gene has also been found to be associated with BP response to ACE inhibitors in several studies (Table). However, a recent study with larger sample size did not show any significant association of this variant with BP response to β blockers (Schelleman et al., 2007). Su et al., 2007 have reported the association of other AGT SNPs with BP response to benazepril, an ACE Inhibitor. These authors also found a significant association of AGT gene polymorphisms, C11537A (rs7079), rs2638362 (C/T) and rs2640543 (G/A) with BP response to ACE inhibitors (Su et al., 2007). AGTR1, which is an important receptor in the RAAS system and plays a crucial role in BP control (Atlas, 2007), is an important candidate for study of genetic variation-pharmacological associations. Its genetic variant, A1166C has been extensively evaluated for an effect on BP lowering by ACE inhibitors (Redon, Luque-Otero, Martell, & Chaves, 2004; Scharplatz et al., 2004) but recent studies have not found any significant effect of this variant with BP lowering ability of ACE inhibitors (Brunner et al., 2007; Filigheddu et al., 2008; Konoshita, 2011; Nordestgaard et al., 2010; Redon, Luque-Otero, Martell, & Chaves, 2004; H. Yu et al., 2009). Besides these commonly studied polymorphisms, the bradykinin B1 receptor gene (BDKRB1) SNP (rs12050217) and the ABO gene polymorphisms (rs495828 and rs8176746) have been also found to be significantly associated with blood pressure response to ACE inhibitors (Brugts et al., 2010; Chung et al., 2010).

### 2.4 Angiotensin Receptor Blockers (ARB)

Angiotensin receptor blockers (ARBs), also known as sartans, block the activation of angiotensin type 1 receptors and have a recognized role in the treatment of blood pressure. Studies on ARB pharmacogenetics have commonly focused on genes of RAAS system. A small-scale study investigated the role of AGTR1- A1166C polymorphism in patients with heart failure who were taking ARB (candesartan) in addition to the ACE inhibitor for BP control. This study observed that AGTR1 A1166C polymorphism significantly influenced the BP response to candesartan (de Denus et al., 2008). However, studies on larger cohorts could not replicate association of AGTR1 A1166C and C573T polymorphisms on the efficacy of ARBs (Konoshita, 2011; Nordestgaard et al., 2010). Variants of other RAAS genes such as ACE (I/D), AGT (M235T) and AT2 variants have not been found to be significantly associated with the action of ARB in BP lowering (Konoshita, 2011; Nordestgaard et al., 2010). A recent study has reported that C-5312T polymorphism of the renin gene (REN) was associated with pharmacogenetics of ARBs (Konoshita, 2011). Additionally, some pilot studies have been conducted on small sample sizes (n=31 to 49) that show significant associations but they need to be reproduced in larger cohorts. In one of these small-scale study, for example, Cytochrome P450 CYP2C9 enzyme (CYP2C9) that metabolizes angiotensin II type 1 (AT (1)) receptor antagonists losartan and irbesartan, has been found to be associated with the DBP response to irbesartan (Hallberg et al., 2002). In another study, AGTR1 5245 TT genotype was found to be associated with plasma concentrations of irbesartan, a specific angiotensin II type 1 receptor

(AGTR1) antagonist and the blood pressure response in hypertensive patients (Kurland et al., 2008). However, these results can't be considered reliable on account of the small sample sizes and need to be validated with larger sample sizes.

### 2.5 Calcium channel blockers

The large-conductance calcium and voltage-dependent potassium (BK) channel found in vascular smooth muscle is comprised of pore-forming-α and regulatory-β1 subunits (Fernández-Fernández et al., 2004). The BK channel, particularly the β1 subunit, functions in a negative feedback mechanism to enhance calcium sensitivity, decrease cell excitability, and limit smooth muscle contraction (Fernández-Fernández et al., 2004). Calcium channels are present in the smooth muscles that line the blood vessels. By relaxing these smooth muscles, calcium channel blockers dilate the blood vessels and reduce the BP (Jun et al., 2010). Calcium channel blockers are commonly used in the treatment of hypertension and angina but the response is widely variable (Nguyen, Parker, Noujedehi, Sullivan, & J A Johnson, 2000). This variability may be best explained by genetic variation and identifying the exact cause of this varied response to calcium channel blockers is important in personalizing treatment for hypertension. The gene that encodes the β1 subunit of the BK channel is KCNMB1, which is likely to carry polymorphisms, which affect the efficacy of calcium channel blockers. Glu65Lys and Val110Leu are the two commonly studied polymorphisms in this gene (Brunner et al., 2007; Plüger et al., 2000). In the INVEST-GENE study, BP response to Verapamil SR was not found to differ by KCNMB1 genotypes. However, individuals with Lys65 allele were found to achieve BP control earlier and were found to be less likely to require multiple drugs for BP control than those with Glu65Glu genotype (Beitelshees et al., 2007). In another analysis of the INVEST GENE study, Verapamil efficacy was investigated for association with the SNPs of endothelial NO synthase (eNOS) gene. Nitric Oxide (NO), the product of NOS gene is a critical mediator of vascular tone and also has antiplatelet, antiproliferative and antimitogenic effect and eNOS activity is important in cardiovascular outcomes and response to treatment. Two commonly studied SNPs are NOS3 -786T>C in promoter region, which reduces gene expression (Cattaruzza et al., 2004; Iwai et al., 2003; Nakayama et al., 1999) and a nonsynonymous SNP (894G>T), which increases its susceptibility to proteolytic cleavage (Tesauro et al., 2000), reducing NO bioavailability (Leeson et al., 2002; Persu et al., 2002; Savvidou, Vallance, Nicolaides, & Hingorani, 2001). The -786T>C genotype was shown to be significantly associated with response to Verapamil; -786C allele carriers showed the greatest reduction in SBP/DBP. However, eNOS 894G>T genotypes were not found to significantly affect the BP response (M. A. Pacanowski, Zineh, Rhonda M. Cooper-DeHoff, Carl J. Pepine, & Julie A. Johnson, 2009). Amlodipine, a dihydropyridine (DHP) class calcium channel blocker is another drug routinely prescribed for BP control. In the ALLHAT study conducted in the USA and Canada, NPPA T2238C allele was found to be significantly associated with the action of this drug. It was seen that TT allele carriers responded better to calcium channel blockers (Lynch et al., 2008). However, in order to be useful in clinical settings, these studies need to be conducted in wider regions of the world covering more ethnic populations.

## 3. Conclusion and future perspectives

Despite the availability of several effective anti hypertensive drug therapies, optimal control of blood pressure remains elusive in a large set of patients. Pharmacogenetics of antihypertensive therapy has the potential to tailor therapy according to patients genetic make up as is evidenced by the above Meta analysis. However, prediction of the right drug for optimum BP control requires large-scale studies on ethnically diverse populations. Most of the studies till date have focused on candidate genes and sample size has ben small. Individual groups were only able to detect small effects in their individual population but collaborating with other groups conducting GWAS and also focusing on relevant pathways will make this more tractable approach and lead to successful clinical translation. Replicating these findings across multiple ethnic populations will also be an be an important aspect of personalizing treatment on genetic basis and increased international collaboration among hypertension pharmacogenomics investigators will be very important to achieve this goal. Additionally whole genome mapping of hypertension and blood pressure traits and understanding the pharmacogenetics of current drugs will enable the discovery of new drug targets in future.

| Drug Class | Drug | Area | Ethnicity | Sample size, N | Genetic variants | Significant difference? | Reference |
|---|---|---|---|---|---|---|---|
| Diuretic | Hydrochloro-thiazide | USA | Non-Hispanic white (50%) Non-Hispanic Black (50%) | 389 | LYZ (rs317689) | Yes | (Turner et al., 2008) |
| | | | | | YEATS4 (rs315135) | Yes | |
| | | USA | White Caucasian (190) African American (197) | 387 | GNB3 C825T (rs5443) | Yes | (Turner et al., 2001) |
| | Chlorthalidone | USA | | 13,860 | NPPA T2238C | Yes | (Lynch et al., 2008) |
| | Hydrochloro-thiazide | Taiwan | Taiwanese | 90 | Renin (rs11240688) | Yes | (C. -C. Huang et al., 2011) |
| | Hydrochloro-thiazide | Netherlands | Dutch | 613 | ADD1 Gly460Trp (rs4961) | No | (van Wieren-de Wijer et al., 2009) |
| β Blockers | Dobutamine | USA | White | 163 | ADRB1 (Ser49Gly) | No | (Aquilante et al., 2008) |
| | | | | | ADRB1 (Arg389Gly)-rs1801253 | No | |
| | | | | | ADRB2 (Arg16Gly) | No | |
| | | | | | ADRB2 (Gln27Glu) | No | |
| | Fluoxetine and paroxetine | USA | White | 122 | ADRB1 (Arg389Gly)-rs1801253 | Yes | (Turner, Bailey, Fridley, Chapman, Schwartz, Chai, Sicotte, Kocher, Rodin, & Boerwinkle, 2008b) |
| | Carvedilol | USA | Caucasian | 110 | ADRB2 (Gln27Glu) | Yes | (Sehrt, Meineke, Tzvetkov, Gültepe, & |
| | | | | | CYP2D6 | No | |

| Drug Class | Drug | Area | Ethnicity | Sample size, N | Genetic variants | Significant difference? | Reference |
|---|---|---|---|---|---|---|---|
| | | | | | | | Brockmöller, 2011) |
| | Atenolol | USA | African Americans (69) and Caucasian White (85) | 151 | GRK5-Leu41 (rs17098707) | No | (Kurnik et al., 2009) |
| | Bisoprolol | Finland | Finnish | 233 | ADRB1 (Ser49Gly)(145A>G)-rs1801252 | No | (Suonsyrjä et al., 2010) |
| | | | | | ADRB1 (Arg389Gly)-rs1801253 | No | |
| | Amlodipine | USA | Multi-ethnic | 8174 | T2238C | Yes | (Lynch et al., 2008) |
| | Metoprolol | China | Chinese | 61 | ADRB1 (Ser49Gly)(145A>G)-rs1801252 | Yes | (J. Liu et al., 2003) |
| | | | | | ADRB1 (Arg389Gly)-rs1801253 | Yes | |
| | Atenolol | Italy | Italians | 1112 | ADRB1 (Arg389Gly) | No | (Fabiana Filigheddu et al., 2010) |
| | | | | | ADRB1 (Ser49Gly)-(145A>G)-rs1801252 | | |
| | | | | | ADRB2 (Cys19Arg) | | |
| | | | | | ADRB2 (Gly16Arg) | | |
| | | | | | ADRB2 (Gln27Glu) | | |
| | | | | | GNB3 (A3882C) | | |
| | | | | | GNB3 (G5249A) | | |
| | | | | | GNB3 (C825T) | | |
| | Trandolapril and/or Atenolol | USA and Puerto Rico | Multiethnic | 5,979 | ADRB1 Ser49Gly (145A>G)-rs1801252 | Yes | (Pacanowski et al., 2008) |
| | | | | | ADRB1 Arg389Gly (1165C>G)-rs1801253 | Yes | |
| ACEI | Imidapril or benazepril | China | Chinese | 517 | ACE (I/D) | No | (Yu, Zhang, & Liu, 2003) |
| | Imidapril or benazepril | China | Chinese | 501 | AGT (M235T) | No | (H. Yu et al., 2005) |
| | Lisinopril | USA | White Caucasians (61%) | 7,528 | ACE (I/D) | No | (D. K Arnett et al., 2005) |
| | | | African Americans (35%) | | | | |
| | Benazepril | China | Chinese | 1,447 | AGT (rs7079 (C/T)) | Yes | (Su et al., 2007) |
| | | | | | AT1 (multi loci, H2 & H3) | Yes | |
| | | | | | AT2 (multi loci) | No | |
| | Trandolapril | USA | White (35%) | 551 | AT1 (A1166C) | No | (Brunner et al., 2007) |
| | | | Hispanic (44%) | | | | |
| | Captopril | China | Chinese | 624 | ACE2 (rs2106809) | Yes | (Fan et al., |

| Drug Class | Drug | Area | Ethnicity | Sample size, N | Genetic variants | Significant difference? | Reference |
|---|---|---|---|---|---|---|---|
| | | | | | | | 2007) |
| | Fosinopril | USA | White | 191 | ACE (I/D) | No | (F. Filigheddu et al., 2008) |
| | | | | | AGT (A-6G) | No | |
| | | | | | AT1 (A1166C) | No | |
| | Imidapril benazepril | China | Chinese | 509 | AT1 (A1166C) | No | (H. Yu et al., 2009) |
| | Lisinopril | USA | White non-Hispanic (47%) | 30,076 | FGB-455 | Yes | (Lynch et al., 2009) |
| | ACEI | Taiwan | Taiwanese | 623 | ACE (rs4343) | Yes | (Chung et al., 2010) |
| | | | | | ABO (rs495828) | Yes | |
| | | | | | ABO (rs8176746) | Yes | |
| | Perindopril | Europe | Caucasians | 8907 | AGTR1 (rs275651) | Yes | (Brugts, Boersma, & Simoons, 2010) |
| | | | | | AGTR1 (rs5182) | | |
| | | | | | BDKRB1 (rs12050217) | | |
| | Enalapril | Europe | Caucasians | 98 | AGT (M235T) | Yes | (Bozec et al., 2003) |
| | Telmisartan | Europe | Caucasians | 206 | AGT (A-6G) | No | (Redon, Luque-Otero, Martell, & Chaves, 2004) |
| | | | | | ACE (I/D) | | |
| | | | | | AT1 (A1166C) | | |
| | | | | | AT1 (C573T) | | |
| ARB | Telmisartan | Spain | Spanish | 206 | ACE (I/D) | No | (Redon, Luque-Otero, Martell, & Chaves, 2004) |
| | | | | | AGT (A-6G) | No | |
| | | | | | AT1 (A1166C) | No | |
| | | | | | AT1 (C573T) | No | |
| | Valsartan | Japan | Japanese | 231 | ACE (I/D) | No | (Konoshita, 2011) |
| | | | | | AGT (M235T) | No | |
| | | | | | AT1 (A1166C) | No | |
| | | | | | AT2 (C3123A) | No | |
| | | | | | REN (C-5312T) | Yes | |
| | Losartan | Scandinavia | White (92%) | 1,774 | ACE (I/D) | No | (Nordestgaard et al., 2010) |
| | | | | | AGT (M235T) | No | |
| | | | | | AT1 (A1166C) | No | |
| Calcium channel blockers | Verapamil SR | USA | Hispanics, White Caucasians and Afro Americans | 5979 | KCNMB1 (Glu65Lys) | No | (Beitelshees et al., 2007) |
| | | | | | KCNMB1 (Val110Leu) | No | |
| | Verapamil SR | USA | Hispanics, White Caucasians and Afro Americans | 1025 | NOS3 (-786T>C)(rs2070744) | Yes | (M. Pacanowski et al., 2008) |
| | | | | | NOS3 Glu298>Asp (rs1799983) | No | |
| | Amlodipine | USA and Canada | Multi-ethnic | 8174 | NPPA (T2238C) | Yes | (Lynch et al., 2008) |

Table 1.

## 4. References

Abdollahi, M. R., Huang, S., Rodriguez, S., Guthrie, P. A. I., Smith, G. D., Ebrahim, S., Lawlor, D. A., et al. (2008). Homogeneous assay of rs4343, an ACE I/D proxy, and an analysis in the British Women's Heart and Health Study (BWHHS). *Disease Markers, 24*(1), 11–17.

Aquilante, C. L., Yarandi, H. N., Cavallari, L. H., Andrisin, T. E., Terra, S. G., Lewis, J. F., Hamilton, K. K., et al. (2008). $\beta$-Adrenergic receptor gene polymorphisms and hemodynamic response to dobutamine during dobutamine stress echocardiography. *The Pharmacogenomics Journal, 8*(6), 408–415.

Arnett, D. K., Claas, S. A., & Glasser, S. P. (2006). Pharmacogenetics of antihypertensive treatment. Vascular Pharmacology, 44(2), 107-118. doi: 10.1016/j.vph.2005.09.010

Atlas, S. A. (2007). The renin-angiotensin aldosterone system: pathophysiological role and pharmacologic inhibition. *Journal of managed care pharmacy, 13*(8), 9.

Beitelshees, A. L., Gong, Yan, Wang, D., Schork, N. J., Cooper-Dehoff, R. M., Langaee, Taimour Y, Shriver, M. D., et al. (2007). KCNMB1 genotype influences response to verapamil SR and adverse outcomes in the INternational VErapamil SR/Trandolapril STudy (INVEST). *Pharmacogenetics and Genomics, 17*(9), 719-729. doi: 10.1097/FPC.0b013e32810f2e3c

Bozec, E., Fassot, C., Tropeano, A. I., Boutouyrie, P., Jeunemaitre, X., Lacolley, P., Dabire, H., et al. (2003). Angiotensinogen gene M235T polymorphism and reduction in wall thickness in response to antihypertensive treatment. *Clinical Science, 105*(5), 637.

Brugts, J. J., Boersma, E., & Simoons, M. L. (2010). Tailored therapy of ACE inhibitors in stable coronary artery disease: pharmacogenetic profiling of treatment benefit. *Pharmacogenomics, 11*(8), 1115-1126. doi: 10.2217/pgs.10.103

Brugts, J. J., Isaacs, A., Boersma, E., Van Duijn, C. M., Uitterlinden, A. G., Remme, W., Bertrand, M., et al. (2010). Genetic determinants of treatment benefit of the angiotensin-converting enzyme-inhibitor perindopril in patients with stable coronary artery disease. *European heart journal, 31*(15), 1854.

Brunner, M., Cooper-DeHoff, R. M, Gong, Y., Karnes, J. H., Langaee, T. Y, Pepine, C. J, & Johnson, J. A. (2007). Factors influencing blood pressure response to trandolapril add-on therapy in patients taking verapamil SR (from the International Verapamil SR/Trandolapril [INVEST] Study). *The American journal of cardiology, 99*(11), 1549–1554.

Brunner, M., Cooper-DeHoff, R. M., Gong, Y., Karnes, J. H., Langaee, T. Y., Pepine, C. J., & Johnson, J. A. (2007). Factors influencing blood pressure response to trandolapril add-on therapy in patients taking verapamil SR (from the International Verapamil SR/Trandolapril [INVEST] Study). *The American journal of cardiology, 99*(11), 1549–1554.

Carretero OA, O. S., & Carretero OA, Oparil S. (2000). Essential hypertension. Part I: definition and etiology. *[[Circulation (journal) | Circulation]], 101*(3), 329–35.

Cattaruzza, M., Guzik, T. J., Słodowski, W., Pelvan, A., Becker, J., Halle, M., Buchwald, A. B., et al. (2004). Shear stress insensitivity of endothelial nitric oxide synthase expression as a genetic risk factor for coronary heart disease. *Circulation Research, 95*(8), 841-847. doi: 10.1161/01.RES.0000145359.47708.2f

Centre for Genetics Education. (2007). PHARMACOGENETICS/PHARMACOGENOMICS. Resource, . Retrieved April 14, 2011, from http://www.genetics.edu.au/factsheet/fs25?searchterm=pharmacogenetics

Chung, C. M., Wang, R. Y., Chen, J. W., Fann, C. S. J., Leu, H. B., Ho, H. Y., Ting, C. T., et al. (2010). A genome-wide association study identifies new loci for ACE activity: potential implications for response to ACE inhibitor. *The Pharmacogenomics Journal, 10*(6), 537–544.

Chung, C.-M., Wang, R.-Y., Chen, J.-W., Fann, C. S. J., Leu, H.-B., Ho, H.-Y., Ting, C.-T., et al. (2010). A genome-wide association study identifies new loci for ACE activity: potential implications for response to ACE inhibitor. *The Pharmacogenomics Journal, 10*(6), 537-544. doi: 10.1038/tpj.2009.70

Cody, R. J. (1997). The integrated effects of angiotensin II. The American Journal of Cardiology, 79(5A), 9-11.

Cowley, A. W. (2006). The genetic dissection of essential hypertension. *Nature Reviews Genetics, 7*(11), 829–840.

Cushman, W. C., Ford, C. E., Cutler, J. A., Margolis, K. L., Davis, B. R., Grimm, R. H., Black, H. R., et al. (2002). ALLHAT Collaborative Research Group. Success and predictors of blood pressure control in diverse North American settings: the antihypertensive and lipid-lowering treatment to prevent heart attack trial (ALLHAT). *J Clin Hypertens, 4*(6), 393–404.

de Denus, S., Zakrzewski-Jakubiak, M., Dubé, M.-P., Bélanger, F., Lepage, S., Leblanc, M.-H., Gossard, D., et al. (2008). Effects of AGTR1 A1166C gene polymorphism in patients with heart failure treated with candesartan. *The Annals of Pharmacotherapy, 42*(7), 925-932. doi: 10.1345/aph.1K657

Dominiczak, A. F., & Munroe, P. B. (2010). Genome-Wide Association Studies Will Unlock the Genetic Basis of Hypertension: Pro Side of the Argument. *Hypertension, 56*(6), 1017-1020. doi: 10.1161/HYPERTENSIONAHA.110.156208

Erdos, E. G., Tan, F., & Skidgel, R. A. (2010). Angiotensin I-converting enzyme inhibitors are allosteric enhancers of kinin B1 and B2 receptor function. *Hypertension, 55*(2), 214.

Ezzati, M., Lopez, A. D., Rodgers, A., Vander Hoorn, S., & Murray, C. J. L. (2002). Selected major risk factors and global and regional burden of disease. *The Lancet, 360*(9343), 1347–1360.

Fan, X., Wang, Y., Sun, K., Zhang, W., Yang, X., Wang, S., Zhen, Y., et al. (2007). Polymorphisms of ACE2 gene are associated with essential hypertension and antihypertensive effects of Captopril in women. *Clinical Pharmacology & Therapeutics, 82*(2), 187–196.

Fernández-Fernández, J. M., Tomás, M., Vázquez, E., Orio, P., Latorre, R., Sentí, M., Marrugat, J., et al. (2004). Gain-of-function mutation in the KCNMB1 potassium channel subunit is associated with low prevalence of diastolic hypertension. *The Journal of Clinical Investigation, 113*(7), 1032-1039. doi: 10.1172/JCI20347

Filigheddu, F., Argiolas, G., Bulla, E., Troffa, C., Bulla, P., Fadda, S., Zaninello, R., et al. (2008). Clinical variables, not RAAS polymorphisms, predict blood pressure response to ACE inhibitors in Sardinians. Pharmacogenomics, 9(10), 1419–1427.

Filigheddu, F., Argiolas, G., Degortes, S., Zaninello, R., Frau, F., Pitzoi, S., Bulla, E., et al. (2010). Haplotypes of the adrenergic system predict the blood pressure response to beta-blockers in women with essential hypertension. Pharmacogenomics, 11(3), 319-325. doi: 10.2217/pgs.09.158

Frazer, K. A., Ballinger, D. G., Cox, D. R., Hinds, D. A., Stuve, L. L., Gibbs, R. A., Belmont, J. W., et al. (2007). A second generation human haplotype map of over 3.1 million SNPs. *Nature, 449*(7164), 851–861.

Gerhard, T., Gong, Y., Beitelshees, A. L., Mao, X., Lobmeyer, M. T., Cooper-DeHoff, R. M., Langaee, T. Y., et al. (2008). Alpha-adducin polymorphism associated with increased risk of adverse cardiovascular outcomes: results from Genetic Substudy of the INternational Verapamil SR-trandolapril STudy (INVEST-GENES). *American Heart Journal, 156*(2), 397-404. doi: 10.1016/j.ahj.2008.03.007

Group, P. C. (2001). Randomized trial of a perindopril-based blood-pressure-lowering regimen among 6105 individuals with previous stroke or transient ischaemic attack. *Lancet, 358*, 1033–1041.

Gu, C. C., Hunt, S. C., Kardia, S., Turner, S. T, Chakravarti, A., Schork, N., Olshen, R., et al. (2007). An investigation of genome-wide associations of hypertension with microsatellite markers in the family blood pressure program (FBPP). *Human genetics, 121*(5), 577–590.

Hall, J. E.; G., & Hall, John E.; Guyton, Arthur C. (2006). *Textbook of medical physiology*. St. Louis, Mo: Elsevier Saunders.

Hallberg, P., Karlsson, J., Kurland, L., Lind, L., Kahan, T., Malmqvist, K., Ohman, K. P., et al. (2002). The CYP2C9 genotype predicts the blood pressure response to irbesartan: results from the Swedish Irbesartan Left Ventricular Hypertrophy Investigation vs Atenolol (SILVHIA) trial. *Journal of Hypertension, 20*(10), 2089-2093.

Han, Y.-F., Fan, X.-H., Wang, X.-J., Sun, K., Xue, H., Li, W.-J., Wang, Y.-B., et al. (2011). Association of intergenic polymorphism of organic anion transporter 1 and 3 genes with hypertension and blood pressure response to hydrochlorothiazide. *American Journal of Hypertension, 24*(3), 340-346. doi: 10.1038/ajh.2010.191

Hingorani, A. D., Stevens, P. A., Brown, M. J., Jia, H., Hopper, R., & Claire Dickerson, J. E. (1995). Renin-angiotensin system gene polymorphisms influence blood pressure and the response to angiotensin converting enzyme inhibition. *Journal of hypertension, 13*(12), 1602.

Huang, C.-C., Chung, Chia-Min, Hung, S.-I., Leu, Hsin-Bang, Wu, T.-C., Huang, P.-H., Lin, Shing-Jong, et al. (2011). Genetic variation in renin predicts the effects of thiazide diuretics. *European Journal of Clinical Investigation, 41*(8), 828-835. doi:10.1111/j.1365-2362.2011.02472.x

Iwai, C., Akita, H., Kanazawa, K., Shiga, N., Terashima, M., Matsuda, Y., Takai, E., et al. (2003). Arg389Gly polymorphism of the human beta1-adrenergic receptor in patients with nonfatal acute myocardial infarction. *American Heart Journal, 146*(1), 106-109. doi: 10.1016/S0002-8703 (03) 00110-8

Julie A Johnson. (2010, March 29). Pharmacogenomics of antihypertensive drugs: past, present and future. Retrieved August 31, 2010, from http://www.futuremedicine.com/doi/abs/10.2217/pgs.10.34

Jun, P., Ko, N. U., English, J. D., Dowd, C. F., Halbach, V. V., Higashida, R. T., Lawton, M. T., et al. (2010). Endovascular Treatment of Medically Refractory Cerebral Vasospasm Following Aneurysmal Subarachnoid Hemorrhage. *AJNR Am J Neuroradiol, 31*(10), 1911-1916. doi:<p>10.3174/ajnr.A2183</p>

Kearney, P. M., Whelton, M., Reynolds, K., Muntner, P., Whelton, P. K., & He, J. (2005). Global burden of hypertension: analysis of worldwide data. *The Lancet, 365*(9455), 217–223.

Konoshita, T. (2011). Do Genetic Variants of the Renin-Angiotensin System Predict Blood Pressure Response to Renin-Angiotensin System-Blocking Drugs? A Systematic Review of Pharmacogenomics in the Renin-Angiotensin System. *Current Hypertension Reports*. doi:10.1007/s11906-011-0212-0

Kurland, L., Hallberg, P., Melhus, H., Liljedahl, U., Hashemi, N., Syvänen, A.-C., Lind, L., et al. (2008). The relationship between the plasma concentration of irbesartan and the antihypertensive response is disclosed by an angiotensin II type 1 receptor polymorphism: results from the Swedish Irbesartan Left Ventricular Hypertrophy

Investigation vs. Atenolol (SILVHIA) Trial. *American Journal of Hypertension, 21*(7), 836-839. doi: 10.1038/ajh.2008.190

Lander, E. S., Linton, L. M., Birren, B., Nusbaum, C., Zody, M. C., Baldwin, J., Devon, K., et al. (2001). Initial sequencing and analysis of the human genome. *Nature, 409*(6822), 860–921.

Leeson, C. P. M., Hingorani, A. D., Mullen, M. J., Jeerooburkhan, N., Kattenhorn, M., Cole, T. J., Muller, D. P. R., et al. (2002). Glu298Asp endothelial nitric oxide synthase gene polymorphism interacts with environmental and dietary factors to influence endothelial function. *Circulation Research, 90*(11), 1153-1158.

Lewington, S., Clarke, R., Qizilbash, N., Peto, R., & Collins, R. (2002). Age-specific relevance of usual blood pressure to vascular mortality: a meta-analysis of individual data for one million adults in 61 prospective studies. *Lancet, 360*(9349), 1903.

Liggett, S. B., Cresci, S., Kelly, R. J., Syed, F. M., Matkovich, S. J., Hahn, H. S., Diwan, A., et al. (2008). A GRK5 polymorphism that inhibits [beta]-adrenergic receptor signaling is protective in heart failure. Nat Med, 14(5), 510-517. Doi: 10.1038/nm1750

Lindholm, L. H., Carlberg, B., & Samuelsson, O. (2005). Should [beta] blockers remain first choice in the treatment of primary hypertension? A meta-analysis. *The Lancet, 366*(9496), 1545–1553.

Liu, J., Liu, Z. Q., Yu, B. N., Xu, F. H., Mo, W., Zhou, G., Liu, Y. Z., et al. (2006). β1-Adrenergic receptor polymorphisms influence the response to metoprolol monotherapy in patients with essential hypertension&ast. *Clinical Pharmacology & Therapeutics, 80*(1), 23–32.

Liu, J., Liu, Z.-Q., Tan, Z.-R., Chen, X.-P., Wang, L.-S., Zhou, G., & Zhou, H.-H. (2003). Gly389Arg polymorphism of beta1-adrenergic receptor is associated with the cardiovascular response to metoprolol. *Clinical Pharmacology and Therapeutics, 74*(4), 372-379. doi: 10.1016/S0009-9236 (03) 00224-8

Luft, F. C. (2001). Twins in cardiovascular genetic research. *Hypertension, 37*(2 Part 2), 350-356.

Luo, F., Wang, Y., Wang, X., Sun, K., Zhou, X., & Hui, R. (2009). A functional variant of NEDD4L is associated with hypertension, antihypertensive response, and orthostatic hypotension. *Hypertension, 54*(4), 796-801. doi: 10.1161/HYPERTENSIONAHA.109.135103

Lynch, A. I., Boerwinkle, E., Davis, B. R., Ford, C. E., Eckfeldt, J. H., Leiendecker-Foster, C., & Arnett, D. K. (2008). Pharmacogenetic association of the NPPA T2238C genetic variant with cardiovascular disease outcomes in patients with hypertension. *JAMA: the journal of the American Medical Association, 299*(3), 296.

Manunta, P., Cusi, D., Barlassina, C., Righetti, M., Lanzani, C., D/'Amico, M., Buzzi, L., et al. (1998). α-Adducin polymorphisms and renal sodium handling in essential hypertensive patients. *Kidney Int, 53*(6), 1471-1478.

Materson, B. J., Reda, D. J., Cushman, W. C., Massie, B. M., Freis, E. D., Kochar, M. S., Hamburger, R. J., et al. (1993). Single-drug therapy for hypertension in men–a comparison of six antihypertensive agents with placebo. *New England Journal of Medicine, 328*(13), 914–921.

Mellen, P. B., & Herrington, D. M. (2005). Pharmacogenomics of blood pressure response to antihypertensive treatment. *Journal of hypertension, 23*(7), 1311.

Nakayama, M., Yasue, H., Yoshimura, M., Shimasaki, Y., Kugiyama, K., Ogawa, H., Motoyama, T., et al. (1999). T-786-->C mutation in the 5′-flanking region of the endothelial nitric oxide synthase gene is associated with coronary spasm. *Circulation, 99*(22), 2864-2870.

Nguyen, B. N., Parker, R. B., Noujedehi, M., Sullivan, J. M., & Johnson, J A. (2000). Effects of COER-verapamil on circadian pattern of forearm vascular resistance and blood pressure. *Journal of Clinical Pharmacology, 40*(12 Pt 2), 1480-1487.

Nordestgaard, B. G., Kontula, K., Benn, M., Dahlöf, B., de Faire, U., Edelman, J. M., Eliasson, E., et al. (2010). Effect of ACE insertion/deletion and 12 other polymorphisms on clinical outcomes and response to treatment in the LIFE study. *Pharmacogenetics and Genomics, 20*(2), 77-85. doi: 10.1097/FPC.0b013e328333f70b

Nozaki, Y., Kusuhara, H., Kondo, T., Hasegawa, M., Shiroyanagi, Y., Nakazawa, H., Okano, T., et al. (2007). Characterization of the uptake of organic anion transporter (OAT) 1 and OAT3 substrates by human kidney slices. *The Journal of Pharmacology and Experimental Therapeutics, 321*(1), 362-369. doi: 10.1124/jpet.106.113076

Oparil S, Z. M., & Oparil S, Zaman MA, Calhoun DA. (2003). Pathogenesis of hypertension. *[[Ann. Intern. Med.]], 139*(9), 761–76.

Pacanowski, M. A., Zineh, I., Cooper-DeHoff, Rhonda M., Pepine, Carl J., & Johnson, Julie A. (2009). Genetic and Pharmacogenetic Associations Between NOS3 Polymorphisms, Blood Pressure, and Cardiovascular Events in Hypertension. *American journal of hypertension, 22*(7), 748-753. doi: 10.1038/ajh.2009.81

Pacanowski, M., Gong, Y, Cooper-DeHoff, R., Schork, N., Shriver, M., Langaee, T., Pepine, C., et al. (2008). β-Adrenergic Receptor Gene Polymorphisms and β-Blocker Treatment Outcomes in Hypertension. *Clinical pharmacology and therapeutics, 84*(6), 715-721. doi: 10.1038/clpt.2008.139

Padmanabhan, S., Melander, O., Johnson, T., Di Blasio, A. M., Lee, W. K., Gentilini, D., Hastie, C. E., et al. (2010). Genome-Wide Association Study of Blood Pressure Extremes Identifies Variant near UMOD Associated with Hypertension, *6*(10). doi: 10.1371/journal.pgen.1001177

Padmanabhan, S., Paul, L., & Dominczak, A. F. (2010). The Pharmacogenomics of Anti-Hypertensive Therapy. *Pharmaceuticals, 3*(6), 1779-1791. doi: 10.3390/ph3061779

Persu, A., Stoenoiu, M. S., Messiaen, T., Davila, S., Robino, C., El-Khattabi, O., Mourad, M., et al. (2002). Modifier effect of ENOS in autosomal dominant polycystic kidney disease. *Human Molecular Genetics, 11*(3), 229-241.

Plüger, S., Faulhaber, J., Fürstenau, M., Löhn, M., Waldschütz, R., Gollasch, M., Haller, H., et al. (2000). Mice with disrupted BK channel beta1 subunit gene feature abnormal Ca(2+) spark/STOC coupling and elevated blood pressure. *Circulation Research, 87*(11), E53-60.

Redon, J., Luque-Otero, M., Martell, N., & Chaves, F. J. (2004). Renin-angiotensin system gene polymorphisms: relationship with blood pressure and microalbuminuria in telmisartan-treated hypertensive patients. *Pharmacogenomics J, 5*(1), 14-20.

Reiter, M. J. (2004). Cardiovascular drug class specificity:[beta]-blockers. *Progress in cardiovascular diseases, 47*(1), 11–33.

Savvidou, M. D., Vallance, P. J., Nicolaides, K. H., & Hingorani, A. D. (2001). Endothelial nitric oxide synthase gene polymorphism and maternal vascular adaptation to pregnancy. *Hypertension, 38*(6), 1289-1293.

Schelleman, H., Klungel, O. H., Witteman, J. C. M., Breteler, M. M. B., Yazdanpanah, M., Danser, A. H. J., Hofman, A., et al. (2007). Angiotensinogen M235T polymorphism and the risk of myocardial infarction and stroke among hypertensive patients on

ACE-inhibitors or $\beta$-blockers. *European Journal of Human Genetics, 15*(4), 478–484.

Sciarrone, M. T., Stella, P., Barlassina, C., Manunta, P., Lanzani, C., Bianchi, G., & Cusi, D. (2003). ACE and alpha-adducin polymorphism as markers of individual response to diuretic therapy. *Hypertension, 41*(3), 398-403. doi: 10.1161/01.HYP.0000057010.27011.2C

Sehrt, D., Meineke, I., Tzvetkov, M., Gültepe, S., & Brockmöller, J. (2011). Carvedilol pharmacokinetics and pharmacodynamics in relation to CYP2D6 and ADRB pharmacogenetics. *Pharmacogenomics, 12*(6), 783-795. doi: 10.2217/pgs.11.20

Shin, J., & Johnson, Julie A. (2007). Pharmacogenetics of β-Blockers. *Pharmacotherapy, 27*(6), 874-887. doi: 10.1592/phco.27.6.874

Su, X., Lee, L., Li, X., Lv, J., Hu, Y., Zhan, S., Cao, W., et al. (2007). Association between angiotensinogen, angiotensin II receptor genes, and blood pressure response to an angiotensin-converting enzyme inhibitor. *Circulation, 115*(6), 725-732. doi: 10.1161/CIRCULATIONAHA.106.642058

Svensson-Färbom, P., Wahlstrand, B., Almgren, P., Dahlberg, J., Fava, C., Kjeldsen, S., Hedner, T., et al. (2011). A functional variant of the NEDD4L gene is associated with beneficial treatment response with β-blockers and diuretics in hypertensive patients. *Journal of Hypertension, 29*(2), 388-395. doi: 10.1097/HJH.0b013e3283410390

Tesauro, M., Thompson, W. C., Rogliani, P., Qi, L., Chaudhary, P. P., & Moss, J. (2000). Intracellular processing of endothelial nitric oxide synthase isoforms associated with differences in severity of cardiopulmonary diseases: cleavage of proteins with aspartate vs. glutamate at position 298. *Proceedings of the National Academy of Sciences of the United States of America, 97*(6), 2832-2835.

Thoenes, M., Neuberger, H. R., Volpe, M., Khan, B. V., Kirch, W., & B\öhm, M. (2009). Antihypertensive drug therapy and blood pressure control in men and women: an international perspective. *Journal of human hypertension, 24*(5), 336–344.

Turner, S. T, Schwartz, G. L, Chapman, A. B, & Boerwinkle, E. (2001). C825T Polymorphism of the G Protein ${$beta$}$ 3-Subunit and Antihypertensive Response to a Thiazide Diuretic. Hypertension, 37(2), 739.

Turner, S. T., Bailey, K. R., Fridley, B. L., Chapman, A. B., Schwartz, G. L., Chai, H. S., Sicotte, H., et al. (2008). Genomic Association Analysis Suggests Chromosome 12 Locus Influencing Antihypertensive Response to Thiazide Diuretic. *Hypertension, 52*(2), 359-365. doi: 10.1161/HYPERTENSIONAHA.107.104273

Werner, D., Werner, U., Meybaum, A., Schmidt, B., Umbreen, S., Grosch, A., Lestin, H. G., et al. (2008). Determinants of steady-state torasemide pharmacokinetics: impact of pharmacogenetic factors, gender and angiotensin II receptor blockers. *Clinical pharmacokinetics, 47*(5), 323–332.

Yu, H., Lin, S., Jin, L., Yu, Y., Zhong, J., Zhang, Y., & Liu, G. (2009). Adenine/cytosine1166 polymorphism of the angiotensin II type 1 receptor gene and the antihypertensive response to angiotensin-converting enzyme inhibitors. *Journal of hypertension, 27*(11), 2278.

# 11

# Differential Gene Expression Profile in Essential Hypertension

Ping Yang
*Department of Internal Medicine and Cardiology, China-Japan Union Hospital, Norman Bethune College of Medicine, Jilin University, Changchun, China*

## 1. Introduction

Essential hypertension affects 20-30% of the population worldwide and contributes significantly to mortality and morbidity[1] from cerebrovascular diseases, myocardial infarction, congestive heart failure and renal insufficiency. Essential hypertension is a prevalent disorder that leads to significant morbidity and mortality. Essential hypertension is defined as chronically elevated arterial pressure resulting from an unknown etiology. Intrinsically, it is a complex, heterogeneous, multifactorial syndrome to which environmental factors are partly responsible for. A lineup of aberrant environmental factors, including dietary salt intake[2,3,4], body weight[5,6], physical inactivity[7.8], physical stress[9.10], cigarette smoking [11-14], alcohol consumption[15-18] and inadequate potassium consumption[19,20] contribute to essential hypertension, possibly by infuriating genetically programmed susceptibilities. Results from twins, adoptive and population studies suggest high degree of similarity of blood pressure values, thus indicating the importance of genetic variables in essential hypertension etiology[21-25]. It is assumed that blood pressure is under the control of a large number of genes each of which has only relatively mild effects.

Despite progress in genomic and statistical tools, identification of genes involved in complex cardiovascular traits such as hypertension remains a major challenge. Several strategies have been developed so far. Of these approaches developed, gene expression techniques hold vast promises as functional roles of gene products are determined among diverse biological processes[26]. Gene expression profiling has become an overshadowing tool for discovery in medicine. Genes have additive function of working together; therefore expression levels of these groups of gene can be monitored through gene expression studies.

At present, differential gene expression between two sets of biological samples is carried out by utilizing techniques such as Northern blot analysis, serial analysis of gene expression (SAGE), differential display reverse transcription-PCR (DDRT-PCR) and Dot Blot analysis [26,27]. The drawback of these techniques is that large numbers of genes cannot be analyzed simultaneously. What's more, with Northern blot limited number of mRNAs may be examined simultaneously and quality and quantification of expression are negatively affected[28]. Although the strengths of SAGE are remarkable, extensive DNA sequencing is technically difficult and formidable. With DDRT-PCR, simultaneous discovery of multiple differences in gene expression is possible; however, screening is not based on identity but in mRNA length[29]. Dot blot analysis is less time consuming, however, no information on the size of the target biomolecules is offered.

DNA microarray technology has the potential to overcome these limitations, as it has allowed unprecedented analysis of thousands of genes in a high-throughput form. On account of its high-throughput expression profiling, DNA microarray technology has become the predominant assay of choice in clinical medicine. This review, to a great extent looks at studies that used gene expression microarray technology in hypertension research to provide information on the disease specific risk profiles and pathology.

## 2. Methods

A literature search of the PUBMED database, using the medical headings "hypertension," "blood pressure," "gene expression," and" microarray analysis," will be conducted. The search will include published studies in human beings and as well as experimental models. Additionally, a search will be performed using references cited in original study articles and reviews and if copies of articles cannot be accessed, authors will be contacted.

### 2.1 Methods for the study of gene expression

Methods used to profile gene expression include Northern blot analysis, serial analysis of gene expression, differential display, dot blot analysis, subtractive hybridization and microarray hybridization.

### 2.2 Northern blot analysis

Although more sensitive gene expression techniques have emerged over the last decade, Northern blot analysis remains the standard for detection and quantitation of mRNA. Northern blotting has proven very effective in evaluating the expression levels of troponin c in chicken skeleton and cardiac muscles[30], arterial natriuretic factor mRNA and peptide in the human heart during development [31], myosin heavy chain and actin[32]. It is remarkable in that it allows a direct relative comparison of message abundance between samples on a single blot. Regrettably, this technique requires large quantities of RNA and is prone to significant experimental manipulation for each of the genes examined. Taniguchi et al compared Northern blotting analyses with DNA microarrays and discovered Northern blotting to be more sensitive and consistent than DNA microarrays[33]. Despite the fact large-scale transcriptome analysis experiments are not performable with Northern blotting, it is however, conveniently used in studies focused on analysis of small numbers of genes.

### 2.3 Serial analysis of gene expression (SAGE)

Serial analysis of gene expression method was recently discovered at John Hopkins University with the intention to create a global picture of cellular function. SAGE enables tagged short sequences of reverse transcribed cDNA to be prepared and identified by DNA sequencing[34]. The SAGE technique can be used to obtain large-scale cardiac gene expression[35,36]. Even supposing the quantitative and cumulative data this technique presents, one limitation is the identification of the genes reported by the SAGE.

### 2.4 Differential Display (DD)

Differential display was first introduced by Liang and Pardee in 1992[37]. This technique involves the identification and analysis of differentially expressed genes at the mRNA level. The basic principle of differential display is to use short primers in combination with oligo-dT primers to amplify and visualize mRNA in a cell. DD has been a powerful and successful method due to its inherent simplicity to detect changes in mRNA profiles among multiple samples without any prior knowledge of genomic information of the organism studied.

### 2.5 Dot blot analysis

Dot blot is an immunological technique and is a simplification of northern blotting, southern blotting, or western blotting methods[38,39]. This method identifies a known protein in a biological sample. Dot blot differs from western blotting in that protein samples are separated electrophoretically but are spotted through circular templates directly onto the membrane or paper substrate. The characteristic of dot blot is the use of immunodetection to identify a specific protein.

### 2.6 Subtractive hybridization

Subtractive hybridization is a powerful technique that was first described by Sargent and Dawid for creating cDNA libraries and generating probes of genes expressed differentially [40]. This technique is based on the principle that nucleic acid sequences in common with the two populations can form hybrids. It is the first tool used for identifying differentially expressed genes on a global scale. With Subtractive hybridization, the isolation of genes does not require prior knowledge of their sequence or identity.

### 2.7 Microarray hybridization

Microarray analysis, is a high through-put technique that provides an important tool to study the global patterns of gene expression. Two of the most commonly used microarrays for gene-expression measurements are oligonucleotide GeneChip expression arrays by Affymetrix and cDNA microarrays. Oligonucleotide microarrays contain sets of multiple 25 mer oligonucleotide probes specific for each gene or expressed-sequence tag (EST), whereas cDNA microarrays generally contain longer oligonucleotide probes (usually 25 to 60 bases) or cDNA probes (usually 500 to 1,000 bases) that stand for the specific gene, so cDNA microarrays are more commonly used. It permits quantitative analysis of RNAs transcribed from both known and unknown genes. Microarray analysis is based on the principle of complementary, single-stranded, nucleic acid sequences forming double-stranded hybrids. This technology can simultaneously measure the expression levels of thousands of genes within a particular mRNA sample in a high-through put manner[42,43].

### 2.8 Research objects

For the DNA microarrays, we could study human or animal models. The spontaneously hypertensive rats (SHR) are the most popular used animal models for essential hypertension, and the Lyon hypertensive rats[44] follows behind, compared to normotensive Wistar Kyoto rats (WKY).

### 2.9 Samples

We mainly use peripheral blood samples[45] in human and vascular smooth muscle cell (VSMC) [46,47], adrenal[44], heart[2,48,49] and kidney[2,44,53-56,58] in animal models.

### 2.10 Software tools

The large amount of information generated from microarrays has been a great strength, but is sometimes seen as a frustrating weakness because of the inability to process experimental data easily, assess the data quality, manage multiple data sets and mine the data with user-friendly tools. Most of the microarrays have the suite of software to deal with the results, such as the Affymetrix software for the Affymetrix microarrays. The related software is listed as follows. The software was not designed to do complex statistical analyses and visualization. Rather, it was designed to help the researcher narrow their search from tens of thousands of gene candidates to several hundred or fewer that meet specific, but adjustable criteria.

### 2.11 Altered gene expression in blood

Peripheral blood gene expression has the potential to provide information on underlying pathologic states. Several authors have used whole blood as a surrogate tissue for gene expression in patients with essential hypertension. In their study, Korkor et al identified 49 differentially expressed genes; 31 up regulated and 18 down regulated genes. Amongst genes found to be altered include CD36, SLC4A1, NET1, SESN3, ZNF652, PRDX6, HIP1, FOLR3, ERAP1, CFD[45]. Most of the genes that were differentially expressed were related to immune/inflammatory responses. In a study conducted by Chon et al, gene expression patterns of hypertensives revealed 680 genes that were upregulated as compared to patients who were normotensive on medication [52]. Timofeeva AV et al reported that 22 genes were up-regulated and 18 genes down-regulation in atherosclerotic aorta compared with normal vessel through cDNA microarray, among these, CD53, SPI1, FPRL2, SPP1, CTSD, ACP5, LCP1, CTSA and LIPA genes are up-regulated both in peripheral blood leukocytes from EH patients and in atherosclerotic lesions of human aorta. The majority of these genes significantly positively correlated with hypertension stage as well as with histological grading of atherosclerotic lesions[53].

### 2.12 Altered gene expression in the tissues and organs

Koo et al reported altered gene expression in the kidneys of adults of spontaneously hypertension rats[54]. Analyzing mRNA from 8-week-old female SHR and age-matched female WKY, 43 up-regulated and 31 down-regulated genes were revealed. The upregulation of stearoyl-COA desaturase-2 gene and downregulation of taurine/beta-alanine transporter gene in SHR compared with WKY rat were reported and in the SHR group, dysregulations of several genes involved in lipid metabolism was also revealed. Seubert et al investigated renal gene expression profiles in SHR and WKY animals at prehypertensiive (3 wk of age) and hypertensive (9 wk of age) stages and identified 22 genes at 3 wk of age and 104 genes at 9 wk of age that were differentially expressed in SHR compared with WKY[55]. There are some other studies identified differential gene expression in animal models of essential hypertension that are listed in table 2.

| Results | References |
|---|---|
| 49 genes were found differentially expressed in essential hypertension, 31 up regulated and 18 down regulated. | Korkor et al. (45) |
| 680 genes were found differentially expressed in untreated hypertensives compared to normotensive controls. On the other hand, only 7 genes were differentially expressed in treated hypertensives compared to normotensive controls. | Chen et al. (52) |
| 22 genes were up-regulated and 18 genes demonstrated down-regulation in atherosclerotic aorta compared with normal vessel, CD53, SPI1, FPRL2, SPP1, CTSD, ACP5, LCP1, CTSA and LIPA genes are up-regulated in peripheral blood leukocytes from EH patients and in atherosclerotic lesions of human aorta. The majority of these genes significantly ($p<0.005$) positively ($r>0.5$) correlated with AH stage as well as with histological grading of atherosclerotic lesions. | Timofeeva AV et al (53) |

Table 1. Differential gene expression profiling in human blood in essential hypertension.

| **Animal model and the control group** | **Tissue** | **Microarray platform** | **Software** | **Observations** | **References** |
|---|---|---|---|---|---|
| SDR, SHR and WKY | Area postrema | Rat Genechip 230 2.0 microarrys | GeneSpring GX11 | 'hypertension-related' elements revealed genes that are involved in the regulation of both blood pressure and immune function | Hindmarch CC et al. (46) |
| eET-1 and wild-type (WT) mice | mesenteric arteries | Ilumina microarray, validation by qPCR of 4 genes | Flexarray software for the microarray results, and Ingenuity Pathway Analysis for the gene lists. | increased endothelial ET-1 expression results in early changes in gene expression in the vascular wall that enhance lipid biosynthesis and accelerate progression of atherosclerosis. | Simeone SM et al. (47) |
| SHR and BNR for the control | Kidney | Affymetrix U34A-C microarrays, validation by RT-PCR, DNA sequencing and RFLP analyses. | Solexa Tag analysis | 88 transcripts are identified to be differentially expressed between SHRs and BN rats. | Johnson MD et al. (2) |

| Animal model and the control group | Tissue | Microarray platform | Software | Observations | References |
|---|---|---|---|---|---|
| normal (normotensive) Wistar rats, DOCA-salt hypertensive (DH) rats, DH rats treated with AG1478, and DH rats treated with FPTIII | kidney | Codelink Uniset Rat 1Bioarrays | Affymetrix Scanner 428, Imagene and Genowiz softwares by Ocimum Biosolutions (India) and subjected to arsinh transformation | 2398 genes were upregulated and only 50 genes were downregulated by more than 2-fold in hypertensive rat kidneys compared to non-diseased controls. | Benter IF et al. (44) |
| SHR | aorta | GeneChip® Affymetrix Rat Genome Rat Genome 230 2.0 Array | GeneChip®Operating Software Version 1.4, Affymetrix analyzer. | Thirty-nine genes that showed more than a 2-fold increase in expression after administration of VPP and IPP, Fourteen genes that showed less than a 0.5-fold decrease in expression | Yamaguchi N et al. (48) |
| SHR and WKY | brain, heart, kidney and liver | UniSet Rat I Expression Bioarray, validation by RT-PCR of 9 genes | F-test and unpaired t test. CodeLink Expression Analysis Software, GenePix Pro 6.0 Software, GeneSpring software | 60 genes were differentially expressed in the heart of SHRSP rats. Of these, five genes were up-regulated and 55 genes were down-regulated. | Kato N et al. (51) |
| SHR, LHR, heterozygous TGR(mRen2)27 rat, and their respective controls | heart | Affymetrix GeneChip Rat Expression Array RAE230A, validation by qPCR of 6 genes. | Affymetrix Microarray Suite 5.0 software, significance analysis of microarrays (SAM) 1.21 software | Only four genes had significantly modified expression in the three hypertensive models among which a single gene, coding for sialyltransferase 7A, was consistently overexpressed | Cerutti C et al. (49) |
| WKY | Kidney and aorta. | Affymetrix rat genome 230A array, validation by RT-PCR | software R together with its bioinformatics packages collected in the Bioconductor project | Six functionally known genes (Igfbp1, Xdh, Sult1a1, Mawbp, Por, and Gstm1) and two expressed sequence tages (BI277460 and AI411345) were significantly upregulated | Westhoff TH et al. (56) |

| Animal model and the control group | Tissue | Microarray platform | Software | Observations | References |
|---|---|---|---|---|---|
| Female C57Bl/6J mice | Blood, heart and liver | Mouse NIH 15K cDNA microarrays | Expression Profiler tool EPCLUST | L-NNA and BSO both caused hypertension. Gene expression was regulated in cytoskeletal components in both models, protein synthesis in L-NNA-treated mice, and energy metabolism in BSO-treated mice. | Chon H et al. (41) |
| SHR and WKY | kidney | Affymetrix rat RG-U34A array | Normalisation and scaling using GeneChip suite. | 20 genes were down-regulated and 7 genes were up-regulated in SHR | Hinojos CA et al. (50) |
| SHR and WKY | heart | Affymetrix Rat Genome U34A GeneChips | Affymetrix software, GeneSpring software | Comparison of LV RNA profiles from 20- and 12-month-old SHR identified 61 known genes and 20 ESTs, whose expression was upregulated >1.5-fold, and 31 known genes and 15 ESTs, whose expression was downregulated >1.5-fold. | Rysä J et al. (57) |
| Sabra rat | kidney | Affymetrix Rat Genome RAE230 GeneChip, validation by RT-PCR of 7 genes. | Affymetrix software | 2470 transcripts were differentially expressed between the study groups. Cluster analysis identified genome-wide 192 genes that were relevant to salt-susceptibility and/or hypertension, 19 of which mapped to chromosome 1. | Yagil C et al. (58) |
| *Nppa*+/+ and *Nppa*−/- mice | Heart, Lung, kidney, brain, liver, and spleen | mouse microarray membranes (GeneFilter GF-400 membranes) | software package | Expression of 80 genes was elevated >2-fold and expression of 10 was reduced to <0.5 in 7-day TAC *Nppa*+/+ compared with control | Dajun Wang et al. (59) |

| Animal model and the control group | Tissue | Microarray platform | Software | Observations | References |
|---|---|---|---|---|---|
| SHR and WKY | Kidney, spleen, and liver | Affymetrix Rat U34 array set validation by qRT-PCR | Affymetrix MAS 5.0 | There was a significant reduction in expression of glutathione S-transferase mu-type 2, a gene involved in the defense against oxidative stress | Martin W. McBride et al. (60) |
| SHR | kidney | Affymetrix Rat Genome U34A arrays | Software packge | Of the 8,799 known genes and expressed sequence tag (EST) clusters of Affymetrix Rat Genome U34A arrays, 74 differentially expressed transcripts, of which 43 were up-regulated and 31 were down-regulated in SHR. | Koo et al. (54) |
| SHR and WKY | kidney | cDNA Rat version 2.0 Chip, validation by Northern blot and RT-PCR | ArraySuite version 2.0 | 22 genes at 3 weeks of age and 104 genes at 9 weeks of age were differentially expressed in SHR compared with WKY in renal gene expression. | Seubert et al. (55) |

SHR, spontaneously hypertensive rats. WKY, Wistar-Kyoto rats, usually used for the control the experimental group. WTR, wild-type rats. BNR, Brown Norway rats. LHR, Lyon hypertensive rats. SDR, Sprague-Dawley rats.

Table 2. Animals' microarray studies utilizing target organ tissue.

## 3. Summary and conclusions

Gene expression profiling provides a phenotypic resolution not feasible with standard clinical criteria. Differences in the gene expression profiles found in these studies identify markers useful for diagnostic, prognostic and therapeutic purposes. These findings emphasize the utility of whole blood and target organs as surrogate tissues for gene expression profiling. Gene expression profiling of different animal models of essential hypertension, and comparison of these profiles with human essential hypertension, will assist in determining the complex pathways that comprise the pathobiology of essential hypertension and help with the diagnostic, prognostic and therapeutic purposes in the future.

## 4. References

[1] Delles C, McBride MW, Graham D, Padmanabhan S, Dominiczak AF. Genetics of hypertension: from experimental animals to humans. Biochim Biophys Acta. 2010;1802(12):1299-308.

[2] Ashitate T, Osanai T, Tanaka M, Magota K, Echizen T, Izumiyama K, Yokoyama H, Shibutani S, Hanada K, Tomita H, Okumura K Overexpression of coupling factor 6 causes cardiac dysfunction under high-salt diet in mice. J Hypertens. 2010; 28(11):2243-51.
[3] Denton D. The Hunger for Salt: An Anthropological, Physiological and Medical Analysis. Berlin, Germany: Springer Verlag; 1982.
[4] Elliott P. The intersalt study: an addition to the evidence on salt and Blood pressure and some implications. J Hum Hypertens. 1989; 3: 289–298.
[5] Goodfriend TL, Ball DL, Egan BM, Campell WB, Nithipatikan K, Obesity; Sleep apnea, and aldosterone: theory and therapy. Hypertension. 2004; 43:518-524.
[6] Delva, P., Pastori, C, Provoli, E., Degan, M., Arosio, E., Montesi, G., Steele, A. & Lechi, A. Erythrocyte Na(-i-)-H-H exchange activity in essential hypertensive and obese patients: role of excess body weight. J Hypertens. 1993; 11, 823.
[7] Chintanadilok, J., Exercise in Treating Hypertension, PhysSports Med. 2002; 11-23.
[8] Urata, H., Antihypertensive and volume-depleting effects of mild exercise on essential hypertension. Hypertension. 1987; 9: 245-52.
[9] Sanders, B.J. & Lawler, J.E. The borderline hypertensive rat (BHR) as a model for environmentally- induced hypertension: a review and update. Neurosci Biobehav Rev. 1992;16, 207.
[10] Schnall, P.L., Pieper, C, Schwartz, J.E., Karasek, R.A., Schlussel, Y., Devereux, R.B., Ganau, A., Alderman, M., Warren, K. & Pickering, T.G. The relationship between 'job strain,' workplace diastolic blood pressure, and left ventricular mass index. Results of a case-control study [published erratum appears in JAMA 1992 Mar 4;267(9): 12091 [see comments]. Jama, 1990; 263, 1929.
[11] Tuomilehto J, Elo J, Nissmen A. Smoking among patients with malignant hypertension. BMJ. 1982; 1:1086.
[12] Beevers G et al. The pathophysiology of Hypertension. BMJ 2001; 322: 912-916.
[13] Keamey PM et al. Global burden of hypertension: analysis of worldwide data. Lancet 2005;365:217-223.
[14] Perry IJ, Whincup PH, Shaper AG. Environmental factors in the development of essential hypertension, Brisitsh medical Bulletin 1994; 50: 246-259.
[15] Beilin, L.J. Alcohol and hypertension. Clin Exp Pharmacol Physiol, 1995; 22, 185.
[16] Chen L, Smith GD, Harbord RM, Lewis SJ. Alcohol intake and Blood pressure: A systematic Review implementing a Mendelian Randomization Approach. PLOS Med 2008;s(3):e s2.
[17] Klatsky, A.L. Alcohol and hypertension. Clin Chim Acta, 1996; 246,91.
[18] Klatsky AL. Blood pressure and alcohol intake. In: Laragh JH, Brenner BM, eds. Hypertension: pathophysiology, diagnosis, and management. 2nd ed. New York: Raven Press, 1995:2649-67.
[19] Grobbee, D.E. Electrolytes and hypertension: results from recent studies. Am J Med Sci, 1994; 307 Suppl 1, S17.
[20] Krishna, G.G. Role of potassium in the pathogenesis of hypertension. Am J Med Sci, 1994; 301 Suppl 1,S2.
[21] Feinleib M, Garrison RJ, Fabsitz R, Christian JC, Hrubec Z, Borhani NO, et al. The NHLBI twin study of cardiovascular disease risk factors: methodologyand summary of results. Am J Epidemiol. 1977; 106:284-5.

[22] Trevisan, C, Saia, A., Schergna, E. & Mantero, F. The Prader-Willi syndrome: neuroendocrine study of identical twins. Ital J Neurol Sci, 1983; 4, 79.

[23] Longini IM Jr, Higgins MW, Hinton PC, Moll PP, Keller JB. Environmental and genetic sources of familial aggregation of blood pressure in Tecumseh, Michigan. Am J Epidemiol. 1984; 120:131-44.

[24] Carmelli, D., Robinette, D. & Fabsitz, R. Concordance, discordance and prevalence of hypertension in World War II male veteran twins. J Hypertens, 1994; 12,323.

[25] True, W.R., Romeis, J.C, Heath, A.C, Flick, L.H., Shaw, L., Eisen, S.A., Goldberg, J. & Lyons, M.J. Genetic and environmental contributions to healthcare need and utilization: a twin analysis. Health Serv. Res, 1997; 32, 37.

[26] Rishi AS, Nelson ND, Goyal A. DNA microarrays: gene expression profiling in plants. Reviews in Plant Biochemistry and Biotechnology 1:81-100.

[27] van Hal NLW, Vorst O, van Houwelingen AMML, Kok ET, Peijinenburg A, Aharoni A, van Tune AJ, Keijer J. The application of DNA microarrays in gene expression analysis. Journal of Biotechnology; 78:271-280.

[28] Streit S, Michalski CW, Erkan M, Kleff J, Fries H. Northern blot analysis for detection and quantification of RNA in Pancreatic cancer cells and tissues. Natrue protocols. 2009; 4(1): 37-43.

[29] Bertioli, D. J., U. H. Schlichter, M. J. Adams, P. R. Burrows, H. H. Steinbiss,and J. F. Antoniw. An analysis of differential display shows a strong bias towards high copy number mRNAs. Nucleic Acids Res. 1995; 23:4520–4523.

[30] Berezowsky C, Bag J, Developmentally regulated slow troponin C messenger RNA in chicken skeleton and cardiac muscles.Biochem cell Biol. 1988; 66:880-888.

[31] Mercadier JJ, Zongazo MA, Wisnewsky C, Butler-Brown G. Atrial natriuretic factor mRNA and peptide in the human heart during ontogenic development. Biochem Biophys Res. Comm.1989;159:777-782.

[32] Swynghedauw B, Moalic JM, Bouveret P, Bercovici J, de la Bastie D, Schwartz. mRNA content and complexity in animal and overloaded rat heart: a preliminary report. Eur Heart J.1984; 5suppl:211-217.

[33] Chen H, Yu SL, Chen WJ, Yang PC, Chien CT, Chou HY, Li HN, Peck K, Huang CH, Lin FY, Chen JJ, Lee YT. Dynamic changes of gene expression profiles during post-natal development of the heart in mice. Heart. 2004;90:927-934.

[34] Velculescu, V. E., Zhang, L., Vogelstein, B., and Kinzler, K. W. Serial Analysis Of Gene Expression. Science. 1995; 270:484-487.

[35] Ye SQ, Lavoie T, Usher DC, Zhang LQ. Microarray, SAGE and their application to cardiovascular disease. Cell Res. 2002;12:705-115.

[36] Anisimov SV, Boheller KR. Aging-associated changes in cardiac gene expression:large-scale transcriptome analysis. Adv. Gerontol.2003;11:67-75.

[37] Liang, P., Pardee, A.B., Differential display of eukaryotic messenger RNA by means of the polymerase chain reaction. Science1992; 257, 967–971.

[38] Spinola S, Cannon J. J Immunol Methods1985; 81:161-5.

[39] Craig PS, Rogan MT, Campos-Ponce M. Parasitology. 2003;127 Suppl: S5-20.

[40] Sargent TD, Dawid IB. Differential gene expression in the gastrula of xenopus laevis. Science. 1983;222:135-139.

[41] Chon et al. Broadly Altered Gene Expression in Blood Leukocytes in Essential Hypertension is Absent During Treatment. Hypertension 2004;43:947-951.

[42] Schena M, Shalon D, Davis RW, Brown PO. Quantitative monitoringof gene expression patterns with a complementary DNA microarray. Science 1995;270:467-70.
[43] Schena M. Microarray biochip technology. Sunnyvale, CA: EatonPublishing; 2000.
[44] Friese RS, Mahboubi P, Mahapatra NR, Mahata SK, Schork NJ, Schmid-Schonbein GW, O'Connor DT. Common genetic mechanisms of blood pressure elevation in two independent rodent models of human essential hypertension. Am J Hypertens. 2005;18:633-652.
[45] Korkor MT, Meng FB, Xing SY, Zhang MC, Guo JR, Zhu XX, Yang P. Microarray Analysis of Differential Gene expression profile in peripheral Blood Cells of Patients with Human Essential Hypertension. Int.J. Med Sci.2011;8(2):168-179.
[46] Simeone SM, Li MW, Paradis P, Schiffrin EL. Vascular gene expression in mice overexpressing human endothelin-1 targeted to the endothelium. Physiol Genomics. 2011; 11;43(3):148-60.
[47] Barchiesi F, Lucchinetti E, Zaugg M, Ogunshola OO, Wright M, Meyer M, Rosselli M, Schaufelberger S, Gillespie DG, Jackson EK, Dubey RK. Candidate genes and mechanisms for 2-methoxyestradiol-mediated vasoprotection. Hypertension. 2010 56(5):964-72.
[48] Rysa J, Leskinen H, Ilves M, Ruskoaho H. Distinct upregulation of extracellular matrix genes in transition from hypertrophy to hypertensive heart failure. Hypertension. 2005;45:927-933.
[49] Cerutti C, Kurdi M, Bricca G, Hodroj W, Paultre C, Randon J, Gustin MP. Transcriptional alterations in the left ventricle of three hypertensive rat models. Physiol Genomics. 2006;27:295-308.
[50] Hinojos CA, Boerwinkle E, Fornage M, Doris PA. Combined genealogical, mapping, and expression approaches to identify spontaneously hypertensive rat hypertension candidate genes. Hypertension. 2005;45(4):698-704.
[51] Kato N, Liang YQ, Ochiai Y, Jesmin S. Systemic evaluation of gene expression changes in major target organs induced by atorvastatin. Eur J Pharmacol. 2008;28;584(2-3):376-89. Epub 2008 Feb 8.
[52] Clemitson JR, Dixon RJ, Haines S, Bingham AJ, Patel BR, Hall L, Lo M, Sassard J, Charchar FJ, Samani NJ. Genetic dissection of a blood pressure quantitative trait locus on rat chromosome 1 and gene expression analysis identifies SPON1 as a novel candidate hypertension gene. Circ Res. 2007;100:992-999.
[53] Timofeeva AV, Goriunova LE, Khaspekov GL, Il'inskaia OP, Sirotkin VN, Andreeva ER, Tararak EM, Bulkina OS, Buza VV, Britareva VV, Karpov IuA, Bibilashvili RSh. Comparative transcriptome analysis of human aorta atherosclerotic lesions and peripheral blood leukocytes from essential hypertension patients. Kardiologiia. 2009;49(9):27-38.
[54] Koo JR, Liang KH, Vaziri ND. Microarray Analysis of Altered Gene Expression in Kidneys of Adult spontaneously Hypertensive Rats. The journal of Applied Research. 2004;4:111-126.
[55] Seubert JM, XU F, Graves JP, Collins JB, Sieber SO, Paules RS, Kroetz DL, Zeldin DC. Differential renal gene expression in prehypertensive and hypertensive spontaneously hypertensive rats. AmJ Physiol Renal Physiol. 2005; 289: 552-561.

[56] Westhoff TH, Scheid S, Tölle M, Kaynak B, Schmidt S, Zidek W, Sperling S, van der Giet M. A physiogenomic approach to study the regulation of blood pressure.Physiol Genomics. 2005; 21;23(1):46-53.
[57] Rysä J, Leskinen H, Ilves M, Ruskoaho H. Distinct upregulation of extracellular matrix genes in transition from hypertrophy to hypertensive heart failure.Hypertension. 2005; 45(5):927-33.
[58] Yagil C, Hubner N, Monti J, Schulz H, Sapojnikov M, Luft FC, Ganten D, Yagil Y. Identification of hypertension-related genes through an integrated genomic-transcriptomic approach.Circ Res. 2005;96(6):617-25.
[59] Wang D, Oparil S, Feng JA, Li P, Perry G, Chen LB, Dai M, John SW, Chen YF. Effects of pressure overload on extracellular matrix expression in the heart of the atrial natriuretic peptide-null mouse. Hypertension. 2003; 42(1):88-95.
[60] Liang M, Yuan B, Rute E, Greene AS, Olivier M, Cowley AW Jr. Insights into Dahl salt-sensitive hypertension revealed by temporal patterns of renal medullary gene expression. Physiol Genomics. 2003; 12(3):229-37.

# 12

# Potential Roles of TGF-β1 and EMILIN1 in Essential Hypertension

Masanori Shimodaira[1,2] and Tomohiro Nakayama[2,3]
[1]*Department of Internal Medicine, Tokyo Metropolitan Hiroo Hospital, Tokyo,*
[2]*Division of Laboratory Medicine, Department of Pathology and Microbiology, Nihon University School of Medicine, Tokyo,*
[3]*Divisions of Nephrology and Endocrinology, Department of Medicine, Nihon University School of Medicine, Tokyo, Japan*

## 1. Introduction

Essential hypertension (EH), which in general increases the arterial blood pressure, is a major health concern and risk factor for other diseases such as myocardial infarction and kidney failure (Barri, 2006; Stokes et al., 1989; Mosterd et al., 1999). EH development is known to be multifactorial, with both genetic determinants, such as allelic variation in the genes that are involved in renal salt absorption, and environmental factors that involve the diet (Lifton et al., 2001). The two widely recognized hallmarks of EH are resistance artery narrowing and large artery stiffening, which increase peripheral resistance and compromise vascular compliance, respectively. Both are known to contribute to the progression and cardiovascular morbidity and mortality associated with EH. However, despite decades of study, the initial causes that lead to these vascular abnormalities have yet to be completely elucidated. Moreover, the question remains as to whether these abnormalities exist prior to, and thus participate in, the initial phase of blood pressure elevation, or are a consequence of it.

The extracellular matrix (ECM) in the vascular wall has been found to be a critical determinant, and therefore it is thought that EH is associated with both an increased cardiovascular deposition and an increased systemic turnover of ECM proteins (Diez et al., 1995). Thus, vessel compliance dictated by the ECM is also involved in modulating the blood pressure.

Transforming growth factor (TGF)-β1 is an extracellular polypeptide member of the TGF-β superfamily of cytokines. It is a secreted protein that performs many cellular functions including control of cell growth, cell proliferation, cell differentiation and apoptosis. TGF-β1 acts bifunctionally to elevate blood pressure by first altering levels of vasoactive mediators and then by changing the vessel wall architecture to increase the peripheral resistance. In the cardiovascular system, TGF-β1 may play a key role in the regulation of the mechanical strain-induced matrix synthesis by the human vascular smooth muscle (VSM) cells. If so, this suggests that TGF-β1 may also play an important role in the development of hypertension-induced cardiovascular fibrosis (O'Callaghan&Williams, 2000).

Elastin microfibril interface-located protein 1 (EMILIN1) is a glycoprotein expressed in the vascular tree that binds to the TGF-β1 precursor and prevents processing by furin. Emilin 1 knockout mice display increased TGF-β1 signaling in their vessel walls. These animals develop peripheral vasoconstriction and arterial hypertension, which can be prevented by inactivation of one TGFB1 allele (Zacchigna, et al., 2006). These matrix-dependent changes in the vascular hemodynamics caused by TGF-β1 and EMILIN1 are important because they ultimately affect the cardiovascular morbidity and mortality rates.

This brief review focuses on the important roles of TGF-β1 and EMILIN1 in human hypertension, and in addition, evaluates the available data within the context of the current knowledge that has been collected from animal models of this disease.

## 2. Transforming growth factor-β1

### 2.1 The family of TGFs

The family of transforming growth factor (TGF) β belongs to a superfamily that consists of over 25 diverse dimeric extracellular polypeptides of 110-140 amino acids. These polypeptides include bone morphogenetic proteins, activins, and inhibitors (Massague et al., 1994). After discovery of the initial member of the TGF family in 1980 (Roberts et al., 1980), these important molecules have subsequently been shown to have complex effects on organ development, cell growth and differentiation. However, they are particularly important with regard to the expression of ECM proteins. There are three cytokine isoforms of TGF-β in mammals, TGF-β1, TGF-β2, and TGF-β3. All of these isoforms bind to the same receptors. In addition, they are encoded by separate genes sharing 60-80% homology and thus are most likely derived from a common ancestor. The major difference between the isoforms appears to be the spatiotemporal control of their expression patterns. While in vitro TGF-β isoforms have a similar effect on biologic tissues, they are generally characterized in vivo by varied degrees of expression and different functions. Their biologic activity depends on quantitative relationships between the individual isoforms (Cho et al., 2004; Li et al., 1999; Nakamura et al., 2004).

### 2.2 TGF-β1 in human hypertension

TGF-β1 is recognized as the most pivotal TGF-β isoform for the cardiovascular system, as it is present in VSM cells, endothelial cells, myofibroblasts, macrophages, and other hematopoietic cells (Annes et al., 2003). TGF-β1 strongly up-regulates the production of ECM proteins including fibronectin and collagen (Ignotz&Massague, 1986), and inhibits the degradation of the ECM by tissue proteinases (Laiho&Keski-Oja, 1989). Although TGF-β1 acts in wound healing via its effects on the ECM, excessive TGF-β can cause several fibrotic diseases including glomerulonephritis and diabetic nephropathy (Okuda et al., 1990). While TGF-β1 has long been thought to have only paracrine and autocrine effects, it has now been shown to have wide-ranging systemic (endocrine) effects (Sporn, 1997).

Lin et al. examined the association between serum TGF-β1 levels and gender, age, and selected lifestyle factors in a large number of healthy Japanese control subjects (Lin et al., 2009). They found that serum TGF-β1 levels appear to be modulated in part by gender, age and lifestyle factors such as obesity, cigarette smoking, and alcohol drinking (Lin et al., 2009). Overproduction of TGF-β1 clearly underlies the tissue fibrosis noted in numerous experimental and human diseases, including EH. Li et al. demonstrated for the first time that a positive correlation exists between circulating TGF-β1 levels and blood pressure in humans (Li et al., 1999). In another previous study, they also reported that the TGF-β1 protein concentration in hypertensive subjects ($n$=61) was 261±9 ng/ml as compared to 188±7 ng/ml in normotensive controls ($n$=90) ($P$<0.0001) (Suthanthiran et al., 2000). Obesity is an independent risk factor for EH and cardiovascular diseases. A strong relationship exists between the body mass index and blood pressure. Porreca et al. have reported that TGF-β1 levels are independently associated with obesity in hypertensive patients (Porreca et al., 2002). In addition, TGF-β1 is positively correlated with the body mass index and creatinine clearance in EH patients (Torun et al., 2007). In adipose tissue from both obese mice and humans, the levels of tissue TGF-β1 antigen have been shown to be well correlated with BMI (Alessi et al., 2000). Moreover, the *TGF-β1* gene was reported to be associated with obesity phenotypes such as BMI, fat mass, and lean mass in a large Caucasian population sample (Long et al., 2003). Likewise, an association was also observed between the TGF-β1 polymorphism and both the BMI and abdominal obesity in Swedish men (Rosmond et al., 2003). These data suggest that elevated levels are not just simply a marker of a similar disease production mechanism, but in fact indicate that elevated levels of circulating TGF-β1 lead to disease production and to the synergy of risk factors that are seen during EH production.

### 2.3 The synthesis of TGF-β1

TGF-β1 is synthesized by many cell types, including the endothelium, and is secreted as a latent dimeric ~75-kDa protein complex. While the enzyme furin cleaves a latency-associated peptide from the active TGF-β molecule during intracellular processing, it remains noncovalently complexed to the mature peptide after secretion. In addition, latent TGF-β-binding proteins, which are members of the fibrillin/latent TGF-β-binding protein family, bind to this complex and then direct it to the adjacent interstitium. Once in the extracellular space, removal of the latent TGF-β frees the mature, ~24-kDa biologically active form of TGF-β (Annes et al., 2003). Thus, endothelium-derived TGF-β1 is typically a locally acting molecule that has autocrine and paracrine actions on the neighboring endothelium and VSM. There are several known mechanisms of activation for TGF-β1. Thrombospondin-1 is secreted by the endothelial cells and appears to be the major regulatory factor involved in this activation (Schultz-Cherry et al., 1994). However, other factors have been identified that stimulate TGF-β1. For example, increased vascular wall stress that occurs in hypertensive individuals can sufficiently promote a strain "dose-dependent" increase in the TGF-β1 production by VSM cells, which leads to an associated increase in the matrix accumulation (O'Callaghan&Williams, 2000). Norepinephrine (Briest et al., 2004), hypoxia (Lee et al., 2009), oxidative stress (Zhao et al., 2008) and high glucose levels (Iglesias-de la Cruz et al., 2002) have also been shown to induce TGF-β1 production. Most of the information known about TGF-β1 has been collected from in vitro and in vivo animal models. Since human TGF-β1 and its nonhuman counterparts share a sufficiently high degree of homology, this makes it possible to extrapolate relevant data from animals to humans.

The Smad proteins (Smad2, Smad3 and Smad7) are essential components of the downstream TGF-β signaling. Positive signaling via activation of Smad2/3, along with negative signaling via the negative feedback mechanism of Smad7, are able to regulate the biological activities of TGF-β1 (Kretzschmar&Massague, 1998). Activation of Smad3, but not Smad2, is one of the key and absolute necessary mechanisms required for Angiotensin (Ang) II-induced vascular fibrosis. This is because the Ang II-induced Smad3/4 promoter activities and collagen matrix expression are abolished in VSMCs null for Smad3 but not Smad2. There are several phases that promote Smad signaling in Ang II. During the first phase, Ang II directly activates an early Smad signaling pathway at approximately 15 to 30 minutes. During the second phase, Ang II subsequently activates the late Smad2/3 signaling pathway at 24 hours. This pathway is TGF-β1 dependent, as it can be blocked by the anti-TGF-β antibody (Wang W et al., 2006).

### 2.4 TGF-β1 and the renin-angiotensin system

Ang II promotes sodium retention, cell growth and fibrosis, in addition to the classical effects it has on blood pressure and fluid homeostasis. Since it is well known that Ang II enhances TGF-β1 expression, TGF-β1 signaling pathways, and cardiac remodeling, which includes cardiac hypertrophy and cardiac fibrosis, the activation of TGF-β1 is considered to be closely associated with an Ang II excess (Ruiz-Ortega et al., 2007).

In the hypertrophic myocardium, TGF-β1 tissue levels are markedly increased after cardiac stress loading, such as with an Ang II excess (Ikeda et al., 2005; Yagi et al., 2008). Furthermore, the stimulus that is associated with the increase in the activity of Ang II in heart tissue can repeatedly trigger the expression of TGF-β1 and lead to continual injury. Therefore, it is thought that there is a biologically rich and complex interaction that occurs between the renin-angiotensin system (RAS) and TGF-β1 in which both act at various points to regulate the actions of the other. This interaction might be the key to understanding the vital roles that RAS and TGF-β1 play in EH development.

Another interplay between RAS and TGF-β1 involves the level of aldosterone. Ang II normally stimulates the production and release of aldosterone from the adrenal gland. Conversely, TGF-β1 suppresses production and strongly blocks the ability of Ang II to stimulate aldosterone by reducing the number of Ang II receptors expressed in the adrenal gland (Gupta et al., 1992). Furthermore, it has been shown that TGF-β1 can block the effects of aldosterone on sodium reabsorption in cultured renal collecting duct cells (Husted et al., 1994). It has also been shown that after an infusion of aldosterone into rats with a remnant kidney, there is an increase in blood pressure, proteinuria, and glomerulosclerosis along with a neutralization of the beneficial effects of the Ang II blockade (Greene et al. 1996). Although the mechanism of aldosterone's pathological effects is still unknown, it might be due to stimulation of TGF-β1 production in the kidney.

EH is the most common cause of hypertension. The second most common cause of hypertension is primary aldosteronism (PA), which has recently been implicated in the alterations of the immune system and progression of cardiovascular disease. As compared to EH controls, PA patients have lower TGF-β1 levels (17.6+/-4.1 vs. 34.5+/-20.5 pg/ml, $p<0.001$). In addition, TGF-β1 levels were shown to exhibit a remarkable correlation with the serum-aldosterone/plasma-renin-activity ratio in the total group (PA+EH) (Carvajal et al., 2009). Therefore, a chronic aldosterone excess in PA patients appears to modify the TGF-β1 levels. If so, this could lead to an imbalance in the immune system homeostasis, thereby leading to an early proinflammatory cardiovascular phenotype in these patients.

### 2.5 TGF-β1 and endothelin 1

Endothelin-1 (ET-1) is a vasoconstricting peptide that is produced primarily in the endothelium and which seems to play a key role in vascular homeostasis, tissue remodelling and fibrogenesis. These effects are mediated via two receptor types, $ET_A$ and $ET_B$. In blood vessels, $ET_A$ receptors are found in VSM cells, whereas $ET_B$ receptors are mainly localized on endothelial cells and, to some extent, in VSM cells and macrophages. ET-1, which acts predominantly via the $ET_A$ receptors, promotes vasoconstriction, cell growth, adhesion, fibrosis, and thrombosis. TGF-β1 induces ET-1 expression by a functional cooperation between Smads and activator protein-1 via activation of the Smad signaling pathway (Yang et al., 2010). Moreover, TGF-β1 enhances NO generation in the endothelium, which in turn suppresses TGF-β1 production. When NO production is impaired, such as with hypertension, aging, and other systemic diseases, unopposed excess vascular TGF-β1 production results in reduced vascular compliance and augmented peripheral arterial constriction and hypertension. Thus, NO functions as both a regulator for TGF-β1 production and as a physiological antagonist of ET-1.

Data from clinical trials have already demonstrated significant blood pressure lowering effects that occur after the combined use of $ET_A$-$ET_B$ receptor blockers. ET-1 receptor blockade diminishes TGF-β production in cardiac, vascular, and renal tissues (Kowala et al., 2004). While the role that ET-1 plays in normal cardiovascular homeostasis and in mild EH is still unclear, plasma ET-1 levels are increased in EH patients with atherosclerosis or nephrosclerosis when compared with patients with uncomplicated EH (Lariviere&Lebel, 2003). Thus, targeting the endothelin system might potentially be an important therapeutic treatment for EH, particularly for preventing target organ damage and managing cardiovascular disease.

### 2.6 TGF-β1 and organ damage-induced hypertension

Several in vitro and in vivo studies have confirmed the role of TGF-β1 in the development of heart muscle hypertrophy. An in vivo model has demonstrated there is an increase in mRNA and protein levels of TGF-β1 in the cardiomyocytes of hypertrophied heart (Kobayashi et al., 2001). Overexpression of TGF-β1 in transgenic mice has been shown to result in cardiac hypertrophy that is characterized by both interstitial fibrosis and hypertrophic growth of the cardiomyocytes (Rosenkranz, et al., 2002). These findings indicate that local production of TGF-β1 in the hypertrophic myocardium and the link between the RAS and TGF-β1 signaling pathway are involved in the hypertrophic response.

Hypertensive subjects can be considered to be at a higher risk of end-stage renal disease (ESRD). Scaglione et al. evaluated the relationship between circulating TGF-β1 and the progression of renal damage in a population of EH subjects. They evaluated the albumin excretion rate in EH patients and found there was a strong relationship between the progressive increase of TGF-β1 levels and the progression of renal damage (Scaglione et al., 2002). Thus, it is possible that TGF-β1 overproduction may be the pathogenetic mechanism for the excess burden of hypertension and hypertensive renal damage. August et al. demonstrated that African Americans with ESRD had higher circulating levels of TGF-β1 protein as compared to Caucasians with ESRD. They also found that hyperexpression of TGF-β1 was more frequent in African Americans with EH than in Caucasian Americans (August et al., 2000). Based on their findings, TGF-β1 is a treatment target that might be especially pertinent in hypertensive African Americans. In addition, anti-TGF-β1 therapy could also be efficacious in preventing or slowing the progression of target organ damage.

## 2.7 TGF-β1 gene polymorphisms, hypertension and organ damage

The *TGF-β1* gene, is located in the 19q13 chromosome and has 7 exons and 6 introns. Molecular biology research has confirmed that there are gene variations and polymorphisms in the *TGFB1* that are associated with EH. A meta-analysis that was performed in the Chinese population and which included 5 separate studies with 2708 subjects showed there was a relationship between the +869T/C polymorphism of *TGFB1* and EH. The pooled odds ratio (OR) for the CC/TC+TT genotype was 2.50, while the pooled OR for the frequency of the C allele was 1.43 (Yan-Yan, 2011). In Japanese individuals, Yamada et al. found that the frequency of the C allele in hypertensive women was higher than that seen in normotensive women, although there were no significant differences noted between hypertensive and normotensive men (Yamada et al., 2002). This research demonstrated that the association of the *TGFB1* polymorphism and EH was most likely influenced by the gender factor. Another study suggested that the prevalence of the TC or CC genotypes of the +29T/C polymorphism in the gene was significantly higher in hypertensives versus normotensives. In addition, there was a higher prevalence of subjects with microalbuminuria and left ventricular hypertrophy (LVH) in hypertensives having these genotypes as compared to the hypertensives with the TT genotype (Argano et al., 2008).

To investigate the linkage between the *TGFB1* polymorphism and the progression of atherosclerosis, Sie et al. conducted a population-based study that investigated five functional polymorphisms in *TGFB1* (-800 G/A, -509 C/T, codon 10 Leu/Pro, codon 25 Arg/Pro and codon 263 Thr/Ile) in relation to the arterial stiffness (pulse wave velocity (PWV), distensibility coefficient (DC) and pulse pressure (PP)). However, neither these polymorphisms nor the haplotypes were associated with the PWW, DC or PP (Sie et al., 2007). Conversely, the C allele of TGFB1 rs4803455 in an elderly Chinese man was shown to be significantly associated with the prevalence of carotid plaque (Deng et al., 2011).

As compared to Caucasian Americans, African Americans have a higher incidence and prevalence of hypertension and hypertension-associated target organ damage, which includes hypertensive nephrosclerosis. Suthanthiran et al. demonstrated that TGF-β1 protein levels were the highest in African American hypertensives, and that the TGF-β1 protein as well as the TGF-β1 mRNA levels were higher in hypertensives when compared to normotensives (Suthanthiran et al., 1998) They also showed that the proline allele at codon 10 of *TGFB1* was more frequently observed in African Americans as compared with Caucasian Americans. In addition, its presence was also associated with higher levels of TGF-β1 mRNA and protein. These findings suggest that TGF-β1 hyperexpression might be a risk factor for hypertension and hypertensive complications, in addition to being the basis of the mechanism for the excess burden of hypertension in African Americans.

## 2.8 TGF-β1 and antihypertensive treatment

Laviades et al. reported that the efficient blockade of the $AT_1$ receptors that is observed when using losartan is associated with the inhibition of TGF-β1, normalization of collagen type I metabolism, and reversal of left ventricular hypertrophy and microalbuminuria in hypertensive patients (Laviades et al., 2000). As a similar effect has been reported for captopril, this suggests that both angiotensin converting enzyme inhibitor (ACEI) and Ang II receptor blocker (ARB) attenuate the TGF-β1 expression (Sharma et al., 1999). Furthermore, although high glucose has also been shown to increase the production of Ang II and TGF-β1, both ACEI and ARB attenuated the increase in TGF-β1 production and reduced the cell proliferation caused by exposure to high glucose. These effects were greater when a combination of the two drugs were used (Kyuden et al., 2005). Scaglione et al. evaluated the effects of 24 weeks of losartan and ramipril treatment, both alone and in combination, on the circulating TGF-β1 and left ventricular mass (LVM) in EH patients. Their results showed that the absolute and percent reduction in TGF-β1 and LVM were significantly higher in the combined versus the individual losartan or ramipril groups. Thus, these findings indicate there is an additional cardioprotective effect provided by the dual blockade of renin-angiotensin in EH patients (Scaglione et al., 2007).

Hallberg et al. determined the impact of the + 915G/C polymorphism of *TGFB1* on the response to antihypertensive treatment. In a randomized double-blind study designed to treat EH patients for 48 weeks with either the $AT_1$ receptor antagonist irbesartan or the β1-adrenoceptor blocker atenolol, they examined the association between the TGF-β1 genotype and LVM regression in patients that had been echocardiographically diagnosed with LVH. Irbesartan-treated patients who were carriers of the C allele, which is associated with a low expression of TGF-β1, responded with a markedly greater decrease in the LVM index (LVMI) as compared to subjects with the GG genotype (adjusted mean change in LVMI -44.7 g/m2 vs. -22.2 g/m2, $p = 0.007$). This decrease occurred independent of the blood pressure reduction. However, no association was noted between the genotype and the change in LVMI in the atenolol group. Therefore, they concluded that the *TGF-β1* + 915G/C polymorphism was related to the change in the LVMI in response to the antihypertensive treatment with the $AT_1$ receptor antagonist irbesartan (Hallberg et al., 2004).

Based on these findings and the observations that ACEI and ARB are able to reduce Ang II-mediated stimulation of the TGF-β1 production, treatments using these agents might be efficacious in preventing or slowing the progression of target organ damage in EH, especially in those patients who have LVH or hyperglycemia. Moreover, based on data presented above, it can be speculated that greater disease reduction could perhaps be achieved if TGF-β1 rather than blood pressure was the therapeutic target.

## 3. Emilin 1

### 3.1 EMILINs family

EMILINs are a family of proteins of the extracellular matrix. The first protein of the family, initially named gp115, was isolated from chicken aorta under harsh solubilizing conditions. This protein was particularly abundant in the aortic tissue, and further immunohistochemical studies also showed it to be strongly expressed in blood vessels and in the connective tissues of a wide variety of organs, particularly in association with elastic fibers (Colombatti et al., 1987). At the ultrastructural level, the molecule was detected in elastic fibers, where it was located at the interface between the amorphous core and the surrounding microfibrils (Bressan et al., 1993). On the basis of this finding, the protein was named EMILIN (elastin microfibril interface-located protein). Cloning of the cDNA of chicken EMILIN lead to the isolation in both human and mouse genes, with a total of three genes having been identified in humans and mice at the present time. The cardiovascular system has been demonstrated to be the major site of expression for the *EMILIN* genes (Braghetta et al., 2004).

EMILINs share four protein domains, the C-terminal C1q domain, collagenous domain, coiled-coil domain and N-terminal cysteine-rich domain (EMI domain) (Colombatti et al., 2000). There are also unique domains that are not shared by the EMILIN proteins. For example, EMILIN1 has two leucine zipper regions, multimerin has an endothelial growth factor-like domain, and EMILIN2 contains a proline-rich domain. This domain organization suggests that there are some shared and some specific functions for each of these EMILIN proteins.

### 3.2 EMILIN1 and hypertension

EMILIN1 was originally isolated form the aorta and is intimately associated with elastic fibers and microfibrils in the blood vessels, as well as in the connective tissue of other organs. EMILIN1 is a monomer when it is within the cells, but upon secretion, it oligomerizes via the formation of disulfide bonds. EMILIN1 appears to be more slowly secreted than other ECM components, although the implication of this is unclear (Colombatti et al., 2000). The function of EMILIN1 remained unknown until the gene was finally disrupted in mice. Although EMILIN1 knockout mice are fertile and have no obvious abnormalities, histological and ultrastructural examinations have shown there are alterations of the elastic fibers in the aorta and skin. Formation of elastic fibers by mutant embryonic fibroblasts in cultures has also been found to be abnormal (Zanetti et al., 2004). These mice develop larger lymphangiomas as compared to Wild type mice. Lymphatic vascular morphological alterations in these mice are also accompanied by functional defects, such as mild lymphedema, a highly significant drop in lymph drainage, and enhanced lymph leakage (Danussi et al., 2008).

In 2006, Zacchigna et al. found that *Emilin1* deficient mice become hypertensive (systolic blood pressure: 120±2 versus 101±1, n=46 per group, $P<0.01$), in addition to exhibiting an increased peripheral vascular resistance and a reduced vessel size, all of which were independent of the cardiac output. Strikingly, after inactivation of a single TGF-β allele, the high blood pressure in the mice returned to normal levels. A further study revealed that EMILIN1 inhibits TGF-β signaling by specifically binding to the proTGF-β precursor, thereby preventing its maturation by the furin convertases in the extracellular space (Zacchigna, et al., 2006). This study highlighted the importance of the relationship between EMILIN1 and TGF-β availability in the pathogenesis of hypertension. EMILIN1 may inhibit TGF-β by several different mechanisms. First, it is possible that it could interfere with TGF-β secretion or maturation, or second, it could prevent the presentation or the interaction of the TGF-β ligands with the cognate receptors. Finally, it could also be possible that it acts by sequestering either the immature or mature ligand (Zacchigna, et al., 2006). Therefore, further studies will need to be undertaken that conclusively prove that: 1) EMILIN1 modulates TGF-β availability during the development of the cardiovascular system, 2) EMILIN1 is associated with the pathogenesis of hypertension, and 3) TGF-β maturation is linked to the blood pressure homeostasis that has been identified in animal studies. If these future studies do lead to the discovery of the genetic susceptibility of *EMILIN1* gene to hypertension, this will ultimately lead to a better understanding of the mechanism of human hypertension.

### 3.3 EMILIN1 gene polymorphisms and EH

The human *EMILIN1* gene, which encodes EMILIN1, consists of 955 amino acids and is located on chromosome 2p23.3-p23.2, which overlaps with the promoter region of the ketohexokinase gene (Doliana et al., 2000). The gene is quite small and consists of approximately 7.3 kilo base-pairs that contain eight exons, and which are interrupted by seven introns. In a previous investigation of the association of the *EMILIN1* gene polymorphisms and EH, we genotyped a total of 287 EH patients and 253 age-matched controls for five single-nucleotide polymorphisms (SNPs) used as genetic markers for the human *EMILIN1* gene (rs2289408, rs2289360, rs2011616, rs2304682, and rs4665947). We confirmed that rs2289360, rs2011616, and rs2304682, as well as the haplotype constructed using rs2536512, rs2011616, and rs17881426 were useful genetic markers of EH in Japanese men (Shimodaira et al., 2010). In a Mongolian population, the rs2304682 locus in *EMILIN1*, as well as the haplotypes G-G constructed using rs3754734 and rs2304682, appeared to be associated with the susceptibility of EH. In addition, rs2304682 may also be associated with the level of the diastolic blood pressure (Mi et al., 2011). Conversely, Shen et al. reported finding no significant association between the *EMILIN1* gene and EH, although the interaction of age and genotype variation of rs3754734 and rs2011616 might increase the risk of EH in the northern Han Chinese population (Shen et al., 2009). In order to definitively determine if there is an association between the genetic variation of the *EMILIN1* gene and increases in the blood pressure, further studies that investigate the role of the *EMILIN1* gene in vascular development and blood pressure homeostasis will need to be undertaken. At the present time, however, there have yet to be any reports of human hereditary diseases that are involved with EMILINs. Therefore, the morphological abnormalities revealed in this study constitute the first potential hallmark of EMILIN1 insufficiency, which may prove to be helpful in identifying heritable diseases induced by mutations of this gene in the future.

## 4. Conclusion

Many studies over the last decade have attempted to elucidate the important roles of TGF-β1 and EMILIN1 in the maintenance of normal blood vessel wall architecture in humans. While most of the results reviewed here are consistent with the concept that TGF-β1 and EMILIN1 have similar roles in the vasculature of humans and rodents, direct and conclusive evidence has yet to be found. However, this is not all that surprising when one considers the difficulty of probing complex systems in humans. Although interventional experiments are commonplace in animal models, almost all without exception are impossible to perform in the regulatory systems in the human vasculature. From a therapeutic point of view, understanding the complexities of the interplay between the TGF-β1 signaling pathway and the development of EH are matters of great importance. For the most part, strategies that decrease TGF-β1 activity may very well be able to protect against hypertension and hypertensive organ damage. Once definitive information on the TGF-β1 signaling pathway and human hypertension becomes available, novel therapeutic approaches that modulate the biological actions of TGF-β1 might become available for use in EH patients.

## 5. References

[1] Stokes J 3rd, K.W., Wolf PA, D'Agostino RB, Cupples LA. , *Blood pressure as a risk factor for cardiovascular disease. The Framingham Study--30 years of follow-up*. Hypertension., 1989. 13: p. I13-8.

[2] Mosterd A, D.A.R., Silbershatz H, Sytkowski PA, Kannel WB, Grobbee DE, Levy D. , *Trends in the prevalence of hypertension, antihypertensive therapy, and left ventricular hypertrophy from 1950 to 1989*. N Engl J Med. , 1999. 340: p. 1221-7.

[3] Barri, Y.M., *Hypertension and kidney disease: a deadly connection*. Current cardiology reports, 2006. 8(6): p. 411-7.

[4] Lifton, R.P., A.G. Gharavi, and D.S. Geller, *Molecular mechanisms of human hypertension*. Cell, 2001. 104(4): p. 545-56.

[5] Diez, J., et al., *Increased serum concentrations of procollagen peptides in essential hypertension. Relation to cardiac alterations*. Circulation, 1995. 91(5): p. 1450-6.

[6] O'Callaghan, C.J. and B. Williams, *Mechanical strain-induced extracellular matrix production by human vascular smooth muscle cells: role of TGF-beta(1)*. Hypertension, 2000. 36(3): p. 319-24.

[7] Zacchigna, L., et al., *Emilin1 links TGF-beta maturation to blood pressure homeostasis*. Cell, 2006. 124(5): p. 929-42.

[8] Massague, J., L. Attisano, and J.L. Wrana, *The TGF-beta family and its composite receptors*. Trends in cell biology, 1994. 4(5): p. 172-8.

[9] Roberts, A.B., et al., *Transforming growth factors: isolation of polypeptides from virally and chemically transformed cells by acid/ethanol extraction*. Proceedings of the National Academy of Sciences of the United States of America, 1980. 77(6): p. 3494-8.

[10] Nakamura, H., et al., *RNA interference targeting transforming growth factor-beta type II receptor suppresses ocular inflammation and fibrosis*. Molecular vision, 2004. 10: p. 703-11.

[11] Cho, H.R., et al., *Differential expression of TGF-beta isoforms during differentiation of HaCaT human keratinocyte cells: implication for the separate role in epidermal differentiation*. Journal of Korean medical science, 2004. 19(6): p. 853-8.

[12] Li, D.Q., S.B. Lee, and S.C. Tseng, *Differential expression and regulation of TGF-beta1, TGF-beta2, TGF-beta3, TGF-betaRI, TGF-betaRII and TGF-betaRIII in cultured human corneal, limbal, and conjunctival fibroblasts*. Current eye research, 1999. 19(2): p. 154-61.

[13] Annes, J.P., J.S. Munger, and D.B. Rifkin, *Making sense of latent TGFbeta activation*. Journal of cell science, 2003. 116(Pt 2): p. 217-24.

[14] Ignotz, R.A. and J. Massague, *Transforming growth factor-beta stimulates the expression of fibronectin and collagen and their incorporation into the extracellular matrix*. The Journal of biological chemistry, 1986. 261(9): p. 4337-45.

[15] Laiho, M. and J. Keski-Oja, *Growth factors in the regulation of pericellular proteolysis: a review*. Cancer research, 1989. 49(10): p. 2533-53.

[16] Okuda, S., et al., *Elevated expression of transforming growth factor-beta and proteoglycan production in experimental glomerulonephritis. Possible role in expansion of the mesangial extracellular matrix*. The Journal of clinical investigation, 1990. 86(2): p. 453-62.

[17] Sporn, M.B., *The importance of context in cytokine action*. Kidney international, 1997. 51(5): p. 1352-4.

[18] Lin, Y., et al., *Variations in serum transforming growth factor-beta1 levels with gender, age and lifestyle factors of healthy Japanese adults.* Disease markers, 2009. 27(1): p. 23-8.
[19] Li, B., et al., *TGF-beta1 DNA polymorphisms, protein levels, and blood pressure.* Hypertension, 1999. 33(1 Pt 2): p. 271-5.
[20] Suthanthiran, M., et al., *Transforming growth factor-beta 1 hyperexpression in African-American hypertensives: A novel mediator of hypertension and/or target organ damage.* Proceedings of the National Academy of Sciences of the United States of America, 2000. 97(7): p. 3479-84.
[21] Porreca, E., et al., *Transforming growth factor-beta1 levels in hypertensive patients: association with body mass index and leptin.* American journal of hypertension, 2002. 15(9): p. 759-65.
[22] Torun, D., et al., *The relationship between obesity and transforming growth factor beta on renal damage in essential hypertension.* International heart journal, 2007. 48(6): p. 733-41.
[23] Alessi, M.C., et al., *Plasminogen activator inhibitor 1, transforming growth factor-beta1, and BMI are closely associated in human adipose tissue during morbid obesity.* Diabetes, 2000. 49(8): p. 1374-80.
[24] Long, J.R., et al., *APOE and TGF-beta1 genes are associated with obesity phenotypes.* Journal of medical genetics, 2003. 40(12): p. 918-24.
[25] Rosmond, R., et al., *Increased abdominal obesity, insulin and glucose levels in nondiabetic subjects with a T29C polymorphism of the transforming growth factor-beta1 gene.* Hormone research, 2003. 59(4): p. 191-4.
[26] Schultz-Cherry, S., J. Lawler, and J.E. Murphy-Ullrich, *The type 1 repeats of thrombospondin 1 activate latent transforming growth factor-beta.* The Journal of biological chemistry, 1994. 269(43): p. 26783-8.
[27] Briest, W., et al., *Norepinephrine-induced changes in cardiac transforming growth factor-beta isoform expression pattern of female and male rats.* Hypertension, 2004. 44(4): p. 410-8.
[28] Lee, Y.K., et al., *Hypoxia induces connective tissue growth factor mRNA expression.* Journal of Korean medical science, 2009. 24 Suppl: p. S176-82.
[29] Zhao, W., et al., *Oxidative stress mediates cardiac fibrosis by enhancing transforming growth factor-beta1 in hypertensive rats.* Molecular and cellular biochemistry, 2008. 317(1-2): p. 43-50.
[30] Iglesias-de la Cruz, M.C., et al., *Effects of high glucose and TGF-beta1 on the expression of collagen IV and vascular endothelial growth factor in mouse podocytes.* Kidney international, 2002. 62(3): p. 901-13.
[31] Kretzschmar, M. and J. Massague, *SMADs: mediators and regulators of TGF-beta signaling.* Current opinion in genetics & development, 1998. 8(1): p. 103-11.
[32] Wang, W., et al., *Essential role of Smad3 in angiotensin II-induced vascular fibrosis.* Circulation research, 2006. 98(8): p. 1032-9.
[33] Ruiz-Ortega, M., et al., *TGF-beta signaling in vascular fibrosis.* Cardiovascular research, 2007. 74(2): p. 196-206.
[34] Yagi, S., et al., *Pitavastatin, an HMG-CoA reductase inhibitor, exerts eNOS-independent protective actions against angiotensin II induced cardiovascular remodeling and renal insufficiency.* Circulation research, 2008. 102(1): p. 68-76.

[35] Ikeda, Y., et al., *Androgen receptor gene knockout male mice exhibit impaired cardiac growth and exacerbation of angiotensin II-induced cardiac fibrosis.* The Journal of biological chemistry, 2005. 280(33): p. 29661-6.
[36] Gupta, P., et al., *Transforming growth factor-beta 1 inhibits aldosterone and stimulates adrenal renin in cultured bovine zona glomerulosa cells.* Endocrinology, 1992. 131(2): p. 631-6.
[37] Husted, R.F., K. Matsushita, and J.B. Stokes, *Induction of resistance to mineralocorticoid hormone in cultured inner medullary collecting duct cells by TGF-beta 1.* The American journal of physiology, 1994. 267(5 Pt 2): p. F767-75.
[38] Greene, E.L., S. Kren, and T.H. Hostetter, *Role of aldosterone in the remnant kidney model in the rat.* The Journal of clinical investigation, 1996. 98(4): p. 1063-8.
[39] Carvajal, C.A., et al., *Primary aldosteronism can alter peripheral levels of transforming growth factor beta and tumor necrosis factor alpha.* Journal of endocrinological investigation, 2009. 32(9): p. 759-65.
[40] Yang, F., et al., *Essential role for Smad3 in angiotensin II-induced tubular epithelial-mesenchymal transition.* The Journal of pathology, 2010. 221(4): p. 390-401.
[41] Kowala, M.C., et al., *Novel dual action AT1 and ETA receptor antagonists reduce blood pressure in experimental hypertension.* The Journal of pharmacology and experimental therapeutics, 2004. 309(1): p. 275-84.
[42] Lariviere, R. and M. Lebel, *Endothelin-1 in chronic renal failure and hypertension.* Canadian journal of physiology and pharmacology, 2003. 81(6): p. 607-21.
[43] Kobayashi, N., et al., *Benidipine inhibits expression of ET-1 and TGF-beta1 in Dahl salt-sensitive hypertensive rats.* Hypertension research : official journal of the Japanese Society of Hypertension, 2001. 24(3): p. 241-50.
[44] Rosenkranz, S., et al., *Alterations of beta-adrenergic signaling and cardiac hypertrophy in transgenic mice overexpressing TGF-beta(1).* American journal of physiology. Heart and circulatory physiology, 2002. 283(3): p. H1253-62.
[45] Scaglione, R., et al., *Relationship between transforming growth factor beta1 and progression of hypertensive renal disease.* Journal of human hypertension, 2002. 16(9): p. 641-5.
[46] August, P., B. Leventhal, and M. Suthanthiran, *Hypertension-induced organ damage in African Americans: transforming growth factor-beta(1) excess as a mechanism for increased prevalence.* Current hypertension reports, 2000. 2(2): p. 184-91.
[47] Yan-Yan, L., *Transforming Growth Factor beta1 +869T/C Gene Polymorphism and Essential Hypertension: A Meta-analysis Involving 2708 Participants in the Chinese Population.* Internal medicine, 2011. 50(10): p. 1089-92.
[48] Yamada, Y., et al., *Association of a polymorphism of the transforming growth factor-beta1 gene with blood pressure in Japanese individuals.* Journal of human genetics, 2002. 47(5): p. 243-8.
[49] Argano, C., et al., *Transforming growth factor beta1 T29C gene polymorphism and hypertension: relationship with cardiovascular and renal damage.* Blood pressure, 2008. 17(4): p. 220-6.
[50] Sie, M.P., et al., *TGF-beta1 polymorphisms and arterial stiffness; the Rotterdam Study.* Journal of human hypertension, 2007. 21(6): p. 431-7.

[51] Deng, H.B., et al., *A polymorphism in transforming growth factor-beta1 is associated with carotid plaques and increased carotid intima-media thickness in older Chinese men: the Guangzhou Biobank Cohort Study-Cardiovascular Disease Subcohort.* Atherosclerosis, 2011. 214(2): p. 391-6.

[52] Suthanthiran, M., et al., *Transforming growth factor-beta 1 hyperexpression in African American end-stage renal disease patients.* Kidney international, 1998. 53(3): p. 639-44.

[53] Laviades, C., N. Varo, and J. Diez, *Transforming growth factor beta in hypertensives with cardiorenal damage.* Hypertension, 2000. 36(4): p. 517-22.

[54] Sharma, K., et al., *Captopril-induced reduction of serum levels of transforming growth factor-beta1 correlates with long-term renoprotection in insulin-dependent diabetic patients.* American journal of kidney diseases : the official journal of the National Kidney Foundation, 1999. 34(5): p. 818-23.

[55] Kyuden, Y., et al., *Tgf-beta1 induced by high glucose is controlled by angiotensin-converting enzyme inhibitor and angiotensin II receptor blocker on cultured human peritoneal mesothelial cells.* Peritoneal dialysis international : journal of the International Society for Peritoneal Dialysis, 2005. 25(5): p. 483-91.

[56] Scaglione, R., et al., *Effect of dual blockade of renin-angiotensin system on TGFbeta1 and left ventricular structure and function in hypertensive patients.* Journal of human hypertension, 2007. 21(4): p. 307-15.

[57] Hallberg, P., et al., *Transforming growth factor beta1 genotype and change in left ventricular mass during antihypertensive treatment--results from the Swedish Irbesartan Left Ventricular Hypertrophy Investigation versus Atenolol (SILVHIA).* Clinical cardiology, 2004. 27(3): p. 169-73.

[58] Colombatti, A., et al., *Widespread codistribution of glycoprotein gp 115 and elastin in chick eye and other tissues.* Collagen and related research, 1987. 7(4): p. 259-75.

[59] Bressan, G.M., et al., *Emilin, a component of elastic fibers preferentially located at the elastin-microfibrils interface.* The Journal of cell biology, 1993. 121(1): p. 201-12.

[60] Braghetta, P., et al., *Overlapping, complementary and site-specific expression pattern of genes of the EMILIN/Multimerin family.* Matrix biology : journal of the International Society for Matrix Biology, 2004. 22(7): p. 549-56.

[61] Colombatti, A., et al., *The EMILIN protein family.* Matrix biology : journal of the International Society for Matrix Biology, 2000. 19(4): p. 289-301.

[62] Zanetti, M., et al., *EMILIN-1 deficiency induces elastogenesis and vascular cell defects.* Molecular and cellular biology, 2004. 24(2): p. 638-50.

[63] Danussi, C., et al., *Emilin1 deficiency causes structural and functional defects of lymphatic vasculature.* Molecular and cellular biology, 2008. 28(12): p. 4026-39.

[64] Doliana, R., et al., *Structure, chromosomal localization, and promoter analysis of the human elastin microfibril interfase located proteIN (EMILIN) gene.* The Journal of biological chemistry, 2000. 275(2): p. 785-92.

[65] Shimodaira, M., et al., *Association study of the elastin microfibril interfacer 1 (EMILIN1) gene in essential hypertension.* American journal of hypertension, 2010. 23(5): p. 547-55.

[66] Mi, D.Q., et al., *[Association of EMILIN1 gene polymorphism with essential hypertension in Mongolian].* Zhonghua yi xue yi chuan xue za zhi = Zhonghua yixue yichuanxue zazhi = Chinese journal of medical genetics, 2011. 28(2): p. 160-4.

[67] Shen, C., et al., *Emilin1 gene and essential hypertension: a two-stage association study in northern Han Chinese population.* BMC medical genetics, 2009. 10: p. 118.